The Multi-Dimensional Contributions of Prefrontal Circuits to Emotion Regulation during Adulthood and Critical Stages of Development

The Multi-Dimensional Contributions of Prefrontal Circuits to Emotion Regulation during Adulthood and Critical Stages of Development

Special Issue Editor

Angela Roberts

MDPI • Basel • Beijing • Wuhan • Barcelona • Belgrade

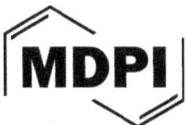

MDPI

Special Issue Editor
Angela Roberts
University of Cambridge
UK

Editorial Office
MDPI
St. Alban-Anlage 66
4052 Basel, Switzerland

This is a reprint of articles from the Special Issue published online in the open access journal *Actuators* (ISSN 2076-0825) from 2018 to 2019 (available at: https://www.mdpi.com/journal/brainsci/special_issues/Neuro_Emotion).

For citation purposes, cite each article independently as indicated on the article page online and as indicated below:

LastName, A.A.; LastName, B.B.; LastName, C.C. Article Title. *Journal Name* **Year**, *Article Number*, Page Range.

ISBN 978-3-03921-702-1 (Pbk)
ISBN 978-3-03921-703-8 (PDF)

Contents

About the Special Issue Editor

Angela Roberts received her degree in Neurobiology from the University of Sussex and her PhD in neuroendocrine control of reproduction from the University of Cambridge under the supervision of Joe Herbert in the Department of Anatomy. She stayed on in Cambridge and did her postdoctoral training in the Department of Experimental Psychology with Trevor Robbins where she held a Royal Society Research Fellowship from 1992–96. She then took up a teaching appointment in the Department of Anatomy and there began her studies on the prefrontal control of emotion regulation. Currently she undertakes the scientific leadership of the marmoset research centre at Cambridge and is Chair of the steering committee for a new Laboratory of Translational Neuroimaging. She also sits on the Executive committee of Cambridge Neuroscience.

She is currently an associate editor for Frontiers in Behavioral Neuroscience, a field Editor for the International Journal of Neuropsychopharmacology and sits on the council of the British Association of Psychopharmacology. In 2016 she was elected to the Fellowship of the Academy of Medical Sciences.

Preface to "The Multi-Dimensional Contributions of Prefrontal Circuits to Emotion Regulation during Adulthood and Critical Stages of Development"

The Multidimensional Contributions of Prefrontal Circuits to Emotion Regulation during Adulthood and Critical Stages of Development.

The prefrontal cortex (PFC) and neighbouring anterior cingulate cortex play a pivotal role in regulating our emotions, as shown by the marked alterations in activity within prefrontal and cingulate circuits that accompany mood and anxiety disorders. These regions are functionally diverse. Thus, a critical step towards better stratification of the symptoms of mood and anxiety disorders and more effective individualised treatment strategies is to define their unique contributions to the regulation of positive and negative emotions.

Since many disorders of emotion have their onset during childhood and adolescence, it is also important to extend our understanding of these prefrontal circuits to the developing brain. This Special Issue brings together the most recent research in humans and other animals that addresses these important questions. Alterations in activity and structural morphology in specific prefrontal circuits identified in adult and adolescent clinical populations are investigated in rodents and monkeys to determine their causal contribution to emotion and cognitive dysregulation. The importance of stress and altered neurodevelopmental trajectories, highlighted as important factors leading to symptoms of anxiety and depression in clinical studies, is explored at the system, cellular, and molecular levels of prefrontal circuits in animals. Together these papers illustrate the importance of the cross-species translation of prefrontal function to inform our understanding of the psychological and physiological mechanisms underlying affective disorders.

The first set of papers consider the adult prefrontal cortex. The functions of area 25 in humans and monkeys and its putative homologue, the infralimbic cortex in rodents, are reviewed in Alexander and colleagues along with their relevance to our understanding of anxiety and anhedonia. One particular cognitive function, occasion setting, is explored in rats by Roughley and Killcross, specifically focussing on the role of the infralimbic and prelimbic cortices. The role of stress in inducing dysregulation within the prefrontal cortex is then discussed by Datta and Arnsten, drawing upon data from humans, monkeys and rats to provide a description of the molecular mechanisms that may mediate such effects and the ensuing loss of hierarchical control. To complete this section, the prospects of using functional magnetic resonance imaging to discover biomarkers that will predict an individual's risk of developing a psychiatric disorder are considered by Nord and colleagues, focussing on fronto-amygdala connectivity. Turning to adolescence, Ernst and colleagues discuss the use of machine learning to test models of brain–behaviour interactions during development. Three papers then describe altered prefrontal function, the first in relation to the neurodevelopmental disorder Williams syndrome, involving reductions in grey matter within area 25 associated with the symptoms of anxiety and hypersociability (Wilder and colleagues). A second reviews the altered intrinsic and extrinsic connectivity of the prefrontal cortex in relation to positive and negative emotion in adolescents suffering from depression (Kaya and McCabe). The ontogeny of strategies to effectively regulate emotion is discussed by Young and colleagues from behavioural, psychophysiological and neural perspectives considering how their dysregulation may underlie symptoms of anxiety and depression in adolescents. The final two papers by Zimmerman and Schipper and their colleagues provide insights into the neurodevelopmental time-course underlying the regulation of threat in rodents focussing on prefrontal–amygdala interactions.

Angela Roberts
Special Issue Editor

brain
sciences

MDPI

Review

A Focus on the Functions of Area 25

Laith Alexander [1,2], Hannah F. Clarke [1,2,*] and Angela C. Roberts [1,2,*]

[1]   Department of Physiology, Development and Neuroscience, University of Cambridge, Cambridge CB2 3DY,
      UK; la326@cam.ac.uk
[2]   Behavioural and Clinical Neuroscience Institute, Department of Psychology, University of Cambridge,
      Cambridge CB2 3EB, UK
*   Correspondence: acr4@cam.ac.uk (A.C.R.); hfc23@cam.ac.uk (H.F.C.); Tel.: +44-1223-339015 (A.C.R.);
      +44-1223-33758 (H.F.C.)

Received: 18 March 2019; Accepted: 29 May 2019; Published: 3 June 2019

Abstract: Subcallosal area 25 is one of the least understood regions of the anterior cingulate cortex, but activity in this area is emerging as a crucial correlate of mood and affective disorder symptomatology. The cortical and subcortical connectivity of area 25 suggests it may act as an interface between the bioregulatory and emotional states that are aberrant in disorders such as depression. However, evidence for such a role is limited because of uncertainty over the functional homologue of area 25 in rodents, which hinders cross-species translation. This emphasizes the need for causal manipulations in monkeys in which area 25, and the prefrontal and cingulate regions in which it is embedded, resemble those of humans more than rodents. In this review, we consider physiological and behavioral evidence from non-pathological and pathological studies in humans and from manipulations of area 25 in monkeys and its putative homologue, the infralimbic cortex (IL), in rodents. We highlight the similarities between area 25 function in monkeys and IL function in rodents with respect to the regulation of reward-driven responses, but also the apparent inconsistencies in the regulation of threat responses, not only between the rodent and monkey literatures, but also within the rodent literature. Overall, we provide evidence for a causal role of area 25 in both the enhanced negative affect and decreased positive affect that is characteristic of affective disorders, and the cardiovascular and endocrine perturbations that accompany these mood changes. We end with a brief consideration of how future studies should be tailored to best translate these findings into the clinic.

Keywords: area 25; infralimbic; autonomic; emotion; anhedonia; negative affect; anticipatory arousal

---

1. Introduction

Area 25 is found within the subcallosal cortex and is one of the least understood regions of the anterior cingulate cortex (ACC). It is variably included with adjacent regions of the subcallosal zone (scACC), also referred to as subgenual, and more broadly, the ventromedial prefrontal cortex (vmPFC), which includes medial PFC regions anterior to the genu of the corpus callosum. Although there is variation in the precise extent of area 25 within current architectonic maps of this area, particularly in the macaque [1,2], there is consensus with respect to its extreme caudal position within the subcallosal region, lying adjacent to the lateral septum of the basal forebrain. Where maps in the macaque differ is with respect to whether area 25 extends onto the orbital surface or not. Area 25 is characterized as agranular cortex in humans, with no identified granular layer IV [3], and dysgranular cortex in monkeys [1] with a very thin granular layer IV, anteriorly. The overall layering within area 25 is relatively undifferentiated, with fusion of layers II and III into a broad supragranular layer and fusion of layers V and VI into a much narrower, but dense infragranular layer. Based on tracing studies in rhesus macaques (Figure 1A), area 25 is densely connected with neighboring ventromedial and posterior orbitofrontal cortex (OFC), involved in affective evaluation and a moderate pathway linking it to fronto-polar area 10 and cognition. Outside of the PFC, area 25 has strong connections with the interoceptive regions of the anterior insula, the medial temporal lobe memory system, the auditory association cortex in the superior temporal gyrus and the multimodal superior temporal sulcus [1]. As described in [1], the propensity of area 25 projections to originate in deep layers and end within superficial layers of eulaminate brain regions is a pattern normally associated with feedback organization. However, its connectivity with agranular regions, including neighboring posterior OFC, vmPFC, medial temporal lobe (MTL) and anterior insula, appears feedforward in nature, suggesting that activity is initiated in area 25. Subcortically, area 25 has by far the strongest reciprocal connectivity with the amygdala compared to all other prefrontal regions. It also has dense projections to the ventral striatum, a number of nuclei within the hypothalamus (including the preoptic area, lateral hypothalamus and dorsomedial hypothalamus), bed nucleus of the stria terminalis, medial septum, diagonal band of Broca and substantia innominata. In the brainstem there are also projections to the monoamine systems as well as the periaqueductal grey and parabrachial nucleus [1,2]. This connectivity pattern positions area 25 at the intersection between emotion, visceromotor function and memory.

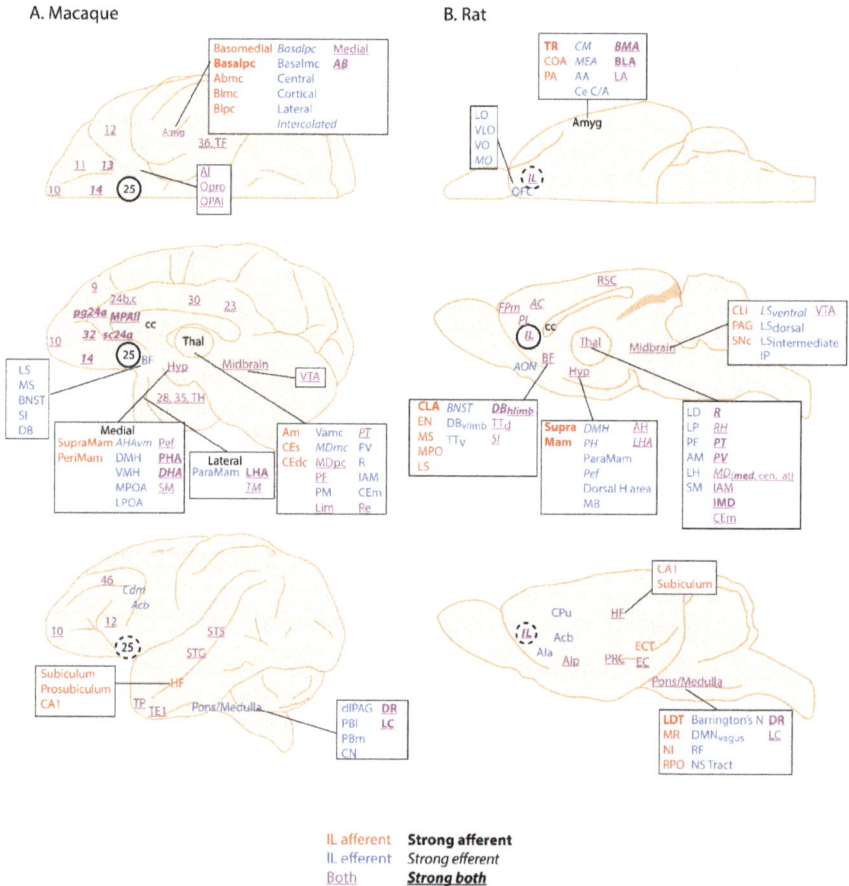

Figure 1. The connectivity of area 25 in macaques and the infralimbic cortex (IL) in rodents. In the macaque (**A**) area 25 has widespread efferent and afferent connections with many cortical and subcortical regions that are comparable to the efferent and afferent connections of IL in the rat (**B**). Afferents and

efferents are depicted superimposed on orbital, medial and lateral views of the macaque and rat brains based on anterograde and retrograde tracing studies. Macaque: [1,4–15]. Rat: [4,6,9]. Abbreviations: AC, Anterior Cingulate; Acb, Accumbens; AIa/p, Agranular Insula anterior/posterior; Amyg, Amygdala (AA, anterior amygdala; AB, Accessory Basal; BMA, basomedial; BLA, basolateral; Bpc/mc, Basal parvicellular/magnocellular; CE, CM, centromedial; central; COA, cortical; LA, lateral; MEA, medial; PA, posterior; TR, Amygdalo-piriform transition zone); AON, Anterior Olfactory Nucleus; BF, Basal Forebrain (BNST, Bed Nucleus of the Stria Terminalis; DB, Diagonal Band of Broca; EN, endopiriform nucleus; LS, Lateral Septum; MPO, Medial Preoptic Area MS, Medial Septum; SI, Substantia Innominata; TTv/d, ventral/dorsal Taenia Tecta); cc, Corpus Callosum; Cdm, medial Caudate; CLA, Claustrum; CLi, Central linear nucleus; CPu, CaudatePutamen; EC, Entorhinal Cortex; ECT, Ectorhinal Cortex; FPm, Frontal Polar Cortex, medial; HF, Hippocampal Formation, Hyp, Hypothalamus (AH, anterior nucleus; AHAvm, Anterior Hypothalamic area, ventromedial) DILA, Dorsal Hypothalamic area; DMH, Dorsomedial, LHA, Lateral Hypothalamic area; LPOA, lateral Preoptic area; MB, Mammillary bodies; MPOA, medial Preoptic area; Pef, Periformical; PH, Posterior nucleus; PHA, Posterior Hypothalamic area; PeriMam, Peri-mammillary; SupraMam, Supra-mammillary; TM, Tubero-mammillary; ParaMam, Paramammillary); IL, Infralimbic;; IP, interpeduncular nucleus; OFC, Orbitofrontal cortex (LO, lateral orbital; VLO, ventrolateral orbital; VO, ventral orbital; MO, medial orbital); Opro, Orbital proisocortex; OPAl, Orbital periallocortex; Pons/Medulla (Barrington's N, Barrington's Nucleus; CN, Cuneiform nucleus; dlPAG, dorsolateral Periaqueductal Grey; DMNvagus, Dorsal Motor Nucleus of Vagus; DR, Dorsal Raphe; LC, Locus Coeruleus; LDT, Laterodorsal tegmental nucleus; MR, Median Raphe; NI, Nucleus Incertus; NSTract, Nucleus of the Solitary Tract; PBl/m, Parabrachial lateral/medial; RF, Reticular Formation); pg, perigenual; PL, Prelimbic; PRC, Perirhinal Cortex; RPO, Nucleus pontis oralis; RSC, Retrosplenial Cortex; SNc, Substantia nigra pars compacta; Thalamus: (Am, medial Anterior; CEs/m/dc, Central superior/medial/ densocellular; IAM, Interanteriomedial; IMD, Intermediodorsal; LD, Lateral dorsal; LH, Lateral Habenula; Lim, Limitans; LP, Lateral posterior; MDpc/mc, Mediodorsal parvocellular.magnocellular; PF, parafascicular; PM, medial Pulvinar; PT, Parataenial; PV, Paraventricular, R, Reuniens; RH, Rhomboid; sc, subcallosal; SM, Submedial; Vamc, Ventral Anterior magnocellular); STG, Superior Temporal Gyrus, STS, Superior Temporal Sulcus; TEI, TF, TH, TP, Temporal pole; VTA, Ventral Tegmental Area; Brodmann's Areas, 9, 10, 11, 12, 13, 14, 23, 24, 25, 28, 30, 32, 35, 36, 46, TE1, TF, TH. Nomenclature of prefrontal cortex parcellation in macaque based on [15].

According to Vogt [16], area 25 can be identified across humans, monkeys, rats and mice which should facilitate inter-species translation of findings across experimental studies. However, structural homology does not necessarily equate to functional homology. In rodents, the area identified as area 25 by Vogt, is commonly called infralimbic cortex (IL) and so will be referred to as IL in this review. As would be expected if primate area 25 and rodent IL are homologous, IL projects to many of the same cortical and subcortical projection areas linked to emotion, visceromotor control and memory as area 25 in the macaque [4] (Figure 1B). Certainly, Haber and colleagues have confirmed the similarity of the IL-25-striatal projection pattern across rats and macaques [5]. In contrast, Barbas and colleagues [17] suggest that IL-amygdala projections of the rat more closely resemble the posterior OFC-amygdala projections of a macaque because of the similarity of the projections onto the GABAergic inhibitory intercalated masses of the amygdala. Notably absent in rats [4,6] are connections with auditory association and polymodal sensory association cortices that have been described in macaques. Conversely, in rats, IL projects to the accessory olfactory nucleus involved in olfactory processing and the Nucleus of the Solitary Tract and other autonomic effector regions in the brainstem, which are not innervated directly by the primate area 25 [1]. Moreover, as will be seen later in the descriptions of functional effects of the rodent IL compared to the monkey area 25, potential differences do emerge, suggesting that the assumption of functional homology between these regions may be premature. Another issue hampering translation is that, often when describing activation foci within the subcallosal zone, human neuroimaging studies do not differentiate between the distinct cytoarchitectonic regions present within this zone [18]. Moreover, in some cases, the term vmPFC is used instead to refer to an even broader area that not only includes the subcallosal cortex, but extends rostrally into ventromedial regions lying in front of the genu [19]. As a consequence, activation loci that truly include area 25 are less evident in the human neuroimaging literature [20], highlighting why current understanding of the functions of this region is particularly dependent upon neurobiological studies targeting area 25 in monkeys. By careful comparison with studies of IL in rodents we can begin to piece together the functions of this region, determine the extent of functional homology, and inform future studies in humans.

2. Physiological Function and the Subcallosal Zone

A prominent function of area 25, and one that is perhaps key to our overall understanding of this subcallosal region, is its involvement in visceral control and feedback mechanisms involving cardiovascular, endocrine and immune systems. Area 25 has been implicated in the regulation of autonomic (particularly cardiovascular) and endocrine functions in studies of non-human primates and humans, and significant insight has also been gleaned from studies in rodents exploring the anatomical connectivity and functional importance of its putative homologue, IL, as described in detail below. When reviewing this literature two factors should be taken into account. First, whether the study has employed an awake or anesthetized preparation, since anesthesia is known to alter cardiovascular activity [21]. Second, how the cortex has been manipulated. Several early functional studies employed electrical stimulation [22] and the frequency of stimulation, together with pulse duration, can result in differing magnitudes of effects and activate adjacent fiber pathways [23]. Furthermore, whether the impact of electrical stimulation is analogous to 'activating' or 'inhibiting' a brain region is not always known.

2.1. Area 25 and Cardiovascular Function

In humans, despite the strong connections between area 25 and autonomic control centers, neuroimaging studies investigating heart rate (HR) and blood pressure (BP) regulation have consistently implicated more dorsal and perigenual (pg)ACC regions rather than more ventral area 25 [24–28]. However, investigations of the dynamic adjustment of HR, using measures of heart rate variability, do implicate area 25 activity across cognitive, motor and affective manipulations [29]. In particular, activity in the caudal regions of human vmPFC, that included area 25, correlated positively with vagal tone whilst shifting between affective states [30]. This linked area 25 and vmPFC BOLD activity patterns directly with high frequency band components of heart rate variability, thought to reflect parasympathetic activity [31]. Thus, in particular, area 25 may modulate parasympathetic output [32,33].

More rarely, modulation of cardiovascular function has also been observed following deep brain stimulation of the human vmPFC, including area 25, in patients undergoing electrode implantation as a prelude to surgery to relieve epilepsy [34]. In the four patients with electrodes within scACC, stimulation produced consistent and striking hypotensive changes; specifically, a reduction in systolic BP with more variable changes in diastolic BP. Hypotensive effects were substantially greater in those patients with a more caudal placement in area 25 compared to a more rostral placement (within area 14; Figure 2Ai). However this interpretation is confounded by differences in the laterality of the hemisphere stimulated, and uncertainty over whether the neurophysiological consequence of deep brain stimulation is excitation, inhibition, or a more generalized disruption [35]. Thus, although scACC/25 is implicated in autonomic, particularly parasympathetic, regulation, the precise role area 25 plays in humans is still unclear.

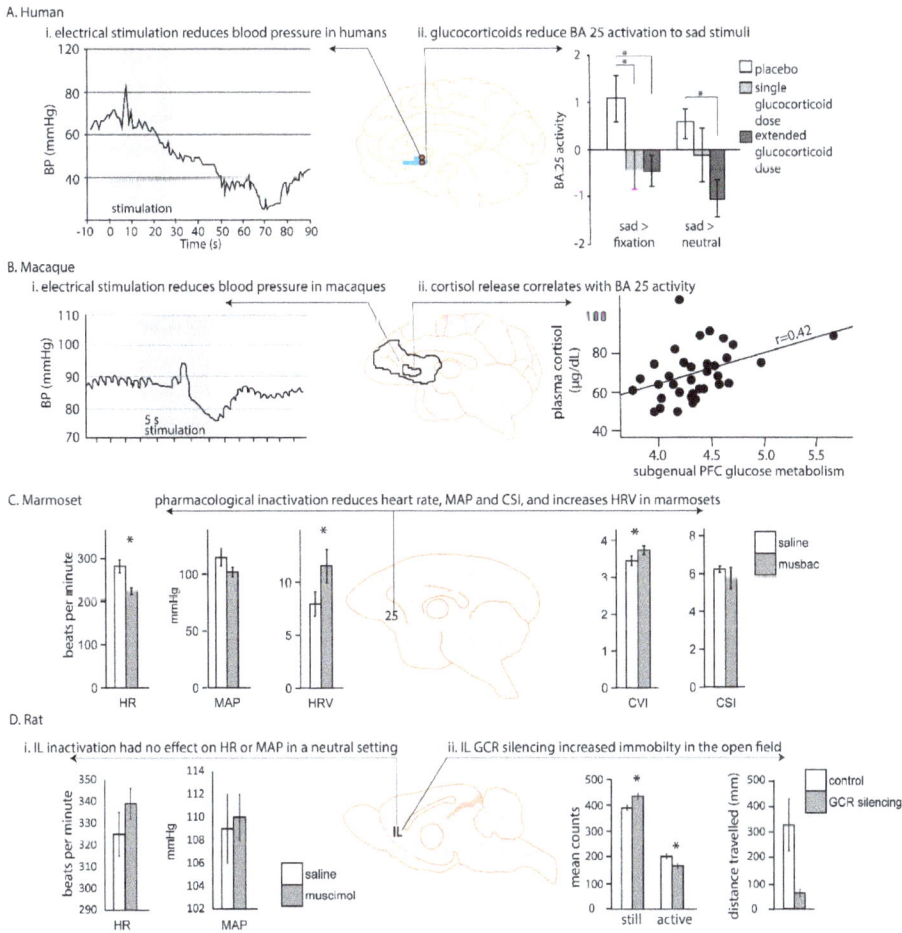

Figure 2. Examples of the relationship between cardiovascular and endocrine responsivity and area 25/infralimbic (IL) activity in emotional and non-emotional conditions in human, macaque, marmoset and rat. (**A**) In humans, (**i**) stimulation of area 25 via deep brain stimulation (red circles indicate stimulation loci) causes a brief hypertension followed by pronounced hypotension in anesthetized humans [34] while (**ii**) the administration of peripheral cortisol decreases area 25 activation to sad stimuli (brain region shaded blue) in the absence of any stressors [36]. (**B**) In macaques (**i**) stimulation of area 25 in anesthetized animals caused a brief hypertension followed by pronounced hypotension [22], similar to humans, and (**ii**) cortisol release correlates with ventromedial prefrontal cortex (vmPFC) activity during neutral conditions (large demarcated area), and specifically with area 25 during both stressful and neutral conditions (small demarcated area; [37]). (**C**) In marmosets, pharmacological inactivation of area 25 with GABA A and B agonists (muscimol and baclofen; 'musbac') in a neutral condition caused a reduction in heart rate (HR) and mean arterial blood pressure (MAP) that was accompanied by an increase in heart rate variability (HRV). Subdivision of the cardiac vagal and cardiac sympathetic indices (CVI and CSI) revealed that this HRV change was caused by a selective increase in the parasympathetic CVI [38]. (**D**) In rats (**i**) inactivation of IL had no effect on HR and MAP [39], unlike humans and non-human primates, but (**ii**) selective glucocorticoid receptor (GCR) silencing within the IL reduced activity within the open field test indicating that cortisol can modulate IL's impact on emotional behavior [40]. Thus, whereas manipulation of area 25 in a neutral setting consistently

modulates cardiovascular function in humans and non-human primates, such changes are not apparent after IL manipulation in the rat. However, glucocorticoids appear to modulate negative emotion in both area 25 and IL indicating similarities in some functional domains, but not others.

Consistent with humans, anatomical tracing of area 25 connectivity in macaque monkeys shows dense projections to the hypothalamic autonomic nuclei which then project to the nucleus of the solitary tract and spinal autonomic centers [41]. Regions of non-human primate vmPFC, including area 25, also diffusely innervate multiple amygdala nuclei, meaning there is dual access to an emotional-visceral motor system [42,43]. Consistent with these anatomical connections, selective manipulations of non-human primate area 25 have shown the importance of this area in contributing to autonomic regulation.

Early functional work, much of which was carried out in macaques, largely focused on determining the contributions of the cingulate gyrus to cardiovascular regulation, rather than the involvement of area 25 specifically [44]. Nevertheless, evidence for a role of ventral subregions came when Kaada and colleagues applied electrical stimulation to regions of pgACC and scACC in anesthetized macaques [22]. Stimulation throughout these regions induced cardiovascular changes, with the most prominent cardiovascular change observed in 'posterior subcallosal cortex,' corresponding to area 25. In addition to having a respiratory effect, application of electrical current in this region produced a BP response, characterized by a transient hypertension followed by a more prolonged—but still short-lived—refractory hypotension (Figure 2Bi). These data support the findings in humans, in which hypotension was observed following deep brain stimulation in caudal vmPFC regions [34]. However, apart from the observation that enhanced activity within scACC/25 is seen during vegetative states such as sleeping (which potentially also reflects an influence on parasympathetic activity [45]), there has been little further electrophysiological investigation of the role of the primate vmPFC in autonomic regulation.

More recently, targeted pharmacological manipulations within the non-human primate vmPFC have specifically dissected out area 25's role in autonomic regulation [38]. Inactivation of area 25 (using a cocktail of GABA A and B agonists) in marmosets, New World monkeys, whilst in an emotionally neutral, quiet resting state, was found to have profound effects on cardiovascular activity, reducing HR and BP and increasing heart rate variability. When effects on heart rate variability were fractionated into vagal (parasympathetic) and sympathetic contributions, area 25 inactivation selectively increased cardiac vagal tone. These effects should be contrasted with the very limited effects on baseline cardiovascular activity, in the form of a modest increase in BP, which followed inactivation of area 32. Area 25 inactivation also reduced the learned HR increases associated with a stressful outcome, while area 32 inactivation elevated them [38], and area 25, but not area 32, activity mediated the normalization effects of hippocampal activation on the autonomic correlates of high-trait anxious responses [46]. Together, these pharmacological studies suggest that non-human primate area 25 has a critical causal role in modulating activity within a central autonomic network during both neutral and emotional states.

These findings do have some apparent similarity to a large body of work in rodents that supports a role for rodent vmPFC, including IL, in the regulation of cardiovascular function. Like in humans and non-human primates, the anatomical connectivity of IL points to a role in autonomic regulation. The IL projects to many autonomic control regions (the hypothalamus, amygdala, insula and periaqueductal gray [4,23]) which in turn project to the autonomic effector regions in the brainstem (Figure 1B). The IL and ventral aspects of the PL also project directly to these brainstem systems including the nucleus of the solitary tract [47] and the spinal cord (intermediolateral nucleus) [48]. These direct projections have led some researchers to coin the term 'visceral motor cortex' for these regions [23,47].

The anatomy is supported by functional studies of cardiovascular regulation which clearly demonstrate that IL manipulations can alter cardiovascular function. Nevertheless, it is difficult to compare these findings with those of non-human primates due to differences in the pharmacological compounds used, and variations in behavioral paradigms and types of stressor. Furthermore, only a few studies have investigated the consequences of IL manipulation in baseline, emotionally neutral conditions. Thus, inactivation of IL with a localized muscimol microinfusion had no effect on cardiovascular control during baseline conditions [39], whilst IL disinhibition with bicuculline increased respiratory and cardiac outflow [49]. In stressful situations the IL does appear to regulate cardiovascular responses, but in a stressor-specific manner [50]. Cobalt chloride injection in the IL (which silences inputs and outputs and 'inactivates' the brain region) reduces tachycardia associated with restraint stress [51]. In contrast, IL inactivation with muscimol did not alter the cardiovascular responses induced by air puff stress, indicating that there are either functional differences in the mechanism of inactivation, or behavioral differences as a consequence of different stressors [39]. Different again, activation of IL with the excitatory amino acid, N-Methyl-D-Aspartate (NMDA) did decrease the HR and BP responses induced by the same air puff [39]. Although both these stressors are unconditioned, air puff is considered a milder stressor compared to restraint stress.

In studies that have investigated the involvement of the IL in regulating conditioned (learned) cardiovascular responses it has been shown that excitotoxic lesions primarily targeting the IL (with variable involvement of the more dorsal prelimbic [PL] subregion) decreased HR responses to a tone predicting shock [52]. This is similar to the reduction in conditioned HR responses seen after area 25 inactivation in the marmoset [38].

In summary, non-human primate area 25 manipulations can clearly modulate cardiovascular function during both neutral and stressful conditions, particularly within the parasympathetic domain. IL manipulation in rodents also modulates cardiovascular function indicating some degree of functional conservation across species, but the direction and consistency of these cardiovascular alterations differ, depending upon the nature of the manipulation and the type of stressor, making it difficult to compare directly with primates. Further investigations that control for these variables are required to fully compare the autonomic influences of rodent IL function with that of primate area 25.

2.2. Area 25 and Endocrine Function

As well as the autonomic component of visceral control, there is strong evidence that area 25, and associated prefrontal regions, also regulates the endocrine component via interactions with the hypothalamic–pituitary–adrenal (HPA) axis, the body's primary stress response system. Unfortunately, as discussed below, surprisingly few studies have examined the neural correlates of HPA axis regulation in humans. Those that have, identify area 25 as an important contributor because it not only shows sensitivity to circulating cortisol levels but appears to be able to directly regulate HPA axis function.

Exogenous cortisol administration directly modulates the response of area 25 to sad picture stimuli, blunting sadness-induced activation [36]. This indicates that area 25 is sensitive to circulating cortisol. Furthermore, in young adolescents, salivary cortisol measurements during social stress positively correlate with elevated functional connectivity between area 25 and the salience network, including the dACC and bilateral anterior insula [53]. However, it is unclear whether this correlation specifically reflects the actions of cortisol on activity within this network, or the effects of the stressor per se or the effects of area 25 on HPA axis function. Stronger negative functional connectivity has also been observed between a region of the vmPFC (encompassing area 25, subcallosal area 24 and perigenual area 32) and the amygdala that was associated with higher cortisol levels [54]. It was proposed that this negative functional connectivity reflects the top-down regulation of the amygdala during stress, which subsequently modulates HPA axis activity. Conversely, however, the correlation could reflect the impact of elevated cortisol on network activity. Nevertheless, together, these findings highlight the complex interactions between prefrontal (including area 25) top-down regulation of the HPA axis, and its regulation by cortisol.

This complex relationship between area 25, the HPA axis and sensitivity to cortisol is also seen in non-human primates. High densities of glucocorticoid and mineralocorticoid receptors, which are sensitive to cortisol and other stress hormones, have been found in the vmPFC (including area 25) and lateral PFC of squirrel monkeys [55], indicating that these areas are sensitive to cortisol. The macaque also shows direct projections to central autonomic centers such as the hypothalamus, but also indirect projections to the adrenal medulla itself, through which it can regulate HPA axis activity. Recent anatomical tracing studies have used injections of rabies virus into the adrenal medulla and a survival time series analysis method to identify the third and fourth order neurons from areas 24c, 25 and 32 as the densest projections to the adrenal medulla. These regions are broadly similar to regions identified in human functional imaging studies related to autonomic modulation, negative affect and cognitive control, indicating that this medial region may mediate the effects of chronic stress on visceral function [56]. Consistent with this, metabolic activity within area 25 has been related to individual differences in HPA axis regulation in macaque monkeys [37]. Having been exposed to four situations of increasing stress for 30 minutes (home with cage-mate, home alone, human intruder exposure or foreign cage alone), macaques then underwent femoral venipuncture for cortisol levels together with - 2-deoxy 2 [^{18}F]fluoro-Dglucose (^{18}F-FDG) Positron Emission tomography (PET) scan. Area 25 was the only brain region in which activity correlated with cortisol output across different contexts. However, as already described for humans, the directionality of the relationship between area 25 activity and circulating cortisol remains unclear. This is because a positive relationship could reflect both stimulatory and inhibitory (negative feedback) processes co-occurring within the HPA axis. For example, area 25 activity could be correlated with cortisol output if it were providing a direct stimulatory input to the HPA axis, or if it were activated by increasing concentrations of circulating cortisol to exert negative feedback.

As in non-human primates, high densities of glucocorticoid receptors are found in the rodent vmPFC, and importantly, the directionality of the relationship between IL activity and cortisol levels has been identified in rodents, as IL manipulations have been shown to alter stress hormone activity in response to a stressor. Thus, after restraint stress, radiofrequency ablation of caudal IL increases adrenocorticotropic hormone (ACTH/corticosterone) levels, while corticosterone implants into IL reduce ACTH/corticosterone levels [57]. Neither manipulation had effects on baseline levels. Clearly therefore, the IL is acting to regulate the HPA axis. It should be noted that combined manipulations of IL and PL have also been shown to modulate corticosterone responses to some stressors, albeit in a different manner to IL alone, but these results are difficult to interpret as the precise area responsible for the effect is not known [58,59]. There is also evidence that glucocorticoids acting directly on IL can regulate the behavioral correlates of acute and chronic stress. Thus, a selective knockdown of glucocorticoid receptors within IL (not PL) increases immobility time in the forced swim test, a commonly used assay of depression-like behavior [40] (Figure 2Dii). However, it remains to be seen if administration of cortisol also directly alters IL activity, as seen in humans.

2.3. Area 25 and Immune Function

In addition to the role that area 25 plays in the release and regulation of physiological factors such as stress hormones, emerging evidence also implicates area 25 as a key player in the orchestrated responses to immune challenges. In humans, elevated activity within area 25 and subcallosal area 24 has been associated with increased levels of interleukin-1β during grief elicitation [60]. Injection of the typhoid vaccine increases interleukin-6 levels and negative mood compared to placebo, and inflammation-associated mood-deterioration directly correlates with elevated activity in area 25, subcallosal area 24 and pgACC area 32 [61]. Depressed patients also show significantly increased numbers of microglial cells in area 25, suggestive of increased inflammation within area 25 itself [62]. However, further work is necessary—particularly in preclinical rodent and non-human primate models—to elucidate whether there is a clinically significant interplay between area 25 and the immune system.

2.4. Summary

To conclude, area 25 clearly contributes to the regulation of the cardiovascular, endocrine and immune components of a co-ordinated visceral response, and as such, holds a vital integrative role across humans, non-human primates and rodents. Despite this, this visceral integration appears to be unconnected to the level of the intrinsic resting connectivity network related to internal processing in the brain. Thus, in healthy subjects, area 25 and the caudal scACC are generally not included within the default mode network; an intrinsic, distributed network of brain regions, including the posterior cingulate and rostral vmPFC, which shows correlated activity at rest, together with correlated task-dependent modulations [63–65] (but see [65–67] which do suggest area 25 involvement). However, it should be noted that area 25 can be preferentially recruited into the default mode network in depressed states. In these situations, the integrative visceral roles of area 25 could assume undue prominence [68] manifesting as suppression of parasympathetic outflow, elevated baseline HR and reduced baseline heart rate variability [29,69]. This is consistent with the preferential modulation of cardiovascular parasympathetic regulation after area 25 manipulations in humans and non human primates, the evidence for autonomic dysregulation in depression, and the preferential effects of the novel antidepressant ketamine on the scACC, including area 25 [38,65,70,71]. Area 25 may therefore be a key node in the integration of negative mood and abnormal visceral regulation, a premise supported by two recent meta-analyses of neuroimaging data that have associated area 25 activity with functions attributed to the default mode network, including emotion processing, attribution of affective meaning and autonomic function, as well as mentalization and autobiographical memory [19,72–74]. If so, area 25 is in a unique position to subconsciously link bioregulatory states with their mnemonic and emotional mood states.

3. Emotional Function and the Subcallosal Zone

3.1. Human Area 25 and Its Association with Negative Emotion and Anhedonia

3.1.1. Non-Pathological Mood States

The subcallosal region of the ACC, including area 25, has received significant attention in the context of negative mood and depression. This is due to the high frequency at which functional and morphological changes within this region have been identified in studies of negative affect, and the function of this region as a point of integration between visceral, attentional and affective information important for homeostasis and allostasis.

Suggestions that elevated area 25 activity may be relevant to disorders of enhanced negative emotion, in part, derive from studies implicating subregions of the scACC in transient states of sadness induced in healthy control subjects. In a comprehensive meta-analysis of earlier work that included 55 PET and fMRI emotion-induction studies across both positive and negative valence, induction of sadness was significantly associated with activation/increases in rCBF of an scACC region which partly encompassed area 25 [75]. Two important issues should be highlighted. First, only 46% of studies using sadness induction paradigms reported increased activity within the subcallosal region. This may be because of differences in the sadness provocation methods used. Earlier studies scanned participants during active generation of the sad state and yielded variable subcallosal activation [76–78]. In contrast, studies which scanned participants once the sad state was attained reported more consistent subcallosal activation [79,80]. Second, when subcallosal activation was reported to include area 25, closer inspection revealed activity to be focused in a more rostral area encompassing subcallosal area 24 rather than area 25.

Nevertheless, studies subsequent to this meta-analysis have identified elevated activity associated with negative affect in area 25. For example, increased activity within a region bordering areas 10 m, 32 m and 25 m positively correlated with an aggregate self-report score of individuals' experience of negative affect over the previous month [81]. Moreover, assessment of the neural responses to sad pictures in healthy elderly individuals revealed elevated activity within the subcallosal region, extending along the rostro-caudal extent to include area 25, subcallosal area 24 and area 14 [82]. Of particular interest, is a recent study [36] in which area 25 was not only selectively activated in participants viewing sad stimuli, but this activity was reduced by hydrocortisone, highlighting the sensitivity of this region to circulating cortisol.

In addition to the use of pictorial or autobiographical stimuli to induce negative mood states, several studies have explored regional metabolism in the context of affective verbal processing. In these studies, regions of the medial PFC are robustly engaged by emotional words, irrespective of valence. However, these regions are typically more rostral than area 25, corresponding to the area 25/24 border zone, subcallosal area 24 and area 32 [83,84]. Tryptophan depletion has also been used to induce negative mood states in healthy controls [85]. Tryptophan is the precursor of serotonin (5-hydroxytryptamine; 5-HT), and rapid depletion of tryptophan reduces brain 5-HT. The effects of tryptophan depletion span cognitive and affective domains, although the magnitude of the affective change is variable, with some studies showing that healthy controls—even if given selective serotonin reuptake inhibitor (SSRI) medication—do not show any mood changes [86]. In one such study, acute tryptophan depletion increased rCBF bilaterally in area 25 that correlated with reduced mood, and simultaneously decreased rCBF in dACC/area 24 in a mood-independent manner [87].

An additional cluster of studies have implicated scACC in negative affect derived from social exclusion and rejection in adolescents and young adults. In these studies, social exclusion is typically induced using a virtual game termed Cyberball [88], in which participants are excluded from a ball-tossing game by other pre-programmed virtual participants. However, a meta-analysis of fMRI-measured brain activations during social exclusion, predominantly using the Cyberball task, identified positive correlations between social exclusion and activity centered on subcallosal area 24, rather than area 25 [89].

In summary, the location of activation within the scACC during negative mood states, including sadness, is quite variable and only sometimes is area 25 included. Indeed, a recent study used the cytoarchitectonic and chemoarchitectonic profile of ten human post-mortem brains to construct continuous and maximum probability maps of the distinct subcallosal fields for areas 25, 24, 32 and 33. Using a forward inference approach, the functional connectivity profile of each area was assessed and it was the subcallosal portion of area 24, rather than area 25, that showed consistent activation in psychological processes encompassing 'sadness' [18].

3.1.2. Pathological Mood States

In one of the earliest studies to report a relationship between reduced volume of the scACC in both unipolar and bipolar depressed subjects [90], the region of interest lay relatively rostral, at the border between subcallosal area 24 and perigenual area 32. Indeed, in an extension of this initial study, the region of interest still lay anterior to area 25 [91]. A subsequent study measured the volumes of both an 'anterior' region corresponding to subcallosal area 24, and a 'posterior' region corresponding to area 25 [92]. Here, the volume of left area 25 was smallest for patients with psychotic major depression compared to schizophrenics and healthy controls, whereas volumes of the subcallosal area 24 did not differ between groups. More recently, several studies have identified reductions in subcallosal volume encompassing varying portions of area 24 [93], area 25 [94], or both [95–97].

Besides reports of volume change, there have also been reports of functional abnormalities. In early studies, hypoperfusion in broad regions encompassing the scACC was consistently reported in Single Photon Emission Computed Tomography (SPECT) and PET studies [98–102]. However, these studies are in part confounded by the influence of volumetric changes within area 25 of patients suffering from Major Depressive Disorder [92]. When corrected for regional atrophy, area 25 does not show reduced activity—instead, rCBF measurements suggest activity is normal [80] or elevated [103]—although in the latter study the subjects were treatment resistant and the elevated activity appeared more rostral than area 25. However, more consistent are the reductions seen in area 25 activity in treatment responders following deep brain stimulation [103], fluoxetine [80], and the placebo effect [104].

Primary increases within subregions of the scACC in depressed populations have also been reported in functional studies. For example, when comparing patients with Major Depressive Disorder to non-depressed individuals, greater activity within area 25 was associated with the processing of sad faces, whereas greater activity within subcallosal area 24 was associated with processing of happy faces [105]. A subsequent meta-analysis of resting-state and emotion-activation studies found increased activity within right area 25 of depressed patients when exposed to positive emotional stimuli [106], and decreased activity following SSRI treatment. However, a more recent meta-analysis found decreases in area 25 associated with emotional processing tasks in depressed patients, although this study did not separate the positive and negative domains of emotion processing [107].

Besides negative mood, a key symptom of depression is anhedonia, the loss of interest and pleasure in all or almost all activities. It is highly prevalent in depression [108] and is a negative prognostic indicator [109,110], often associated with treatment resistant depression. However, area 25 is seldom identified in anhedonia-related neuroimaging studies. Functional activity changes associated with anhedonia are typically more rostral than area 25, encompassing regions such as area 10/24 and perigenual area 32 [111]. A recent study did however investigate abnormal connectivity patterns in a more posterior subcallosal region associated with altered activity in mood and anxiety disorders based, on an activation-likelihood estimation meta-analysis. The connectivity of the ROI with key reward-related regions (including the nucleus accumbens and ventral tegmental area [VTA]) was negatively correlated with anhedonia during pleasant music listening, but not anxiety levels, whereas resting state activity changes within the ROI did not differentiate between the two symptom clusters [112]. However, this ROI mainly included area 24 and was still rostral to area 25.

3.1.3. Neurobiological Models of Depression with a Focus on Human Area 25

There are several influential neurobiological models of depression that directly implicate vmPFC dysfunction in its etiology and/or pathogenesis, namely the limbic-cortical, cortico-striato-pallido-thalamic (CSPT) and default mode network models. These models are not mutually exclusive and are overlapping in terms of the neurobiological substrates being implicated, and the consequences that dysfunction within these structures has on behavior, physiology and cognition. We will focus on the role of area 25 within these models.

The limbic-cortical model was formulated in order to link impairments in cognition to sustained alterations in mood states characteristic of depression [113]. It focused on hypoactivity in a dorsal compartment proposed to be principally involved with the attentional and cognitive features of depression, including dm/dlPFC, area 24, parietal cortex and the dorsal striatum. Hyperactivity in a ventral compartment, consisting of limbic and paralimbic structures including area 25, was proposed to mediate the vegetative and somatic aspects of depression. Finally, the rostral cingulate, corresponding to perigenual areas 24 and 32, [113] was proposed to regulate the interaction between the dorsal and ventral compartments. Depression was then hypothesized to result from a failure of the coordinated interactions within and between compartments.

One of the most promising treatment modalities developed from this model is deep brain stimulation. In 2005, it was reported that deep brain stimulation targeting area 25 ameliorated symptoms of depression in four out of six individuals with treatment refractory depression [103]. Although an industry-sponsored trial utilizing deep brain stimulation of area 25 has failed in recent years [114], this has not stalled further investigation, with subsequent work refining neurosurgical targeting techniques and identifying potential biomarkers which might predict treatment response. Tractography imaging techniques to identify similarities in electrode contacts within deep brain stimulation responders have also highlighted the importance of four white matter bundles underlying area 25 [115]. This approach is proving valuable in identifying optimal deep brain stimulation targets to achieve antidepressant responses [116].

The cortico-striato-pallido-thalamic model posits abnormal activity in the CSPT circuitry to explain, at least in part, the clinical symptoms and cognitive deficits associated with depression. CSPT loops connect regions of the PFC with the basal ganglia and thalamus in a parallel but overlapping manner to support a multitude of behavioral and cognitive functions [117]. Evidence for the importance of

CSPT circuitry in mood disorders includes: (i) structural and functional imaging studies that show evidence of alterations in CSPT components associated with depression [118–120]; and (ii) a higher prevalence of depression associated with neurodegenerative and vascular diseases that involve CSPT circuitry [121–123]. The ventral caudate and nucleus accumbens (forming, together with the olfactory tubercle, the ventral striatum) are arguably the most consistently implicated striatal subregions in depression. Patients with remitted depression show hyperactivation of the caudate and accumbens during negative picture viewing [124], and currently depressed patients show hypoactivation of the accumbens and ventral caudate during rewards [125,126]. Aberrant ventral striatal functional connectivity also predicts future risk for developing depression [127].

Given the anatomical evidence that area 25 and adjacent vmPFC projects strongly to the ventral striatum [117], area 25-ventral striatal limbic circuitry has been explored in the context of CSPT changes associated with depression. Meta-analytic approaches have consistently identified volumetric abnormalities within these limbic CSPT circuits: reduced volume in the PFC—especially area 25 and OFC—together with reduced volume in the ventral caudate and putamen [128,129]. However, a meta-analysis of functional resting-state network connectivity in depression identified reduced connectivity between subcallosal activity rostral to area 25 and the ventral striatum [130].

Finally, in the *default mode network model*, increases in functional connectivity between the caudal vmPFC, specifically area 25 and nodes (rostral vmPFC and posterior cingulate cortex) within the default mode network, have been reported in people with depression [131]. Thalamic involvement is also evident, with increased connectivity between area 25, the mediodorsal (MD) thalamus and the default mode network, which has also been linked to higher levels of rumination [132–134]. These findings have led to the proposal that increased functional connectivity between this network (involved in biasing towards self-referential thinking processes) and area 25 (supporting negatively affectively-laden behavioral withdrawal) result in pathological rumination: self-focused, negatively valenced and withdrawn thinking processes [132]. However, since area 25 does not directly project to nodes of the network [135], but does project to the MD thalamus (which itself projects to the network nodes) it is suggested that the increased correlation of activity between area 25 and the default mode network is mediated by projections through the MD thalamus.

Altogether, whilst there is considerable correlative evidence for a role of area 25 in negative mood states in humans, direct evidence is limited. Whilst there have been a number of important studies describing the behavioral effects of varying levels of damage to human vmPFC (for review see [136], the selective contributions of area 25 could not be determined. Perhaps surprisingly, few non-human primate studies have addressed the contributions of area 25 to emotion and its regulation and thus, until recently, the majority of our understanding had come from studies of the IL in rodents. The findings from monkeys and rodents will now be described and their translatability to one another, and to human studies, will be discussed.

3.2. Monkey Area 25 and Its Association with Negative Emotion and Anhedonia

3.2.1. Neurophysiological Correlates of Reward and Punishment

One of the earliest studies in macaques to record in mid to caudal regions of area 25 found that the neurons had very low spontaneous firing rates, and failed to respond to tastes and olfactory cues, or to reward associated stimuli on a visual discrimination reversal task, including faces. Of the 93 recorded neurons, 11 showed an increase in responding from zero to approximately four spikes/sec during slow wave sleep [45]. Consistent with the lack of responsiveness to appetitive cues, a more recent study also showed that area 25 neurons displayed little response to appetitive conditioned stimuli (CSs; i.e., visual cues paired with reward) and unconditioned stimuli (USs; i.e., reward) during appetitive blocks of a Pavlovian task [137]. However, they did signal both aversive CSs and USs, in the form of visual cues paired with an air puff to the face. In contrast, more ventrally located neurons [1,2] were persistently more active in appetitive blocks. When recordings were made more rostrally in perigenual regions of area 25, neurons responded to a wide range of variables during a gambling task, both positive and negative, although there was a bias towards encoding of negative outcomes [138]. An overlapping region of recordings in this perigenual zone identified neurons as being more sensitive to internal factors, such as satiation, rather than external factors, such as visual cues [139]. Whether these differences across studies reflect changes in function between rostral and caudal and dorsal and ventral sectors of area 25 remain to be determined.

3.2.2. Area 25 Manipulations and Threat

Recently, pharmacological studies have been carried out in marmoset monkeys that temporarily inactivate or activate area 25 (see Figure 3). Inactivation with GABA A and B agonists (muscimol and baclofen) (i) reduced the expression of behavioral (orienting/scanning) and cardiovascular (blood pressure and heart rate) conditioned threat responses during Pavlovian discriminative conditioning when a previously neutral stimulus (i.e., an auditory cue) became associated with an aversive event (i.e., a loud noise and (ii) accelerated extinction of conditioned cardiovascular and behavioral responses, when the conditioned stimulus no longer predicted the aversive event (i.e., rubber snake) [38]. These findings suggest that non-human primate area 25 normally acts to drive Pavlovian cardiovascular and behavioral responses during threatening situations.

The directionality of the effects of area 25 manipulations were conserved in the instrumental domain too. Using a touchscreen approach-avoidance decision-making task where marmosets responded for rewards with the potential for punishment, inactivation of marmoset area 25 reduced punishment avoidance. Conversely, enhancing pre-synaptic glutamate release within area 25 (using a combination of $mGlu_{2/3}$ and $GABA_B$ receptor antagonists) enhanced punishment avoidance [140]. The increased sensitivity to punishment seen when glutamate release in area 25 was enhanced, causally relates elevated activity in area 25 to negative decision-making biases observed in individuals with depression [142,143]. Consistent with these findings, increasing activity within marmoset area 25 using an alternative method, namely inhibiting the excitatory amino acid transporter-2 (EAAT2) to reduce glutamate reuptake (using dihydrokainic acid [DHK],) enhanced marmoset responsivity on the human intruder test, a classic method of measuring anxiety-like behavior in a primate which assesses the behavioral responses to an unfamiliar human that elicits uncertainty [141]. Taken together, these data suggest that inhibiting activity within marmoset area 25 reduces the behavioral and cardiovascular correlates of negative affect, whereas increasing activity has the opposite effect, and enhances these correlates. These effects may reflect the behavioral and physiological output of the neural bias in encoding negative outcomes described in electrophysiological studies.

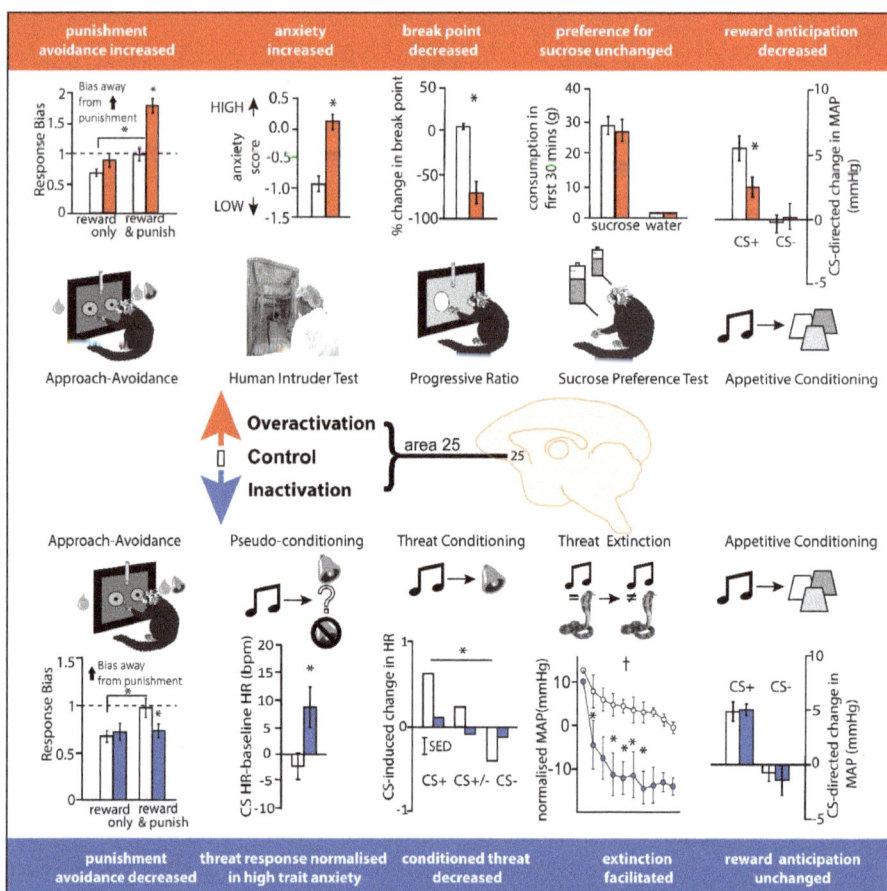

Figure 3. Over-activation and inactivation of area 25 in marmoset has largely opposing effects on tests measuring the regulation of responsivity to rewarding and punishing stimuli. Top from left. Over-activation via presynaptic glutamatergic disinhibition increased the bias away from punishment in an approach-avoidance decision making paradigm [140], and over-activation via inhibition of the excitatory glutamate amino acid transporter (EAAT2; with dihydrokainic acid [DHK]) increased anxiety-like behavior in the human intruder paradigm, increased the break point in a progressive ratio task, left sucrose consumption unaltered, and blunted the anticipation of food reward during appetitive conditioning [141]. Bottom from left. In contrast, inactivation with GABA A and B agonists (muscimol and baclofen) decreased the avoidance of punishment during approach-avoidance decision making [140] and reversed the blunted cardiovascular responsivity to threat in high trait anxious animals [46]. Inactivation also blunted the threat-induced anticipatory increases in heart rate and vigilant scanning (not shown) during Pavlovian threat conditioning and enhanced the rate of threat extinction [38], but had no effect on reward anticipation during appetitive conditioning [141]. *, $p < 0.05$, †, $p < 0.05$, main effect of manipulation; error bars indicate SEM. Thus, in general, over-activation blunted appetitive responses whilst enhancing threat-induced responses whilst inactivation primarily dampened threat-induced responses.

3.2.3. Area 25 Manipulations and Reward

The only lesion study to target area 25 in a non-human primate implicated this region in the maintenance of arousal in anticipation of positive rewarding outcomes. Ablation of area 25 in macaques impaired their ability to sustain autonomic (pupillary dilation) arousal during a trace interval between an appetitive CS and US [144]. Disruption of this function could be relevant to the reduced reward processing associated with depression, broadly referred to as anhedonia (involving a reduced ability to experience pleasure, together with reduced anticipation and motivation). However, as discussed above, reduced activity in this area is more consistently associated with recovery from depression. Moreover, given that this study in macaques used ablations, it is possible that the effects reported were a consequence of damage to fibers of passage, especially since this region is a major conduit for a number of fiber bundles carrying fibers to and from the cortex [115].

More recently, temporary pharmacological manipulations in area 25 of marmoset monkeys that selectively target neurons intrinsic to area 25, without affecting fibers of passage, has revealed that over-activation of area 25 not only enhances negative reactivity but also blunts anticipatory and motivational appetitive arousal (see Figure 3). The measurement of cardiovascular and behavioral responses during the CS 'anticipatory' and US 'consummatory' period of a Pavlovian appetitive conditioning task revealed selective blunting during the anticipatory period only following DHK-induced increases in glutamate release in area 25. The same infusions also caused an earlier breakpoint on an instrumental progressive ratio schedule of reinforcement [141] reflecting a reduction in the willingness to work for reward. The finding that inactivation of area 25 (using the GABA A and B agonists muscimol and baclofen) had no effect on anticipation suggests that area 25 activity is not necessary for reward-related anticipatory arousal but, when activated, has an inhibitory effect. An obvious question arising from these findings is what factor(s) naturally cause(s) activation of area 25? Given the relationship between area 25 and the HPA axis, described above in 'Area 25 and endocrine function', stress may be a key factor.

^{18}F-FDG PET imaging has provided insight into the changes in downstream brain regions caused by area 25 over-activation. These include increases in metabolic activity in the dorsomedial PFC and insula, but decreases in activity within a region encompassing the nucleus of the solitary tract and brainstem 5-HT neurons [141], all regions implicated in the networks of depression [132]. Of particular relevance to our understanding of current treatments of depression, peripheral ketamine, a recently discovered glutamate based anti-depressant with particular efficacy in treating reward-related deficits [145–147], ameliorated the anhedonia-like symptoms induced by area 25 over-activation. Not only did ketamine restore cardiovascular and behavioral anticipatory arousal but it also reversed the changes in the network. Thus, over-activation of area 25 produces both anxiety-like and anhedonia-like behavioral symptoms in a monkey and, consistent with clinical reductions of area 25 activity in treatment responders, ketamine ameliorates the anhedonia-like effects.

3.2.4. Area 25 and Its Interactions with the Anterior Hippocampus

Pharmacological intervention studies in marmosets have also probed the importance of area 25 in the wider network of structures important for regulating affective behavior. Initial studies have focused on the anterior hippocampus (aHipp), given the importance of connectivity between these regions in psychiatric disorders [148]. In one study, aHipp activations in high trait anxious marmosets were shown to reduce the marmosets' anxiety-like behavior to uncertain threat in the form of a human intruder, as well as to normalize their blunted behavioral and cardiovascular response to unpredictable aversive loud noise. Simultaneous inactivation of area 25, but not area 32, however, blocked these anxiolytic effects, areas which, when inactivated independently, reduced or had no effect on anxiety, respectively [46]. Simultaneous inactivations of area 25 have also been shown to block the ability of aHipp activations to reduce punishment avoidance on an approach-avoidance instrumental decision-making paradigm, despite area 25 reducing punishment avoidance when inactivated independently [140]. In both examples, activation of aHipp and inactivation of area 25 independently reduced threat-induced responses, but when occurring simultaneously these anxiolytic effects were abolished, thereby highlighting the importance of the interaction between these two regions in the regulation of negative emotion. However, how their effects are orchestrated within the wider network of structures known to be involved in regulating responsivity to threat is a key question for future studies. For example, the amygdala, striatum, OFC and ventrolateral prefrontal cortex (vlPFC) have all been implicated in approach-avoidance decision making [149–152]. Indeed, using the exact same paradigm, interactions between the OFC and amygdala in marmosets have been shown to contribute to the long-lasting mnemonic effects of punishment on decision making, without influencing decision making at the time of punishment per se [149]. Different again are the effects of inactivation of the vlPFC, which acts to enhance avoidance of punishment on decision making at the time of punishment. Since the aHipp projects to the vlPFC as well as area 25 [14] and there is weak to moderate connectivity between area 25 and vlPFC [1], investigating the nature of the interactions between these structures on approach-avoidance decision making and other threatening contexts is an important next step.

3.3. Rodent Infralimbic Cortex and Its Association with Negative Emotion and Anhedonia

3.3.1. Conditioned Threat and Its Extinction

Experimental studies in rodents have implicated IL in a range of different behavioral functions, but some of the most extensive investigations have focused upon its role in the extinction of conditioned threat. Early experiments in rodents assessed the effects of broad lesions to mPFC (including PL, IL, Medial OFC and ACC) on the extinction of threat memories, as measured by the low level of conditioned freezing displayed to a CS that was no longer paired with foot shock, and found these lesions severely impaired extinction, without an effect on the acquisition of conditioned freezing [153]. Subsequently, lesions restricted to the IL confirmed this region's role in the successful recall of extinction while, lesions that spared most of the IL did not have an effect, suggesting that the IL is the critical mPFC sector necessary for recalling extinction memories [154]. Since this lesion work, electrophysiological, microstimulation and pharmacological inactivation studies have also probed the specific contributions of the IL and PL to threat regulation. In seminal work, reviewed in Milad and Quirk [155], recordings from IL neurons during acquisition, extinction and extinction recall phases revealed that IL neurons fired only when recalling a CS/noUS association on extinction recall days. The degree of firing correlated with successful recall of this association: the more IL neurons fired, the less rodents froze. Pharmacological inactivation studies have since extended this work by causally implicating IL in extinction and extinction recall and indicate that IL is a key player in the inhibitory mechanisms which may 'gate' information flow within downstream structures—such as the amygdala—during CS-noUS learning and retention [156,157]. These effects are not just restricted to conditioned freezing, as IL inactivation also disrupts extinction recall when avoidance is the conditioned response [158] and conversely, IL activation during extinction using d-cycloserine can facilitate re-extinction of the conditioned freezing response the next day [159].

Although neuroimaging studies in humans have been interpreted to support the role of this region in recall of extinction of conditioned threat responses [160–162], as measured by skin conductance responses, the regions of altered activity are far more rostral than area 25, in one case almost at the level of the genu of the corpus callosum. Thus, although a region within vmPFC in humans shows correlated activity with extinction recall, it does not correspond to area 25 (Figure 4A). Moreover, as described above, inactivation of area 25 in marmosets facilitates extinction rather than impairs it, and in contrast to the impaired extinction recall in rodents, has no apparent impact on its recall (compare Figures 4B and 4C). Incidentally, area 32 inactivation in marmosets also produces opposite effects to those reported following inactivation of the putative functionally homologous region in rats, namely, the PL, with area 32 inactivation retarding extinction in marmosets as opposed to the impaired threat recall after PL inactivation in rats. There are at least two explanations for this discrepancy. The first is that the IL in rodents is not functionally homologous to primate area 25. The second is that the task design used in marmosets to study extinction of conditioned threat, although developed to match that of the rodents as close as possible, was not identical and performance relied on different psychological processes to those of the rat, that were differentially sensitive to area 25 inactivation. If the latter, then at the very least these results call into question the hypothesis that area 25 is essential for threat extinction and in particular threat extinction recall. Instead, it suggests that the underlying function of this region, when dysregulated, can have mixed effects on the extinction of conditioned threat responses, e.g., facilitative or antagonistic, presumably depending upon the precise context in which the conditioned threat is learned and modulated. Before considering, however, what the underlying function of IL might be, the contribution of IL to additional behavioral domains will be discussed.

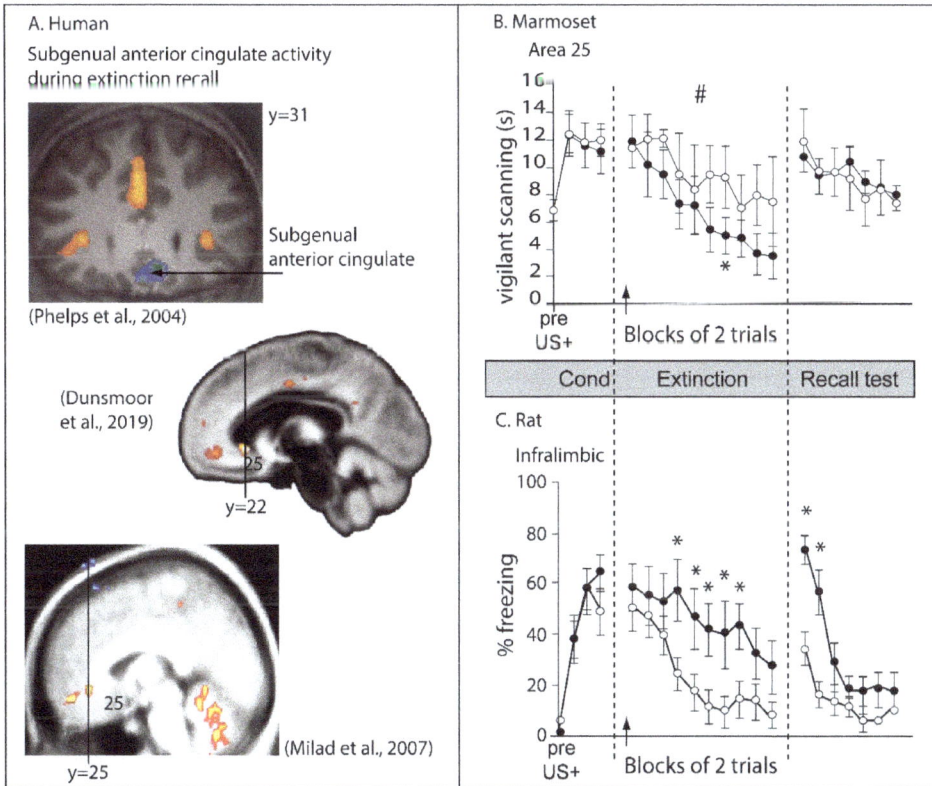

Figure 4. Re-thinking the role of area 25 in threat extinction in humans, marmosets and rats. (**A**) Human neuroimaging of extinction recall has identified regions of the subcallosal zone (scACC) in which the deactivation induced by the conditioned stimulus, CS+ is blocked following successful extinction recall [160–162]. However, these regions of activity are generally more rostral than area 25. (**B**) In marmosets, inactivation of area 25 with GABA A and B agonists (muscimol and baclofen; closed circles) hastened the behavioral extinction of an aversive (rubber snake) Pavlovian conditioned association [38]. In contrast (**C**) IL inactivation in rats (muscimol; closed circles) impeded the behavioral extinction and extinction recall of conditioned footshock. Redrawn from Sierra-Mercado et al., [157]. *, $p < 0.05$; #, $p < 0.05$, manipulation × CS interaction; error bars indicate SEM. Arrow indicates point of inactivation.

3.3.2. Depression-Like and Anxiety-Like Symptoms

Besides extinction of conditioned threat, altered activity in rodent IL has been implicated in putative depression-like (despair) and anxiety-like symptoms, as measured across a range of paradigms including forced swim, tail suspension (despair-like tests) and novelty suppressed feeding, elevated plus maze and open field (anxiety-like tests). Here, however, the findings have been contradictory.

An early report [163] revealed anti-depressant effects of inactivation of IL induced by the GABA agonist, muscimol, on the forced swim test in normal rats and those bred for high anxiety; activation of this area by the GABA antagonist, bicuculline, had no effect. In contrast, more recently, activation of IL induced by DHK [164] produced anti-depressant and anti-anxiety-like effects on the forced swim test and novelty suppressed feeding tests, respectively. A similar effect is seen following an acute optogenetically-induced activation of the pathway between IL and the amygdala [165], or following sustained optogenetically-induced activation of area 25 globally [166]; in which case the anti-anxiety effect is long lasting, being seen 24 h later and beyond. Different again, however, activation of IL induced by a GABA-A antagonist, induced anxiety-like behaviors on elevated plus maze, open field and novelty-suppressed feeding [167], as did an acute optogenetic activation of IL pyramidal neurons [168]. Acute versus more sustained activation of IL may contribute to the variation in the results, with acute effects tending to be anxiogenic whilst prolonged effects are more likely anxiolytic. However, very recently, sustained activation induced by genetic knockdown of the astrocytic glutamate transporter GLAST/GLT-1 expression, induced a depressive-like phenotype on the tail suspension and forced swim tests [169]. Other contributory factors to the variation in findings may therefore include whether the animal was tested in its subjective 'night' or 'day', with the former being likely to enhance the level of stress experienced; however, this information is not always provided. Prior experience with other stressors may also impact on overall subjective experience. Finally, whether IL was targeted via cannulas passing through the PL or not has also been suggested to be an important consideration, since there may be infusion spread up the tract which can only be ruled out by direct comparison with infusions into the PL [170].

The contribution of IL to reward processing domains have also been investigated. Overall, inactivation of the IL tends to increase, and activation of the IL reduce, reward driven behaviors in a variety of contexts. These include the spontaneous recall and reinstatement of Pavlovian and instrumental appetitive responses following extinction (reviewed in [171]) that are increased by lesions/inactivation of IL, comparable to that seen following extinction of Pavlovian threat responses reviewed above. Conversely, activation with d-cycloserine induces the opposite effect [172]. In addition, activation with DHK increases the threshold for lever pressing for electrical brain stimulation and increases the latency to begin consuming sucrose [173], all effects consistent with putative symptoms of anhedonia and opposite to the anti-depressant effects on the forced swim test described above [164]. It should be noted however that in the latter [173], cannulas passed through the PL to reach the IL, but infusions were not compared with equivalent manipulations of the PL. Nevertheless, additional support of a pro-depressant effect of IL activation in the reward domain, sustained activation by knockdown of GLAST/GLT-1 expression reduced sucrose consumption, an effect that was not due to PL involvement [169]. Moreover, IL activation using the GABA antagonist bicuculline dampens the intense eating behavior generated by glutamate disruptions in the nucleus accumbens shell [174]. In contrast, acute inactivation of the IL does not affect the break point of a progressive ratio schedule [175] and excitotoxic lesions of the IL have no effect on acquisition of appetitive Pavlovian conditioned autoshaping [176]. Thus, in summary, as seen in marmosets, activation of IL very often has broader effects on rewarded behaviors than effects of inactivation and in general, activation tends to dampen reward driven responses.

Without direct comparisons across laboratories using identical paradigms and pharmacological doses of drugs such as DHK and muscimol, or light stimulation parameters in the case of optogenetics, it is difficult to reconcile these mixed pro-depressant and anti-depressant findings on tests of learned helplessness and reward, and integrate them with the effects on conditioned threat extinction. Moreover, it is problematic to interpret changes in apparently 'normal' behavioral responses on a given test as anti-depressant, when there is no evidence that performance is 'depressed-like' in the first place. There are many reasons why an animal may spend more time swimming in a forced swim test and more time eating in the novelty suppressed feeding test other than they are displaying, respectively, a less 'depression-like' and 'anxiety-like' phenotype [177]. Future studies should determine whether

IL activation shows similar effects in a variety of other contexts designed to measure depression-like and anxiety-like behaviors to determine the consistency of these effects e.g. anticipatory, motivational and decision-making contexts related to reward processing and cognitive and affective negative biases associated with anxiety. In addition, these studies should include the measurement of multiple indices that extend beyond behavior to include physiological measures such as cardiovascular reactivity and cortisol levels since, as described above, depressive and anxiety-like states have a marked impact on physiology. Moreover, if testing for anti-depressant-like effects, it is more informative if a depressive-like phenotype is induced first, such as that produced by learned helplessness models [178].

Given the marked variation between rodent studies with regards anti-depressant and anxiolytic behavior, it is difficult to compare results with those described in marmosets. Comparisons are really only informative when the same pharmacological manipulation is made across species. Thus, DHK (overactivation)-induced anhedonia-like effects on responding to brain stimulation in rats [173] appear consistent with the anhedonia-like effects of DHK infusion into area 25 on the instrumental progressive ratio test in marmosets. Apparently different though is the deficit in sucrose consumption reported in rats, but not in marmosets. However, it should be noted that sucrose consumption per se was intact in rats and only a DHK-induced increase in the latency to begin drinking was observed. The latter could be interpreted as an anticipatory effect, which would then be consistent with the DHK-induced effects on anticipatory responding in marmosets. Nevertheless, it is still difficult to reconcile the hypothesized anxiolytic/anti-depressant effects of rodent IL DHK in the novelty-suppressed feeding test [164], with the DHK induced increase in anxiety like responses to an uncertain threat in the human intruder test in marmosets [141]. Such discrepancies can only be resolved in future studies using more comparable tests and with detailed comparison of the effects of DHK on network activity across species.

3.3.3. Stress and Its Controllability

Another emotion-related domain that involves both the IL and PL is the behavioral immunization effect of learned control over a stressor. Those animals that learn to run in a wheel to escape tail shock subsequently learn to avoid shock in other apparati (typically a shuttle box), in contrast to animals that learn that their attempts to escape a shock are futile, and then go on to fail to avoid subsequent shuttle box shocks [178]. This immunization effect produced by the experience of control over a stressor is seen across a range of contexts including aggression, social dominance, immobility, neophobia, threat conditioning and extinction [179]. PL appears most central to these effects since inactivation of PL disrupts immunization effects on both social and shuttle box behavior, whereas IL inactivation only blocks immunization effects on social behavior [180]. Enhanced release of serotonin in the dorsal raphe nucleus (DRN) and forebrain terminal regions is implicated in the learned helplessness effect [179], but only neurons in the PL (not IL) projecting to the DRN show selective activation to escapable stress [181]. Thus, the role of the IL in the behavioral immunization effect remains less clear.

However, the sensitivity of the IL to stress per se does appear clear. Whilst chronic stress can induce morphological changes within the PL and IL [182], the IL appears particularly sensitive, with even acute stress causing apical dendritic retraction, reduced spine-induced learning and disrupted threat extinction [183,184]. Moreover, intermittent stress in early adolescence increases the serotoninergic innervation of IL, but not PL, and promotes the emergence of an anxious phenotype in adulthood, although whether these two outputs were related was not investigated [183].

3.3.4. A More Complex Role for IL in Behavioral Control

Given the varied effects of experimental lesions or temporary inactivation of the IL and PL across the appetitive/aversive and cognitive/emotion domains, recent critiques have attempted to integrate these diverse findings [185,186] by taking into account the role of the IL in the ability of well-trained responses to dominate behavior. As summarized by Sharpe and Killcross [186], lesions of IL prevent appetitive instrumental responding becoming habit-like and insensitive to alterations in the valuation of the goal, following over-training [187], and inactivation re-instates goal directed sensitivity of over-trained instrumental responses [188]. They also prevent over-trained responses from disrupting the ability of contextual cues from an under-trained task to resolve response conflict in a rat version of the Stroop task [189]. Accordingly, Sharpe and Killcross [186] propose that a parsimonious explanation for IL function is that it acts to promote performance of well-trained responses that are context independent and reflect the animal's long term experience with the current contingencies. This expands upon a previous synthesis that suggested that IL inhibited previously established goal directed actions [185]. While they acknowledge some caveats with their current account, nevertheless it makes the point that high-order cognitive functions within this region are likely to have variable effects on tests of threat and reward driven behaviors depending upon the range of cues, responses and contingencies that may be in operation. Certainly, a recent study inactivated, independently, neuronal ensembles related to either food seeking or the extinction of food seeking within rat vmPFC, (targeting the IL in particular) and revealed the opposing effects that such manipulations could have on food seeking behavior [171]. It remains to be determined if similar effects can be seen with respect to threat-driven behaviors in rodents.

4. Summary and Future Directions

Fundamental to our understanding of area 25 in disease states is gaining an insight into the physiological, behavioral and cognitive functions requiring an 'on-line' area 25 (summarized in Figure 5). Encouragingly, the finding that area 25 is an important cortical visceral motor center holds across anatomical and functional studies in rodents, non-human primates and humans. This suggests that there are aspects of area 25's function in physiological domains that are conserved across species and given the importance of autonomic activity in the generation of affect, it would not be unreasonable to expect some degree of similarity in the effects of area 25 manipulations on affective behavior. This may indeed be the case when comparing human, non-human primate and rodent findings with respect to reward processing. Area 25 activation in marmosets blunts appetitive anticipatory and motivational arousal, effects reversed by an acute dose of ketamine, thus mirroring the reduction in area 25 activity following successful treatment in patients suffering from treatment-resistant depression. IL activation in rats also tends to reduce rewarded responding. Nevertheless, caution is warranted when drawing comparisons between behavioral and autonomic correlates of anticipatory affect in non-human primates and rodents and subjective states in humans. Future studies in the clinic should include the measurement of additional physiological and behavioral outputs to facilitate translation.

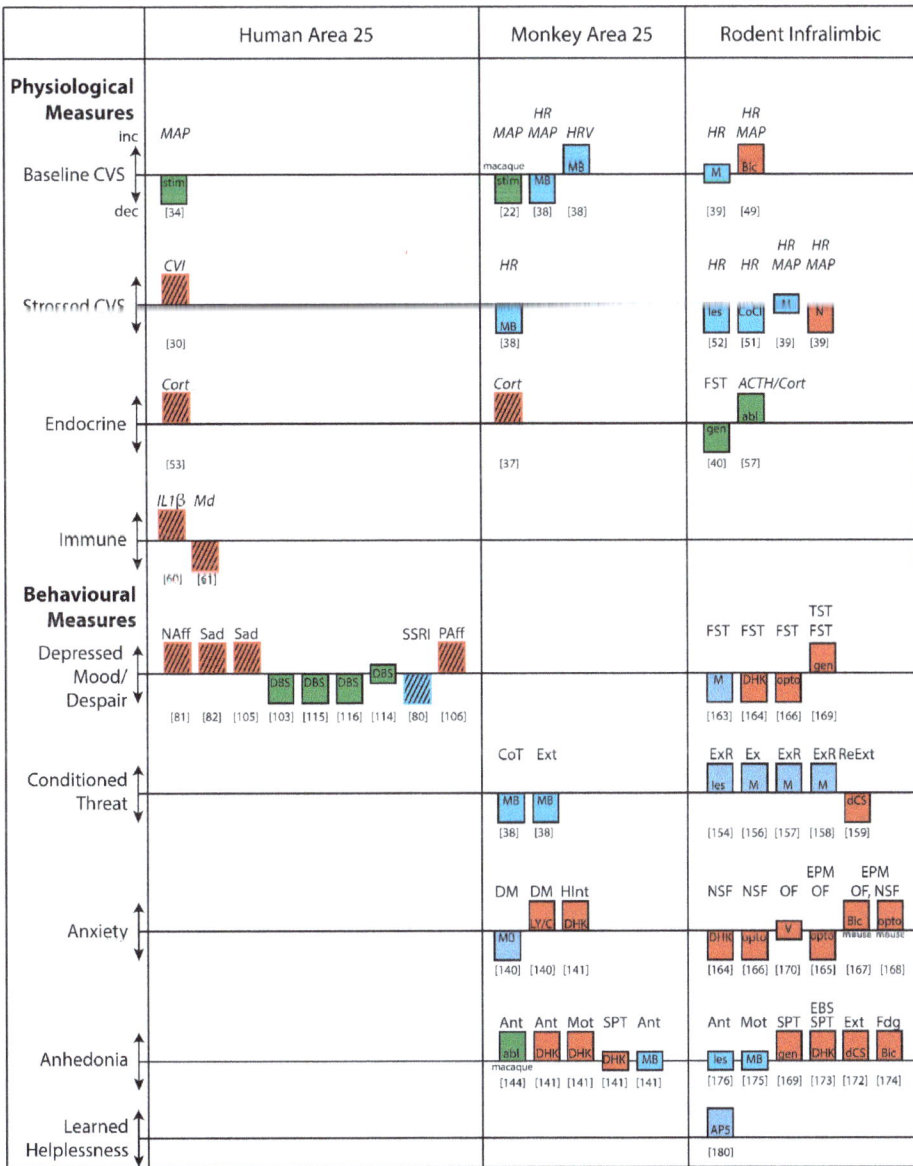

Figure 5. A summary of the physiological and behavioral functions associated with human and monkey area 25 and rodent infralimbic (IL). These representative studies illustrate, (i) the similarities and differences in the functional effects of manipulations of area 25 in monkeys and IL in rodents; (ii) how these map onto effects in humans; and (iii) where there are gaps in our knowledge. Blue bars denote reductions in activity, red bars denote increases in activity whilst green bars denote either that the direction of effects in area 25 are unclear, or that the effects may not be specific to area 25. Thus, if red and blue bars are going in the same direction (as in rodent despair), or if the same colored bars are going in opposite directions (as in rodent anxiety), the results are inconsistent. Headings above the bars indicate physiological measure if in italics, and the behavioral paradigm if non-italic. Hatching indicates correlations rather than manipulations. In terms of physiology, there is reasonable correspondence

between monkey and rodent with respect to the reductions/increases in cardiovascular activity following reductions/increases in area 25/IL activity, especially during stress; although there are exceptions (see [39]). Any correspondence with the effects of stimulation in humans is unclear, however, because the excitatory versus inhibitory effects of stimulation on area 25 activity are unknown; if indeed the effects are due to changes in area 25 at all, since effects on fibers of passage cannot be ruled out. In relation to cortisol, there is agreement between correlatory findings in humans and monkeys that indicate positive correlations between cortisol levels and area 25 activity in monkeys and area 25 functional connectivity in humans. However, this similarity does not extend to rodents [57], as radiofrequency ablation of the IL increases corticosteroids; although whether the ablation effects are specific to the IL cannot be determined. Whilst immune function is related to area 25 activity in humans, this hasn't yet been addressed in monkeys or rodents. With respect to behavior, changes in activity in area 25 in relation to depression can be variable, but successful treatment, especially in treatment resistant patients following DBS, is very often associated with reductions in area 25 activity. In line with this, the most consistent effects in both monkey area 25 and rodent IL are the overactivation-induced anhedonia-like effects. In contrast, the effects in monkeys and rodents of area 25/IL manipulations on conditioned threat responses and their extinction appear opposite, while in rodent studies the effects on despair-like and anxiety-like behaviors are inconsistent. Abl, ablation manipulation; AP5, AP-5 (NMDA antagonist); ACTH, adrenocorticotrophic hormone; Ant, Anticipatory arousal; Bic, Bicuculline (GABA$_A$ antagonist); CoCl, Cobalt chloride (silences activity); CoT, conditioned threat; Cort, Corticosterone; CVI, Cardiac vagal index of heart rate variability; CVS, Cardiovascular system; DBS, Deep brain stimulation; dCS, d-Cycloserine (NMDA co-agonist); DHK, Dihydrokainic acid (EAAT2 inhibitor); DM, Decision making (approach-avoidance); EPM, Elevated plus maze; Ext, Extinction; ExR, Extinction recall; Fdg, Feeding behaviour; FST, Forced Swim Test; Gen, genetic manipulation; HInt, Human intruder test; HR, Heart rate; HRV, heart rate variability; IL1β, Interleukin 1β; Les, lesion manipulation; LY/C, LY341495 (mGluR2/3 antagonist) and CGP52432 (GABA$_B$ antagonist); M, Muscimol (GABA$_A$ agonist); MAP, mean arterial pressure; MB, Muscimol (GABA$_A$ agonist) and baclofen (GABA$_B$ agonist); Md, Mood; Mot, Motivational arousal; NAff, Negative affect; NSF, Novelty suppressed feeding, OF, Open Field test; Opto, Optogenetic manipulation; PAff, Positive affect; ReExt, Re-extinction; Sad, Response to sad faces; SPT, Sucrose preference test; SSRI, Selective serotonin reuptake inhibitor; Stim, Stimulation manipulation; TST, Tail suspension test; V, Veratrine (Sodium channel activator). Numbers indicate the relevant reference.

Critical to overall progress in this field will be closer integration between studies across humans, monkeys and rodents, with monkeys acting to bridge the gap between rodents and humans. Especially important will be identifying under what circumstances area 25 is activated and determining the interaction between cognitive, physiological and behavioral functions associated with this region. From studies so far it can be seen that functional similarities between monkey area 25 and rodent IL are far from clear and in some cases appear opposite. As discussed above, these may be due, in part, to differences in the pharmacological tools used to induce activation and the duration of such effects, along with variations in the psychological/cognitive mechanisms engaged to perform a given task. However, it should also be borne in mind that whilst IL and area 25 are considered structurally homologous, the anatomical framework in which they reside is not. Primate area 25 is operating in concert with the highly developed dorsolateral (dlPFC), ventrolateral and frontopolar cortices, which are likely to be contributing to many of the tasks in which area 25 manipulations have been investigated. Thus, they may contribute to some of the differences observed between area 25 manipulations in primates and rodents. Given the vast expansion of PFC in primates it is more than likely that there has been an expansion and specialization of cognitive functions, in which the rudiments are instantiated in more generic processing modules within the rodent PFC.

Future studies in non-human primates should focus on these higher-order regions and begin to dissect out their interactions with area 25 to advance our understanding of the higher-order control of reward and threat-driven behaviors. By employing novel chemogenetic and optogenetic tools, the investigation of these specific non-human primate pathways descending into area 25 is now possible, alongside similar studies investigating selective efferents of area 25. This will be particularly important in establishing the multitude of functions that area 25 likely contributes to, given its extensive anatomical connectivity.

An additional consideration is how best to translate these findings into the clinic. So far, most targeted area 25/IL manipulations in preclinical animal work involve transient activations or inactivations, but see [169]. However, disease states are associated with chronic, long-term changes in a distributed network of structures. For instance, it is a tonic elevation in area 25 that has been associated with depression, compared to acute changes associated with sadness induction in healthy controls [190]. At a cellular level, sustained changes in neural activity are more likely to cause receptor desensitization and endocytosis, together with functional and structural plasticity. At a circuit level, sustained alterations in activity of a single brain region are more likely to induce compensatory changes in other brain networks, which may be relevant to the disease phenotype. Finally, at a cognitive level, mental illnesses are associated with maladaptive learning over time, which further contributes to the behavioral, subjective and executive sequelae of these disorders. Thus, future studies should also determine the effects of chronic over-activity in area 25. These can be investigated using a variety of techniques that would permit such chronicity without the need for chronic brain interventions. These include the area 25-specific administration of siRNA targeting EAAT2 to inhibit glutamate reuptake or the chronic administration of DREADD (designer receptors exclusively activated by designer drugs) ligands using osmotic minipumps in animals with G_q-coupled DREADDs targeting area 25 to increase neuronal excitability. Such studies should not only be undertaken in adulthood, but also at different stages of development, because disorders such as anxiety and depression very often have their onset during puberty and adolescence (for review see Young et al., this issue). Insight has already been gained into the functional development of rodent vmPFC (including IL) in relation to conditioned threat extinction (reviewed in Zimmermann et al, this Special issue), paving the way for similar studies of primate area 25. Indeed, the unique growth trajectory of area 25 was revealed in a recent study mapping marmoset structural growth trajectories of cortical and subcortical regions. Compared to neighboring prefrontal and ACC areas, area 25 displayed an early onset of grey matter decline (thought to reflect changes in synaptic plasticity, pruning and increased myelination) around the start of puberty which then continued throughout adolescence, with the greatest rate of decline not occurring until the end of adolescence [191]. This prolonged period of structural 'change' may make area 25 particularly vulnerable to external stressors across extended periods of development and may explain its prominent role in models of depression. As reviewed in Datta and Arnsten (this Special issue) prefrontal cellular circuits, as revealed by studies of the cellular mechanisms underlying working memory in dlPFC, appear particularly vulnerable to uncontrollable stress, effects that can be exacerbated during adolescence, but whether similar or different interactions are played out in area 25 during development are as yet unknown.

5. Conclusions

Area 25 plays a key, causal role in physiological and behavioral changes that resemble symptoms of enhanced negative affect and anhedonia, constituting key features of major psychiatric disorders such as depression and anxiety. However, other regions within the vmPFC also play a role, and care must be taken not to equate area 25 with the vmPFC. Further characterization of behavioral and cognitive functions subserved specifically by area 25 in the non-diseased state will aid in delineating the importance of dysfunction within area 25 to the phenotype of these conditions. Work in non-human primates, whose vmPFC is more similar in its overall organization to humans than rodents, is critical to this effort. Success is dependent on far closer integration of studies across species and more readiness to acknowledge differences, as well as similarities, across those species.

Author Contributions: Conceptualization, L.A., H.F.C. and A.C.R.; Methodology, L.A., H.F.C. and A.C.R.; Writing–Original Draft Preparation, L.A., H.F.C. and A.C.R.; Writing–Review & Editing, H.F.C. and A.C.R.; Visualization, H.F.C. and A.C.R.; Funding Acquisition, H.F.C. and A.C.R.

Funding: The marmoset work described here was supported by a Wellcome Trust grant (108089/Z/15/) and MRC grant (MR/M023990/1) to ACR and a MRC career development award (RG62920) to HFC and conducted within the University of Cambridge Behavioral and Clinical Neuroscience Institute, supported by a joint award from the Medical Research Council and the Wellcome Trust (MRCG1000183).

Acknowledgments: We thank Nicole Horst for her artwork.

Conflicts of Interest: The authors declare no conflict of interest.

References

1. Joyce, M.K.P.; Barbas, H. Cortical connections position primate area 25 as a keystone for interoception, emotion, and memory. *J. Neurosci.* **2018**, *38*, 1677–1698. [CrossRef] [PubMed]
2. Ongur, D.; Ferry, A.T.; Price, J.L. Architectonic subdivision of the human orbital and medial prefrontal cortex. *J. Comp. Neurol.* **2003**, *460*, 425–449. [CrossRef] [PubMed]
3. Palomero-Gallagher, N.; Vogt, B.A.; Schleicher, A.; Mayberg, H.S.; Zilles, K. Receptor architecture of human cingulate cortex: Evaluation of the four-region neurobiological model. *Hum. Brain Mapp.* **2009**, *30*, 2336–2355. [CrossRef] [PubMed]
4. Vertes, R.P. Differential projections of the infralimbic and prelimbic cortex in the rat. *Synapse* **2004**, *51*, 32–58. [CrossRef] [PubMed]
5. Heilbronner, S.R.; Rodríguez-Romaguera, J.; Quirk, G.J.; Groenewegen, H.J.; Haber, S.N. Circuit based cortico-striatal homologies between rat and primate. *Boil. Psychiatry* **2016**, *80*, 509–521. [CrossRef]
6. Hoover, W.B.; Vertes, R.P. Anatomical analysis of afferent projections to the medial prefrontal cortex in the rat. *Anat. Embryol.* **2007**, *212*, 149–179. [CrossRef]
7. Yeterian, E.H.; Pandya, D.N.; Tomaiuolo, F.; Petrides, M. The cortical connectivity of the prefrontal cortex in the monkey brain. *Cortex* **2012**, *48*, 58–81. [CrossRef]
8. Ghashghaei, H.; Barbas, H. Pathways for emotion: Interactions of prefrontal and anterior temporal pathways in the amygdala of the rhesus monkey. *Neuroscience* **2002**, *115*, 1261–1279. [CrossRef]
9. Takagishi, M.; Chiba, T. Efferent projections of the infralimbic (area 25) region of the medial prefrontal cortex in the rat: An anterograde tracer PHA-L study. *Brain Res.* **1991**, *566*, 26–39. [CrossRef]
10. Chiba, T.; Kayahara, T.; Nakano, K. Efferent projections of infralimbic and prelimbic areas of the medial prefrontal cortex in the Japanese monkey, Macaca fuscata. *Brain Res.* **2001**, *888*, 83–101. [CrossRef]
11. Freedman, L.J.; Insel, T.R.; Smith, Y. Subcortical projections of area 25 (subgenual cortex) of the macaque monkey. *J. Comp. Neurol.* **2000**, *421*, 172–188. [CrossRef]
12. An, X.; Bandler, R.; Ongür, D.; Price, J.L.; Ongur, D.; Price, J.L. Prefrontal cortical projections to longitudinal columns in the midbrain periaqueductal gray in macaque monkeys [see comments]. *J. Comp. Neurol.* **1998**, *401*, 455–479. [CrossRef]
13. Rempel-Clower, N.; Barbas, H. Topographic organization of connections between the hypothalamus and prefrontal cortex in the rhesus monkey. *J. Comp. Neurol.* **1998**, *398*, 393–419. [CrossRef]
14. Barbas, H.; Blatt, G.J. Topographically specific hippocampal projections target functionally distinct prefrontal areas in the rhesus monkey. *Hippocampus* **1995**, *5*, 511–533. [CrossRef] [PubMed]
15. Petrides, M.; Tomaiuolo, F.; Yeterian, E.H.; Pandya, D.N. The prefrontal cortex: Comparative architectonic organization in the human and the macaque monkey brains. *Cortex* **2012**, *48*, 46–57. [CrossRef] [PubMed]
16. Vogt, B.A.; Paxinos, G. Cytoarchitecture of mouse and rat cingulate cortex with human homologies. *Brain Struct. Funct.* **2014**, *219*, 185–192. [CrossRef]
17. Zikopoulos, B.; Hoistad, M.; John, Y.; Barbas, H. Posterior orbitofrontal and anterior cingulate pathways to the amygdala target inhibitory and excitatory systems with opposite functions. *J. Neurosci.* **2017**, *37*, 5051–5064. [CrossRef]
18. Palomero-Gallagher, N.; Eickhoff, S.B.; Hoffstaedter, F.; Schleicher, A.; Mohlberg, H.; Vogt, B.A.; Amunts, K.; Zilles, K. Functional organization of human subgenual cortical areas: Relationship between architectonical segregation and connectional heterogeneity. *NeuroImage* **2015**, *115*, 177–190. [CrossRef]

19. Hiser, J.; Koenigs, M. The Multifaceted Role of the Ventromedial Prefrontal Cortex in Emotion, Decision Making, Social Cognition, and Psychopathology. *Boil. Psychiatry* **2018**, *83*, 638–647. [CrossRef]

20. Myers-Schulz, B.; Koenigs, M. Functional anatomy of ventromedial prefrontal cortex: Implications for mood and anxiety disorders. *Mol. Psychiatry* **2012**, *17*, 132–141. [CrossRef]

21. Vatner, S.F. Effects of anesthesia on cardiovascular control mechanisms. *Environ. Heal. Perspect.* **1978**, *26*, 193–206. [CrossRef] [PubMed]

22. Kaada, B.R.; Pribram, K.H.; Epstein, J.A. Respiratory and vascular responses in monkeys from temporal pole, insula, orbital surface and cingulate gyrus: A preliminary report. *J. Neurophysiol.* **1949**, *12*, 347–356. [CrossRef] [PubMed]

23. Loewy, A.D.; Spyer, K.M. *Central Regulation of Autonomic Functions*; Oxford University Press: Oxford, UK, 1990; ISBN 978-0-19-976311-5.

24. Critchley, H.D.; Tang, J.; Glaser, D.; Butterworth, B.; Dolan, R.J. Anterior cingulate activity during error and autonomic response. *NeuroImage* **2005**, *27*, 885–895. [CrossRef] [PubMed]

25. Critchley, H.D.; Corfield, D.R.; Chandler, M.P.; Mathias, C.J.; Dolan, R.J. Cerebral correlates of autonomic cardiovascular arousal: A functional neuroimaging investigation in humans. *J. Physiol.* **2000**, *523*, 259–270. [CrossRef] [PubMed]

26. Gianaros, P.J.; Wager, T.D. Brain-Body Pathways Linking Psychological Stress and Physical Health. *Dir. Psychol. Sci.* **2015**, *24*, 313–321. [CrossRef] [PubMed]

27. Gianaros, P.J.; Jennings, J.R.; Sheu, L.K.; Derbyshire, S.W.G.; Matthews, K.A. Heightened functional neural activation to psychological stress covaries with exaggerated blood pressure reactivity. *Hypertension* **2007**, *49*, 134–140. [CrossRef] [PubMed]

28. Gianaros, P.J.; Sheu, L.K.; Matthews, K.A.; Jennings, J.R.; Manuck, S.B.; Hariri, A.R. Individual differences in stressor-evoked blood pressure reactivity vary with activation, volume, and functional connectivity of the amygdala. *J. Neurosci.* **2008**, *28*, 990–999. [CrossRef]

29. Thayer, J.F.; Åhs, F.; Fredrikson, M.; Sollers, J.J.; Wager, T.D. A meta-analysis of heart rate variability and neuroimaging studies: Implications for heart rate variability as a marker of stress and health. *Neurosci. Biobehav. Rev.* **2012**, *36*, 747–756. [CrossRef]

30. Lane, R.D.; Weidenbacher, H.; Smith, R.; Fort, C.; Thayer, J.F.; Allen, J.J. Subgenual anterior cingulate cortex activity covariation with cardiac vagal control is altered in depression. *J. Affect. Disord.* **2013**, *150*, 565–570. [CrossRef]

31. Goswami, R.; Frances, M.F.; Shoemaker, J.K. Representation of somatosensory inputs within the cortical autonomic network. *NeuroImage* **2011**, *54*, 1211–1220. [CrossRef]

32. Porges, S.W. Orienting in a defensive world: Mammalian modifications of our evolutionary heritage. A Polyvagal Theory. *Psychophysiology* **1995**, *32*, 301–318. [CrossRef] [PubMed]

33. Thayer, J.F.; Lane, R.D. A model of neurovisceral integration in emotion regulation and dysregulation. *J. Affect. Disord.* **2000**, *61*, 201–216. [CrossRef]

34. Lacuey, N.; Hampson, J.P.; Theeranaew, W.; Zonjy, B.; Vithala, A.; Hupp, N.J.; Loparo, K.A.; Miller, J.P.; Lhatoo, S.D. Cortical structures associated with human blood pressure control. *JAMA Neurol.* **2018**, *75*, 194–202. [CrossRef] [PubMed]

35. Chiken, S.; Nambu, A. Disrupting neuronal transmission: Mechanism of DBS? *Front. Syst. Neurosci.* **2014**, *3*. [CrossRef] [PubMed]

36. Sudheimer, K.D.; Abelson, J.L.; Taylor, S.F.; Martis, B.; Welsh, R.C.; Warner, C.; Samet, M.; Manduzzi, A.; Liberzon, I. Exogenous glucocorticoids decrease subgenual cingulate activity evoked by sadness. *Neuropsychopharmacology* **2013**, *38*, 826–845. [CrossRef]

37. Jahn, A.L.; Fox, A.S.; Abercrombie, H.C.; Shelton, S.E.; Oakes, T.R.; Davidson, R.J.; Kalin, N.H. Subgenual pfc activity predicts individual differences in hpa activity across different contexts. *Boil. Psychiatry* **2010**, *67*, 175–181. [CrossRef] [PubMed]

38. Wallis, C.U.; Cardinal, R.N.; Alexander, L.; Roberts, A.C.; Clarke, H.F. Opposing roles of primate areas 25 and 32 and their putative rodent homologs in the regulation of negative emotion. *Proc. Natl. Acad. Sci. USA* **2017**, *114*, E4075–E4084. [CrossRef]

39. Müller-Ribeiro, F.C.D.F.; Fontes, M.A.P.; Zaretsky, D.V.; Zaretskaia, M.V.; Santos, R.A.S.; A DiMicco, J. Contribution of infralimbic cortex in the cardiovascular response to acute stress. *Am. J. Physiol. Integr. Comp. Physiol.* **2012**, *303*, R639–R650. [CrossRef]

40. McKlveen, J.M.; Myers, B.; Flak, J.N.; Bundzikova, J.; Solomon, M.B.; Seroogy, K.B.; Herman, J.P. Role of Prefrontal Cortex Glucocorticoid Receptors in Stress and Emotion. *Boil. Psychiatry* **2013**, *74*, 672–679. [CrossRef]

41. Barbas, H.; Saha, S.; Rempel-Clower, N.; Ghashghaei, T. Serial pathways from primate prefrontal cortex to autonomic areas may influence emotional expression. *BMC Neurosci.* **2003**, *4*, 25. [CrossRef]

42. Alheid, G.F.; Heimer, L. Chapter 28 Theories of basal forebrain organization and the "emotional motor system". In *Progress in Brain Research*; Elsevier: Amsterdam, The Netherlands, 1996; Volume 107, pp. 461–484.

43. Holstege, G. Chapter 14 Descending motor pathways and the spinal motor system: Limbic and non-limbic components. In *Progress in Brain Research*; Elsevier: Amsterdam, The Netherlands, 1996; Volume 87, pp. 307–421.

44. Smith, W.K. The functional significance of the rostral cingular cortex as revealed by its responses to electrical excitation. *J. Neurophysiol.* **1945**, *8*, 241–255. [CrossRef]

45. Rolls, E.T.; Inoue, K.; Browning, A. Activity of primate subgenual cingulate cortex neurons is related to sleep. *J. Neurophysiol.* **2003**, *90*, 134–142. [CrossRef] [PubMed]

46. Zeredo, J.L.; Quah, S.K.L.; Wallis, C.U.; Alexander, L.; Cockcroft, G.J.; Santangelo, A.M.; Xia, J.; Shiba, Y.; Dalley, J.W.; Cardinal, R.N.; et al. Glutamate within the marmoset anterior hippocampus interacts with area 25 to regulate the behavioral and cardiovascular correlates of high-trait anxiety. *J. Neurosci.* **2019**, *39*, 3094–3107. [CrossRef] [PubMed]

47. Terreberry, R.R.; Neafsey, E.J. Rat medial frontal cortex: A visceral motor region with a direct projection to the solitary nucleus. *Brain Res.* **1983**, *278*, 245–249. [CrossRef]

48. Hurley, K.M.; Herbert, H.; Moga, M.M.; Saper, C.B. Efferent projections of the infralimbic cortex of the rat. *J. Comp. Neurol.* **1991**, *308*, 249–276. [CrossRef] [PubMed]

49. Hassan, S.F.; Cornish, J.L.; Goodchild, A.K. Respiratory, metabolic and cardiac functions are altered by disinhibition of subregions of the medial prefrontal cortex. *J. Physiol.* **2013**, *591*, 6069–6088. [CrossRef] [PubMed]

50. Myers, B. Corticolimbic regulation of cardiovascular responses to stress. *Physiol. Behav.* **2017**, *172*, 49–59. [CrossRef] [PubMed]

51. Tavares, R.; Corrêa, F.; Resstel, L. Opposite role of infralimbic and prelimbic cortex in the tachycardiac response evoked by acute restraint stress in rats. *J. Neurosci.* **2009**, *87*, 2601–2607. [CrossRef]

52. Frysztak, R.J.; Neafsey, E.J. The effect of medial frontal cortex lesions on cardiovascular conditioned emotional responses in the rat. *Brain Res.* **1994**, *643*, 181–193. [CrossRef]

53. Thomason, M.E.; Hamilton, J.P.; Gotlib, I.H. Stress-induced activation of the HPA axis predicts connectivity between subgenual cingulate and salience network during rest in adolescents. *J. Child Psychol. Psychiatry* **2011**, *52*, 1026–1034. [CrossRef]

54. Veer, I.M.; Oei, N.Y.; Spinhoven, P.; Van Buchem, M.A.; Elzinga, B.M.; Rombouts, S.A. Endogenous cortisol is associated with functional connectivity between the amygdala and medial prefrontal cortex. *Psychoneuroendocrinology* **2012**, *37*, 1039–1047. [CrossRef] [PubMed]

55. Patel, P.D.; Lopez, J.F.; Lyons, D.M.; Burke, S.; Wallace, M.; Schatzberg, A.F. Glucocorticoid and mineralocorticoid receptor mRNA expression in squirrel monkey brain. *J. Psychiatr.* **2000**, *34*, 383–392. [CrossRef]

56. Dum, R.P.; Levinthal, D.J.; Strick, P.L. Motor, cognitive, and affective areas of the cerebral cortex influence the adrenal medulla. *Proc. Natl. Acad. Sci. USA* **2016**, *113*, 9922–9927. [CrossRef] [PubMed]

57. Diorio, D.; Viau, V.; Meaney, M. The role of the medial prefrontal cortex (cingulate gyrus) in the regulation of hypothalamic-pituitary-adrenal responses to stress. *J. Neurosci.* **1993**, *13*, 3839–3847. [CrossRef] [PubMed]

58. Sullivan, R.M.; Gratton, A. Lateralized effects of medial prefrontal cortex lesions on neuroendocrine and autonomic stress responses in rats. *J. Neurosci.* **1999**, *19*, 2834–2840. [CrossRef] [PubMed]

59. Crane, J.W.; Ebner, K.; A Day, T. Medial prefrontal cortex suppression of the hypothalamic-pituitary-adrenal axis response to a physical stressor, systemic delivery of interleukin-1beta. *Eur. J. Neurosci.* **2003**, *17*, 1473–1481. [CrossRef]

60. O'Connor, M.-F.; Irwin, M.R.; Wellisch, D.K. When grief heats up: Pro-inflammatory cytokines predict regional brain activation. *NeuroImage* **2009**, *47*, 891–896. [CrossRef] [PubMed]

61. Harrison, N.A.; Brydon, L.; Walker, C.; Gray, M.A.; Steptoe, A.; Critchley, H.D. Inflammation causes mood changes through alterations in subgenual cingulate activity and mesolimbic connectivity. *Boil. Psychiatry* **2009**, *66*, 407–414. [CrossRef]

62. Steiner, J.; Walter, M.; Gos, T.; Guillemin, G.J.; Bernstein, H.-G.; Sarnyai, Z.; Mawrin, C.; Brisch, R.; Bielau, H.; Zu Schwabedissen, L.M.; et al. Severe depression is associated with increased microglial quinolinic acid in subregions of the anterior cingulate gyrus: Evidence for an immune-modulated glutamatergic neurotransmission? *J. Neuroinflamm.* **2011**, *8*, 94. [CrossRef]

63. Fox, M.D.; Raichle, M.E. Spontaneous fluctuations in brain activity observed with functional magnetic resonance imaging. *Nat. Rev. Neurosci.* **2007**, *8*, 700–711. [CrossRef]

64. Fox, M.D.; Snyder, A.Z.; Vincent, J.L.; Corbetta, M.; Van Essen, D.C.; Raichle, M.E. The human brain is intrinsically organized into dynamic, anticorrelated functional networks. *Proc. Natl. Acad. Sci. USA* **2005**, *102*, 9673–9678. [CrossRef] [PubMed]

65. Menon, V. Large-scale brain networks and psychopathology: A unifying triple network model. *Trends Cogn. Sci.* **2011**, *15*, 483–506.

66. Smith, S.M.; Fox, P.T.; Miller, K.L.; Glahn, D.C.; Fox, P.M.; Mackay, C.E.; Filippini, N.; Watkins, K.E.; Toro, R.; Laird, A.R.; et al. Correspondence of the brain's functional architecture during activation and rest. *Proc. Natl. Acad. Sci. USA* **2009**, *106*, 13040–13045. [PubMed]

67. Uddin, L.Q.; Supekar, K.S.; Ryali, S.; Menon, V. Dynamic reconfiguration of structural and functional connectivity across core neurocognitive brain networks with development. *J. Neurosci.* **2011**, *31*, 18578–18589. [CrossRef] [PubMed]

68. Etkin, A.; Egner, T.; Kalisch, R. Emotional processing in anterior cingulate and medial prefrontal cortex. *Trends Cogn. Sci.* **2011**, *15*, 85–93. [CrossRef] [PubMed]

69. Shoemaker, J.K.; Goswami, R. Forebrain neurocircuitry associated with human reflex cardiovascular control. *Front. Physiol.* **2015**, *6*, 1–14. [CrossRef]

70. Lv, Q.; Yang, L.; Li, G.; Wang, Z.; Shen, Z.; Yu, W.; Jiang, Q.; Hou, B.; Pu, J.; Hu, H.; et al. Large-Scale Persistent Network Reconfiguration Induced by Ketamine in Anesthetized Monkeys: Relevance to Mood Disorders. *Boil. Psychiatry* **2016**, *79*, 765–775. [CrossRef]

71. Lane, R.D.; McRae, K.; Reiman, E.M.; Chen, K.; Ahern, G.L.; Thayer, J.F. Neural correlates of heart rate variability during emotion. *NeuroImage* **2009**, *44*, 213–222. [CrossRef]

72. Roy, M.; Shohamy, D.; Wager, T.D. Ventromedial prefrontal-subcortical systems and the generation of affective meaning. *Trends Cogn. Sci.* **2012**, *16*, 147–156. [CrossRef]

73. Bechara, A.; Damasio, H. Emotion, Decision Making and the Orbitofrontal Cortex. *Cereb. Cortex* **2000**, *10*, 295–307.

74. Spreng, R.N.; Mar, R.A.; Kim, A.S.N. The common neural basis of autobiographical memory, prospection, navigation, theory of mind, and the default mode: A quantitative meta-analysis. *J. Cogn. Neurosci.* **2009**, *21*, 489–510. [CrossRef] [PubMed]

75. Phan, K.; Wager, T.; Taylor, S.F.; Liberzon, I. Functional neuroanatomy of emotion: A meta-analysis of emotion activation studies in pet and fmri. *NeuroImage* **2002**, *16*, 331–348. [CrossRef] [PubMed]

76. Gemar, M.C.; Kapur, S.; Segal, Z.V.; Brown, G.M.; Houle, S. Effects of self-generated sad mood on regional cerebral activity: A PET study in normal subjects. *Depression* **1996**, *4*, 81–88. [CrossRef]

77. George, M.S.; A Ketter, T.; I Parekh, P.; Horwitz, B.; Herscovitch, P.; Post, R.M. Brain activity during transient sadness and happiness in healthy women. *Am. J. Psychiatry* **1995**, *152*, 341–351. [PubMed]

78. Pardo, J.V.; Pardo, P.J.; E Raichle, M. Neural correlates of self-induced dysphoria. *Am. J. Psychiatry* **1993**, *150*, 713–719. [PubMed]

79. Liotti, M.; Woldorff, M.G.; Pérez, R.; Mayberg, H.S. An ERP study of the temporal course of the Stroop color-word interference effect. *Neuropsychologia* **2000**, *38*, 701–711. [CrossRef]

80. Mayberg, H.S.; Liotti, M.; Brannan, S.K.; McGinnis, S.; Mahurin, R.K.; A Jerabek, P.; A Silva, J.; Tekell, J.L.; Martin, C.C.; Lancaster, J.L.; et al. Reciprocal limbic-cortical function and negative mood: Converging PET findings in depression and normal sadness. *Am. J. Psychiatry* **1999**, *156*, 675–682.

81. Zald, D.H.; Mattson, D.L.; Pardo, J.V. Brain activity in ventromedial prefrontal cortex correlates with individual differences in negative affect. *Proc. Natl. Acad. Sci. USA* **2002**, *99*, 2450–2454. [CrossRef]

82. Paradiso, S. Regional cerebral blood flow changes during visually induced subjective sadness in healthy elderly persons. *J. Neuropsychiatry Clin. Neurosci.* **2003**, *15*, 35–44. [CrossRef]

83. Elliott, R.; Rubinsztein, J.S.; Sahakian, B.J.; Dolan, R.J. Selective attention to emotional stimuli in a verbal go/no-go task: An fMRI study. *NeuroReport* **2000**, *11*, 1739–1744. [CrossRef]

84. Maddock, R.J.; Garrett, A.S.; Buonocore, M.H. Posterior cingulate cortex activation by emotional words: fMRI evidence from a valence decision task. *Hum. Brain Mapp.* **2003**, *18*, 30–41. [CrossRef] [PubMed]
85. Young, S.N.; Smith, S.E.; Pihl, R.O.; Ervin, F.R. Tryptophan depletion causes a rapid lowering of mood in normal males. *Psychopharmacology* **1985**, *87*, 173–177. [CrossRef] [PubMed]
86. Barr, L.C.; Heninger, G.R.; Goodman, W.; Charney, D.S.; Price, L.H. Effects of fluoxetine administration on mood response to tryptophan depletion in healthy subjects. *Boil. Psychiatry* **1997**, *41*, 949–954. [CrossRef]
87. Talbot, P.S.; Cooper, S.J. Anterior Cingulate and Subgenual Prefrontal Blood Flow Changes Following Tryptophan Depletion in Healthy Males. *Neuropsychopharmacol* **2006**, *31*, 1757–1767. [CrossRef] [PubMed]
88. Williams, K.D.; Cheung, C.K.T.; Choi, W. Cyberostracism: Effects of being ignored over the Internet. *J. Pers. Soc. Psychol.* **2000**, *79*, 748–762. [CrossRef] [PubMed]
89. Vijayakumar, N.; Cheng, T.W.; Pfeifer, J.H. Neural correlates of social exclusion across ages: A coordinate-based meta-analysis of functional MRI studies. *NeuroImage* **2017**, *153*, 359–368. [CrossRef] [PubMed]
90. Drevets, W.C.; Price, J.L.; Simpson, J.R.; Todd, R.D.; Reich, T.; Vannier, M.; Raichle, M.E. Subgenual prefrontal cortex abnormalities in mood disorders. *Nat. Cell Boil.* **1997**, *386*, 824–827. [CrossRef] [PubMed]
91. Botteron, K.N.; E Raichle, M.; Drevets, W.C.; Heath, A.C.; Todd, R.D. Volumetric reduction in left subgenual prefrontal cortex in early onset depression. *Boil. Psychiatry* **2002**, *51*, 342–344. [CrossRef]
92. Coryell, W.; Nopoulos, P.; Drevets, W.; Wilson, T.; Andreasen, N.C. Subgenual Prefrontal Cortex Volumes in Major Depressive Disorder and Schizophrenia: Diagnostic Specificity and Prognostic Implications. *Am. J. Psychiatry* **2005**, *162*, 1706–1712. [CrossRef]
93. Vassilopoulou, K.; Papathanasiou, M.; Michopoulos, I.; Boufidou, F.; Oulis, P.; Kelekis, N.; Rizos, E.; Nikolaou, C.; Pantelis, C.; Velakoulis, D.; et al. A magnetic resonance imaging study of hippocampal, amygdala and subgenual prefrontal cortex volumes in major depression subtypes: Melancholic versus psychotic depression. *J. Affect. Disord.* **2013**, *146*, 197–204. [CrossRef]
94. Yücel, K.; McKinnon, M.C.; Chahal, R.; Taylor, V.H.; Macdonald, K.; Joffe, R.; MacQueen, G.M. Kinnon Anterior Cingulate Volumes in Never-Treated Patients with Major Depressive Disorder. *Neuropsychopharmacol* **2008**, *33*, 3157–3163. [CrossRef] [PubMed]
95. Hajek, T.; Kozeny, J.; Kopecek, M.; Alda, M.; Höschl, C. Reduced subgenual cingulate volumes in mood disorders: A meta-analysis. *J. Psychiatry Neurosci.* **2008**, *33*, 91–99. [PubMed]
96. Du, M.-Y.; Wu, Q.-Z.; Yue, Q.; Li, J.; Liao, Y.; Kuang, W.-H.; Huang, X.-Q.; Chan, R.C.; Mechelli, A.; Gong, Q.-Y. Voxelwise meta-analysis of gray matter reduction in major depressive disorder. *Prog. Neuro-Psychopharmacol. Boil. Psychiatry* **2012**, *36*, 11–16. [CrossRef]
97. Rodriguez-Cano, E.; Sarró, S.; Monte, G.C.; Maristany, T.; Salvador, R.; McKenna, P.J.; Pomarol-Clotet, E. Evidence for structural and functional abnormality in the subgenual anterior cingulate cortex in major depressive disorder. *Psychol. Med.* **2014**, *44*, 3263–3273. [CrossRef] [PubMed]
98. Baker, S.C.; Frith, C.D.; Dolan, R.J. The interaction between mood and cognitive function studied with PET. *Psychol. Med.* **1997**, *27*, 565–578. [CrossRef] [PubMed]
99. Bench, C.J.; Friston, K.J.; Brown, R.G.; Scott, L.C.; Frackowiak, R.S.J.; Dolan, R.J. The anatomy of melancholia – focal abnormalities of cerebral blood flow in major depression. *Psychol. Med.* **1992**, *22*, 607–615. [CrossRef]
100. Curran, S.M.; Murray, C.M.; Van Beck, M.; Dougall, N.; O'Carroll, R.E.; Austin, M.-P.; Ebmeier, K.P.; Goodwin, G.M. A single photon emission computerised tomography study of regional brain function in elderly patients with major depression and with alzheimer-type dementia. *Br. J. Psychiatry* **1993**, *163*, 155–165. [CrossRef] [PubMed]
101. Ito, H.; Kawashima, R.; Awata, S.; Ono, S.; Sato, K.; Goto, R.; Koyama, M.; Sato, M.; Fukuda, H. Hypoperfusion in the limbic system and prefrontal cortex in depression: SPECT with anatomic standardization technique. *J. Med.* **1996**, *37*, 410–414.
102. Mayberg, H.S.; Lewis, P.J.; Regenold, W.; Wagner, H.N. Paralimbic hypoperfusion in unipolar depression. *J. Med.* **1994**, *35*, 929–934.
103. Mayberg, H.S.; Lozano, A.M.; Voon, V.; McNeely, H.E.; Seminowicz, D.; Hamani, C.; Schwalb, J.M.; Kennedy, S.H. Deep Brain Stimulation for Treatment-Resistant Depression. *Neuron* **2005**, *45*, 651–660. [CrossRef]
104. Mayberg, H.S.; Brannan, S.K.; Mahurin, R.K.; Jerabek, P.A.; Silva, J.A.; Tekell, J.L.; McGinnis, S. The Functional Neuroanatomy of the Placebo Effect. *Am. J. Psychiatry* **2002**, *159*, 728–737. [CrossRef] [PubMed]

105. Gotlib, I.H.; Sivers, H.; Gabrieli, J.D.; Whitfield-Gabrieli, S.; Goldin, P.; Minor, K.L.; Canli, T. Subgenual anterior cingulate activation to valenced emotional stimuli in major depression. *NeuroReport* **2005**, *16*, 1731–1734. [CrossRef] [PubMed]

106. Fitzgerald, P.B.; Laird, A.R.; Maller, J.; Daskalakis, Z.J. A Meta-Analytic Study of Changes in Brain Activation in Depression. *Hum. Brain Mapp.* **2008**, *29*, 683–695. [CrossRef] [PubMed]

107. Palmer, S.M.; Crewther, S.G.; Carey, L.M. The START project team a meta analysis of changes in brain activity in clinical depression. *Front. Hum. Neurosci.* **2015**, *8*, 8. [CrossRef] [PubMed]

108. Keller, M.B.; Klein, D.N.; Hirschfeld, R.M.; Kocsis, J.H.; McCullough, J.P.; Miller, I.; First, M.B.; Holzer, C.P.; I Keitner, G.; Marin, D.B. Results of the DSM-IV mood disorders field trial. *Am. J. Psychiatry* **1995**, *152*, 843–849. [PubMed]

109. Uher, R.; Perlis, R.H.; Henigsberg, N.; Zobel, A.; Rietschel, M.; Mors, O.; Hauser, J.; Dernovsek, M.Z.; Souery, D.; Bajs, M.; et al. Depression symptom dimensions as predictors of antidepressant treatment outcome: Replicable evidence for interest-activity symptoms. *Psychol. Med.* **2012**, *42*, 967–980. [CrossRef] [PubMed]

110. Spijker, J.; Bijl, R.V.; De Graaf, R.; Nolen, W.A. Determinants of poor 1-year outcome of DSM-III-R major depression in the general population: Results of the Netherlands Mental Health Survey and Incidence Study (NEMESIS). *Nat. Psychiatr. Scand.* **2001**, *103*, 122–130. [CrossRef]

111. Keedwell, P.A.; Andrew, C.; Williams, S.C.; Brammer, M.J.; Phillips, M.L. The Neural Correlates of Anhedonia in Major Depressive Disorder. *Boil. Psychiatry* **2005**, *58*, 843–853. [CrossRef] [PubMed]

112. Young, C.B.; Chen, T.; Nusslock, R.; Keller, J.; Schatzberg, A.F.; Menon, V. Anhedonia and general distress show dissociable ventromedial prefrontal cortex connectivity in major depressive disorder. *Transl. Psychiatry* **2016**, *6*, e810. [CrossRef]

113. Mayberg, H.S. Limbic-cortical dysregulation: A proposed model of depression. *J. Psychiatry Clin. Neurosci.* **1997**, *9*, 471–481.

114. E Holtzheimer, P.; Husain, M.M.; Lisanby, S.H.; Taylor, S.F.; A Whitworth, L.; McClintock, S.; Slavin, K.V.; Berman, J.; McKhann, G.M.; Patil, P.G.; et al. Subcallosal cingulate deep brain stimulation for treatment-resistant depression: A multisite, randomised, sham-controlled trial. *Lancet Psychiatry* **2017**, *4*, 839–849. [CrossRef]

115. Riva-Posse, P.; Choi, K.S.; Holtzheimer, P.E.; McIntyre, C.C.; Gross, R.E.; Chaturvedi, A.; Crowell, A.L.; Garlow, S.J.; Rajendra, J.K.; Mayberg, H.S. Defining critical white matter pathways mediating successful subcallosal cingulate deep brain stimulation for treatment-resistant depression. *Boil. Psychiatry* **2014**, *76*, 963–969. [CrossRef] [PubMed]

116. Riva-Posse, P.; Choi, K.S.; Holtzheimer, P.E.; Crowell, A.L.; Garlow, S.J.; Rajendra, J.K.; McIntyre, C.C.; Gross, R.E.; Mayberg, H.S. A connectomic approach for subcallosal cingulate deep brain stimulation surgery: Prospective targeting in treatment-resistant depression. *Mol. Psychiatry* **2018**, *23*, 843–849. [CrossRef] [PubMed]

117. Haber, S.N. Corticostriatal circuitry. *Dialogues Clin. Neurosci.* **2016**, *18*, 7–21.

118. Furman, D.J.; Hamilton, J.P.; Gotlib, I.H. Frontostriatal functional connectivity in major depressive disorder. *Boil. Mood Anxiety Disord.* **2011**, *1*, 11. [CrossRef]

119. Marchand, W.R.; Yurgelun-Todd, D.; Yurgelun-Todd, D. Striatal structure and function in mood disorders: A comprehensive review. *Bipolar Disord.* **2010**, *12*, 764–785. [CrossRef] [PubMed]

120. A Rogers, M.; Bradshaw, J.L.; Pantelis, C.; Phillips, J.G. Frontostriatal deficits in unipolar major depression. *Brain Res. Bull.* **1998**, *47*, 297–310. [CrossRef]

121. Lauterbach, E.C.; Cummings, J.L.; Duffy, J.; Coffey, C.E.; Kaufer, D.; Lovell, M.; Malloy, P.; Reeve, A.; Royall, D.R.; Rummans, T.A.; et al. Neuropsychiatric correlates and treatment of lenticulostriatal diseases: A review of the literature and overview of research opportunities in Huntington's, Wilson's, and Fahr's diseases. A report of the ANPA Committee on Research. American Neuropsychiatri. *J. Neuropsychiatry Clin. Neurosci.* **1998**, *10*, 249–266.

122. Marchand, W.R. Cortico-basal ganglia circuitry: A review of key research and implications for functional connectivity studies of mood and anxiety disorders. *Anat. Embryol.* **2010**, *215*, 73–96. [CrossRef]

123. Walterfang, M.; Evans, A.; Looi, J.C.L.; Jung, H.H.; Danek, A.; Walker, R.H.; Velakoulis, D. The neuropsychiatry of neuroacanthocytosis syndromes. *Neurosci. Biobehav. Rev.* **2011**, *35*, 1275–1283. [CrossRef]

124. Admon, R.; Holsen, L.M.; Aizley, H.; Remington, A.; Whitfield-Gabrieli, S.; Goldstein, J.M.; Pizzagalli, D.A. Striatal hypersensitivity during stress in remitted individuals with recurrent depression. *Biol. Psychiatry* **2015**, *78*, 67–76. [CrossRef] [PubMed]

125. Pizzagalli, D.A.; Holmes, A.J.; Dillon, D.G.; Goetz, E.L.; Birk, J.L.; Bogdan, R.; Dougherty, D.D.; Iosifescu, D.V.; Rauch, S.L.; Fava, M. Reduced caudate and nucleus accumbens response to rewards in unmedicated subjects with major depressive disorder. *Am. J. Psychiatry* **2009**, *166*, 702–710. [CrossRef] [PubMed]

126. Smoski, M.J.; Felder, J.; Bizzell, J.; Green, S.R.; Ernst, M.; Lynch, T.R.; Dichter, G.S. fMRI of alterations in reward selection, anticipation, and feedback in major depressive disorder. *J. Affect. Disord.* **2009**, *118*, 69–78. [CrossRef] [PubMed]

127. Pan, P.M.; Mari, J.; Jackowski, A.; Picon, F.; Leibenluft, E.; Stringaris, A.; Sato, J.R.; Salum, G.A.; Rohde, L.A.; Gadelha, A.; et al. Ventral striatum functional connectivity as a predictor of adolescent depressive disorder in a longitudinal community-based sample. *Am. J. Psychiatry* **2017**, *174*, 1112–1119. [CrossRef] [PubMed]

128. Bora, E.; Harrison, B.J.; Davey, C.G.; Yücel, M.; Pantelis, C. Meta-analysis of volumetric abnormalities in cortico-striatal-pallidal-thalamic circuits in major depressive disorder. *Psychol. Med.* **2012**, *42*, 671–681. [CrossRef]

129. Koolschijn, P.; van Haren, N.; Lensvelt-Mulders, G.; Pol, H.H.; Kahn, R.; Koolschijn, P.C. Brain volume abnormalities in major depressive disorder: A Meta-analysis of magnetic resonance imaging studies. *NeuroImage* **2009**, *47*, S152. [CrossRef]

130. Kaiser, R.H.; Andrews-Hanna, J.R.; Wager, T.D.; Pizzagalli, D.A. Large-scale network dysfunction in major depressive disorder: A meta-analysis of resting-state functional connectivity. *JAMA Psychiatry* **2015**, *72*, 603–611. [CrossRef]

131. Hamilton, J.P.; Chen, G.; Thomason, M.E.; Schwartz, M.E.; Gotlib, I.H. Investigating neural primacy in Major Depressive Disorder: Multivariate Granger causality analysis of resting-state fMRI time-series data. *Mol. Psychiatry* **2011**, *16*, 763–772. [CrossRef]

132. Hamilton, J.P.; Farmer, M.; Fogelman, P.; Gotlib, I.H. Depressive rumination, the default-mode network, and the dark matter of clinical neuroscience. *Boil. Psychiatry* **2015**, *78*, 224–230. [CrossRef]

133. Zhu, X.; Wang, X.; Xiao, J.; Liao, J.; Zhong, M.; Wang, W.; Yao, S. Evidence of a Dissociation Pattern in Resting-State Default Mode Network Connectivity in First-Episode, Treatment-Naive Major Depression Patients. *Boil. Psychiatry* **2012**, *71*, 611–617. [CrossRef]

134. Berman, M.G.; Peltier, S.; Nee, D.E.; Kross, E.; Deldin, P.J.; Jonides, J. Depression, rumination and the default network. *Soc. Cogn. Affect. Neurosci.* **2011**, *6*, 548–555. [CrossRef] [PubMed]

135. Johansen-Berg, H.; Gutman, D.A.; Behrens, T.E.J.; Matthews, P.M.; Rushworth, M.F.S.; Katz, E.; Lozano, A.M.; Mayberg, H.S. Anatomical connectivity of the subgenual cingulate region targeted with deep brain stimulation for treatment-resistant depression. *Cereb. Cortex* **2008**, *18*, 1374–1383. [CrossRef] [PubMed]

136. Schneider, B.; Koenigs, M. Human lesion studies of ventromedial prefrontal cortex. *Neuropsychologia* **2017**, *107*, 84–93. [CrossRef] [PubMed]

137. Monosov, I.E.; Hikosaka, O. Regionally distinct processing of rewards and punishments by the primate ventromedial prefrontal cortex. *J. Neurosci.* **2012**, *32*, 10318–10330. [CrossRef] [PubMed]

138. Azab, H.; Hayden, B.Y. Correlates of economic decisions in the dorsal and subgenual anterior cingulate cortices. *Eur. J. Neurosci.* **2018**, *47*, 979–993. [CrossRef] [PubMed]

139. Bouret, S.; Richmond, B.J. Ventromedial and orbital prefrontal neurons differentially encode internally and externally driven motivational values in monkeys. *J. Neurosci.* **2010**, *30*, 8591–8601. [CrossRef]

140. Wallis, C.U.; Cockcroft, G.J.; Cardinal, R.N.; Roberts, A.C.; Clarke, H.F. Hippocampal interaction with area 25, but not area 32, regulates marmoset approach-avoidance behaviour. *Cereb. Cortex* **2019**. [CrossRef]

141. Alexander, L.; Gaskin, P.L.R.; Sawiak, S.J.; Fryer, T.D.; Hong, Y.T.; Cockcroft, G.J.; Clarke, H.F.; Roberts, A.C. Fractionating blunted reward processing characteristic of anhedonia by over-activating primate subgenual anterior cingulate cortex. *Neuron* **2019**, *101*, 307–320. [CrossRef]

142. Roiser, J.P.; Sahakian, B.J. Hot and cold cognition in depression. *CNS Spectrums* **2013**, *18*, 139–149. [CrossRef]

143. Dickson, J.M.; MacLeod, A.K. Approach and Avoidance Goals and Plans: Their Relationship to Anxiety and Depression. *Cogn. Ther.* **2004**, *28*, 415–432. [CrossRef]

144. Rudebeck, P.H.; Putnam, P.T.; Daniels, T.E.; Yang, T.; Mitz, A.R.; Rhodes, S.E.V.; Murray, E. A role for primate subgenual cingulate cortex in sustaining autonomic arousal. *Proc. Natl. Acad. Sci. USA* **2014**, *111*, 5391–5396. [CrossRef] [PubMed]

145. Lally, N.; Nugent, A.C.; A Luckenbaugh, D.; Ameli, R.; Roiser, J.P.; A Zarate, C. Anti-anhedonic effect of ketamine and its neural correlates in treatment-resistant bipolar depression. *Transl. Psychiatry* **2014**, *4*, e469. [CrossRef] [PubMed]

146. Lally, N.; Nugent, A.C.; Luckenbaugh, D.A.; Niciu, M.J.; Roiser, J.P.; Zarate, C.A. Neural correlates of change in major depressive disorder anhedonia following open-label ketamine. *J. Psychopharmacol.* **2015**, *29*, 596–607. [CrossRef]

147. Parsaik, A.K.; Singh, B.; Khosh-Chashm, D.; Mascarenhas, S.S. Efficacy of ketamine in bipolar depression. *J. Psychiatr. Pr.* **2015**, *21*, 427–435. [CrossRef] [PubMed]

148. Godsil, B.P.; Kiss, J.P.; Spedding, M.; Jay, T.M. The hippocampal–prefrontal pathway: The weak link in psychiatric disorders? *Eur. Neuropsychopharmacol.* **2013**, *23*, 1165–1181. [CrossRef] [PubMed]

149. Clarke, H.F.; Horst, N.K.; Roberts, A.C. Regional inactivations of primate ventral prefrontal cortex reveal two distinct mechanisms underlying negative bias in decision making. *Proc. Natl. Acad. Sci. USA* **2015**, *112*, 4176–4181. [CrossRef]

150. Piantadosi, P.T.; Yeates, D.C.; Wilkins, M.; Floresco, S.B. Contributions of basolateral amygdala and nucleus accumbens subregions to mediating motivational conflict during punished reward-seeking. *Neurobiol. Learn. Mem.* **2017**, *140*, 92–105. [CrossRef]

151. Winstanley, C.A.; Floresco, S.B. Deciphering decision making: Variation in animal models of effort- and uncertainty-based choice reveals distinct neural circuitries underlying core cognitive processes. *J. Neurosci.* **2016**, *36*, 12069–12079. [CrossRef]

152. Gourley, S.L.; Olevska, A.; Zimmermann, K.S.; Ressler, K.J.; Dileone, R.J.; Taylor, J.R. The orbitofrontal cortex regulates outcome-based decision-making via the lateral striatum. *Eur. J. Neurosci.* **2013**, *38*, 2382–2388. [CrossRef]

153. Morgan, M.A.; Romanski, L.M.; LeDoux, J.E. Extinction of emotional learning: Contribution of medial prefrontal cortex. *Neurosci. Lett.* **1993**, *163*, 109–113. [CrossRef]

154. Quirk, G.J.; Russo, G.K.; Barron, J.L.; Lebrón, K. The role of ventromedial prefrontal cortex in the recovery of extinguished fear. *J. Neurosci.* **2000**, *20*, 6225–6231. [CrossRef] [PubMed]

155. Milad, M.R.; Quirk, G.J. Neurons in medial prefrontal cortex signal memory for fear extinction. *Nat. Cell Boil.* **2002**, *420*, 70–74. [CrossRef] [PubMed]

156. Westbrook, R.F.; Laurent, V. Inactivation of the infralimbic but not the prelimbic cortex impairs consolidation and retrieval of fear extinction. *Learn. Mem.* **2009**, *16*, 520–529.

157. Sierra-Mercado, D.; Padilla-Coreano, N.; Quirk, G.J. Dissociable roles of prelimbic and infralimbic cortices, ventral hippocampus, and basolateral amygdala in the expression and extinction of conditioned fear. *Neuropsychopharmacol* **2010**, *36*, 529–538. [CrossRef]

158. Bravo-Rivera, C.; Roman-Ortiz, C.; Brignoni-Perez, E.; Sotres-Bayon, F.; Quirk, G.J. Neural structures mediating expression and extinction of platform-mediated avoidance. *J. Neurosci.* **2014**, *34*, 9736–9742. [CrossRef]

159. Chang, C.-H.; Maren, S. Medial prefrontal cortex activation facilitates re-extinction of fear in rats. *Learn. Mem.* **2011**, *18*, 221–225. [CrossRef] [PubMed]

160. Phelps, E.A.; Delgado, M.R.; Nearing, K.I.; LeDoux, J.E. Extinction learning in humans: Role of the amygdala and vmPFC. *Neuron* **2004**, *43*, 897–905. [CrossRef]

161. Milad, M.R.; Wright, C.I.; Orr, S.P.; Pitman, R.K.; Quirk, G.J.; Rauch, S.L. Recall of fear extinction in humans activates the ventromedial prefrontal cortex and hippocampus in concert. *Biol. Psychiatry* **2007**, *62*, 446–454. [CrossRef]

162. Dunsmoor, J.E.; Kroes, M.C.; Li, J.; Daw, N.D.; Simpson, H.B.; Phelps, E.A. Role of human ventromedial prefrontal cortex in learning and recall of enhanced extinction. *J. Neurosci.* **2019**, *39*, 3264–3276. [CrossRef]

163. A Slattery, D.; Neumann, I.D.; Cryan, J.F. Transient inactivation of the infralimbic cortex induces antidepressant-like effects in the rat. *J. Psychopharmacol.* **2010**, *25*, 1295–1303. [CrossRef]

164. Gasull-Camós, J.; Tarrés-Gatius, M.; Artigas, F.; Castañé, A. Glial GLT-1 blockade in infralimbic cortex as a new strategy to evoke rapid antidepressant-like effects in rats. *Transl. Psychiatry* **2017**, *7*, e1038. [CrossRef] [PubMed]

165. Adhikari, A.; Lerner, T.N.; Finkelstein, J.; Pak, S.; Jennings, J.H.; Davidson, T.J.; Ferenczi, E.; Gunaydin, L.A.; Mirzabekov, J.J.; Ye, L.; et al. Basomedial amygdala mediates top-down control of anxiety and fear. *Nature* **2015**, *527*, 179–185. [CrossRef] [PubMed]

166. Fuchikami, M.; Thomas, A.; Liu, R.; Wohleb, E.S.; Land, B.B.; Dileone, R.J.; Aghajanian, G.K.; Duman, R.S. Optogenetic stimulation of infralimbic PFC reproduces ketamine's rapid and sustained antidepressant actions. *Proc. Natl. Acad. Sci. USA* **2015**, *112*, 8106–8111. [CrossRef] [PubMed]

167. Bi, L.-L.; Wang, J.; Luo, Z.-Y.; Chen, S.-P.; Geng, F.; Chen, Y.-H.; Li, S.-J.; Yuan, C.-H.; Lin, S.; Gao, T.-M. Enhanced excitability in the infralimbic cortex produces anxiety-like behaviors. *Neuropharmacology* **2013**, *72*, 148–156. [CrossRef] [PubMed]

168. Berg, L.; Eckardt, J.; Masseck, O.A. Enhanced activity of pyramidal neurons in the infralimbic cortex drives anxiety behavior. *PLoS ONE* **2019**, *14*, e0210949. [CrossRef]

169. Fullana, M.N.; Ruiz-Bronchal, E.; Ferrés-Coy, A.; Juárez-Escoto, E.; Artigas, F.; Bortolozzi, A. Regionally selective knockdown of astroglial glutamate transporters in infralimbic cortex induces a depressive phenotype in mice. *Glia* **2019**, *67*, 1122–1137. [CrossRef]

170. Suzuki, S.; Saitoh, A.; Ohashi, M.; Yamada, M.; Oka, J.-I.; Yamada, M. The infralimbic and prelimbic medial prefrontal cortices have differential functions in the expression of anxiety-like behaviors in mice. *Behav. Brain* **2016**, *304*, 120–124. [CrossRef]

171. Warren, B.L.; Mendoza, M.P.; Cruz, F.C.; Leao, R.M.; Caprioli, D.; Rubio, F.J.; Whitaker, L.R.; McPherson, K.B.; Bossert, J.M.; Shaham, Y.; et al. Distinct fos-expressing neuronal ensembles in the ventromedial prefrontal cortex mediate food reward and extinction memories. *J. Neurosci.* **2016**, *36*, 6691–6703. [CrossRef]

172. Peters, J.; De Vries, T. d-Cycloserine administered directly to infralimbic medial prefrontal cortex enhances extinction memory in sucrose-seeking animals. *Neuroscience* **2013**, *230*, 24–30. [CrossRef]

173. John, C.S.; Smith, K.L.; Veer, A.V.; Gompf, H.S.; A Carlezon, W.; Cohen, B.M.; Öngür, D.; Bechtholt-Gompf, A.J. Blockade of astrocytic glutamate uptake in the prefrontal cortex induces anhedonia. *Neuropsychopharmacol* **2012**, *37*, 2467–2475. [CrossRef]

174. Richard, J.M.; Berridge, K.C. Prefrontal cortex modulates desire and dread generated by nucleus accumbens glutamate disruption. *Biol. Psychiatry* **2013**, *73*, 360–370. [CrossRef] [PubMed]

175. Riaz, S.; Puveendrakumaran, P.; Khan, D.; Yoon, S.; Hamel, L.; Ito, R. Prelimbic and infralimbic cortical inactivations attenuate contextually driven discriminative responding for reward. *Sci. Rep.* **2019**, *9*, 3982. [CrossRef] [PubMed]

176. Chudasama, Y.; Robbins, T.W. Dissociable contributions of the orbitofrontal and infralimbic cortex to pavlovian autoshaping and discrimination reversal learning: Further evidence for the functional heterogeneity of the rodent frontal cortex. *J. Neurosci.* **2003**, *23*, 8771–8780. [CrossRef] [PubMed]

177. Anyan, J.; Amir, S. Too depressed to swim or too afraid to stop? a reinterpretation of the forced swim test as a measure of anxiety-like behavior. *Neuropsychopharmacology* **2018**, *43*, 931–933. [CrossRef] [PubMed]

178. Seligman, M.E.P. Depression and learned helplessness. In *The Psychology of Depression: Contemporary Theory and Research*; Winston-Wiley: New York, NY, USA, 1974; pp. 83–113.

179. Maier, S.F. Behavioral control blunts reactions to contemporaneous and future adverse events: Medial prefrontal cortex plasticity and a corticostriatal network. *Neurobiol. Psychiatry* **2015**, *1*, 12–22. [CrossRef] [PubMed]

180. Christianson, J.P.; Flyer-Adams, J.G.; Drugan, R.C.; Amat, J.; Daut, R.A.; Foilb, A.R.; Watkins, L.R.; Maier, S.F. Learned stressor resistance requires extracellular signal-regulated kinase in the prefrontal cortex. *Front. Behav. Neurosci.* **2014**, *8*, 348. [CrossRef] [PubMed]

181. Baratta, M.V.; Zarza, C.M.; Gomez, D.M.; Campeau, S.; Watkins, L.R.; Maier, S.F. Selective activation of dorsal raphe nucleus-projecting neurons in the ventral medial prefrontal cortex by controllable stress. *Eur. J. Neurosci.* **2009**, *30*, 1111–1116. [CrossRef] [PubMed]

182. Wellman, C.L.; Moench, K.M. Preclinical studies of stress, extinction, and prefrontal cortex: Intriguing leads and pressing questions. *Psychopharmacology* **2018**, *236*, 59–72. [CrossRef] [PubMed]

183. Moench, K.M.; Maroun, M.; Kavushansky, A.; Wellman, C. Alterations in neuronal morphology in infralimbic cortex predict resistance to fear extinction following acute stress. *Neurobiol. Stress* **2016**, *3*, 23–33. [CrossRef] [PubMed]

184. Izquierdo, A.; Wellman, C.L.; Holmes, A. Brief uncontrollable stress causes dendritic retraction in infralimbic cortex and resistance to fear extinction in mice. *J. Neurosci.* **2006**, *26*, 5733–5738. [CrossRef] [PubMed]

185. Barker, J.M.; Taylor, J.R.; Chandler, L.J. A unifying model of the role of the infralimbic cortex in extinction and habits. *Learn. Mem.* **2014**, *21*, 441–448. [CrossRef] [PubMed]

186. Sharpe, M.J.; Killcross, S. Modulation of attention and action in the medial prefrontal cortex of rats. *Psychol. Rev.* **2018**, *125*, 822–843. [CrossRef] [PubMed]
187. Killcross, S.; Coutureau, E. Coordination of actions and habits in the medial prefrontal cortex of rats. *Cereb. Cortex* **2003**, *13*, 400–408. [CrossRef] [PubMed]
188. Coutureau, E.; Killcross, S. Inactivation of the infralimbic prefrontal cortex reinstates goal-directed responding in overtrained rats. *Behav. Brain* **2003**, *146*, 167–174. [CrossRef]
189. Haddon, J.; Killcross, S. Inactivation of the infralimbic prefrontal cortex in rats reduces the influence of inappropriate habitual responding in a response-conflict task. *Neuroscience* **2011**, *199*, 205–212. [CrossRef]
190. Holtzheimer, P.E.; Mayberg, H.S. Stuck in a rut: Rethinking depression and its treatment. *Trends Neurosci.* **2011**, *34*, 1–9. [CrossRef] [PubMed]
191. Sawiak, S.J.; Shiba, Y.; Oikonomidis, L.; Windle, C.P.; Santangelo, A.M.; Grydeland, H.; Cockcroft, G.; Bullmore, E.T.; Roberts, A.C. Trajectories and milestones of cortical and subcortical development of the marmoset brain from infancy to adulthood. *Cereb. Cortex* **2018**, *28*, 4440–4453. [CrossRef]

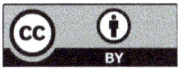

brain
sciences

MDPI

Article

Loss of Hierarchical Control by Occasion Setters Following Lesions of the Prelimbic and Infralimbic Medial Prefrontal Cortex in Rats

Stephanie Roughley and Simon Killcross *

School of Psychology, University of New South Wales, Sydney 2052, Australia; stephanie.kelly@unsw.edu.au
*   Correspondence: s.killcross@unsw.edu.au; Tel.: +61-(2)-9385-3034

Received: 31 January 2019; Accepted: 26 February 2019; Published: 26 February 2019

Abstract: Recent work suggests complementary roles of the prelimbic and infralimbic regions of the rat medial prefrontal cortex in cognitive control processes, with the prelimbic cortex implicated in top-down modulation of associations and the infralimbic cortex playing a role in the inhibition of inappropriate responses. Following selective lesions made to prelimbic or infralimbic regions (or control sham-surgery) rats received simultaneous training on Pavlovian feature negative (A+, XA−) and feature positive (B−, YB+) discriminations designed to lead to hierarchical occasion-setting control by the features (X, Y) over their respective targets (A, B). Evidence for hierarchical control was assessed in a transfer test in which features and targets were swapped (YA, XB). All groups were able to learn the feature negative and feature positive discriminations. Whilst sham-lesioned animals showed no transfer of control by features to novel targets (a hallmark of hierarchical control), rats with lesions of prelimbic or infralimbic regions showed evidence of transfer from the positive feature (Y) to the negative target (A), and from the negative feature (X) to the positive target (B; although this only achieved significance in infralimbic-lesioned animals). These data indicate that damage to either of these regions disrupts hierarchical occasion-setting control, extending our knowledge of their role in cognitive control to encompass flexible behaviours dictated by discrete cues.

Keywords: prelimbic; infralimbic; medial prefrontal cortex; cognitive control; hierarchical control; occasion setting; extinction; Pavlovian

---

1. Introduction

In order to behave appropriately in environments that are complex and changing, operating via simple associative contingencies is often insufficient. Instead, an organism must be able to use task-relevant information to extract specific 'rules' for responding, as well as apply the top-down control necessary to implement and adapt these strategies as required, including both the capacity to promote relevant responses and the capacity to inhibit inappropriate responses. Previous research has implicated the medial prefrontal cortex (mPFC) in this sort of hierarchical control of behavioural responding, in recent years focusing specifically on prelimbic (PL) and infralimbic (IL) subregions. These regions appear to serve separable but complementary functions that together may offer an explanation as to how the mPFC might be organized to accommodate higher-order control processes. The research detailed below provides direct evidence of the involvement of PL and IL regions in the development of hierarchical control in the context of discrete cues controlling Pavlovian conditioning. This expands our understanding of the role of these areas in the flexible control of behaviour, complementing previous research examining contextual control of instrumental behaviours.

For example, in a rodent version of the Stroop task, work by Killcross, Haddon, and colleagues [1,2] provided explicit evidence for differential involvement of PL and IL cortices in hierarchical control of behaviour using contextual cues. Here, rats are trained on two biconditional discrimination tasks in separate contexts. These tasks involved presentations of two discriminable stimuli (auditory for one context: A1 and A2, Visual for the other: V1 and V2), each of which dictated that responding on a particular lever (L1 or L2) would be rewarded. At test, animals were presented with audio-visual compounds of these stimuli in each context, where either both stimuli had stipulated the same response in training (congruent) or had each stipulated an opposing response (incongruent). When presented with incongruent trials, animals are required to use the experimental context in order to disambiguate the conflicting response information and determine where to direct responding (i.e., the lever associated with the stimulus element that had been trained in that context). Results demonstrated that temporary inactivation of the PL cortex impaired the ability of these animals to perform context-appropriate responses on the incongruent trials, suggesting that the PL cortex, in particular, is necessary for using contextual information to guide appropriate responding in situations of cue and response conflict [2]. In contrast, using a version of the task in which the amount of training on the two discriminations was manipulated such that one discrimination received three times the training of the other [1], rats are normally unable to use the undertrained contextual cues to allow expression of the context-appropriate response when presented with an incongruent compound comprising both undertrained and overtrained cues. However, following inactivation of the IL cortex prior to the test, rats were able to overcome the impact of the overtrained discrimination in favour of the contextually appropriate undertrained cue. This suggests that the IL cortex usually functions to promote basic stimulus-response associations (which could be excitatory, inhibitory, or both), regardless of context, and oppose top-down modulation by the contextual cues.

The PL cortex has also been shown to be important for contextual control of responding in aversive Pavlovian conditioning [3]. In a contextual biconditional discrimination task, animals were trained with two cues in two contexts. Both cues were presented in both contexts, but in the first context, one cue was paired with a shock and the other with nothing, while in the second context this was reversed. Thus, the context dictated which cue to fear and which cue was safe. Inactivation of the PL cortex was found to interrupt both acquisition and performance of this discrimination, suggesting that the role of the PL cortex in hierarchical control processes extends to both appetitive and aversive domains.

In both of the situations outlined above, each of the cues has a mixed associative history, sometimes preceding an appetitive or aversive outcome and sometimes not, and the context is required to determine which associative structure is operational at a given time. Another well-documented phenomenon that may involve the same sort of contextual modulation of simple associative structures is extinction. In extinction learning, an organism learns that a cue (CS) that previously predicted an outcome (US) no longer does, resulting in a decrease in conditioned responding to that stimulus. One prevalent model of extinction (Reference [4], but see also Reference [5]) stipulates that this learning can be thought of in terms of a new inhibitory association forming, which exists alongside the original excitatory one. This inhibitory association is context-dependent, such that it is only activated in preference to the original learning in contexts similar to that in which extinction learning occurred [6]. In this way, the context is said to gate the inhibitory association, modulating behavioural performance on the basis of which association is more likely to be valid in a particular environment.

There has been considerable research investigating the roles of PL and IL cortices in acquisition and expression of extinction learning. For example, the IL cortex has been shown to be important for the retrieval and expression of previously acquired extinction of fear learning [7], and lesions to the IL cortex have also been shown to increase recovery, reinstatement, and renewal of an extinguished Pavlovian response in an appetitive conditioning paradigm [8,9]. In contrast, lesions of the PL cortex have been shown to impair renewal of an extinguished fear response, with extinction learning appearing instead to generalize across contexts [10]. Taken together, these findings suggest that the IL cortex is important for facilitating the expression of extinction learning, and the generalization of inhibitory associations across contexts, while one possible function of the PL cortex is to gate the inhibitory extinction association on the basis of contextual features, modulating the expression of extinction based on contextual cues [11]. This is in line with evidence outlined above implicating the PL cortex in contextual modulation of behavior such that features of the organism's current environment are better able to retrieve appropriate associations that come to be expressed in behaviour. Conversely, the IL cortex may be seen as again playing a complementary role by promoting the capacity of learning to be generalized across contexts, independently of higher-order cues or rules.

Many of these studies examining the role of PL and IL in the development of behavioural flexibility, or the implementation of rule-based strategies, have examined the ability of contextual cues to come to control performance. However, recent work has indicated that the PL and IL may also both play a role in the use of discrete cues to provide top-down control of response alternatives. On the one hand, Meyer and Bucci [12] have demonstrated that pre-training lesions of the PL region of the mPFC produce deficits in the acquisition of conditioned inhibition in a compound feature negative discrimination (of the form A+, AX−, where A+ is a 10-s tone followed by pellet reward, and AX- is presentation of a 10-s compound tone and light cue followed by no outcome). Rats with lesions of the IL region produced a level of discrimination that did not differ significantly from either PL-lesioned animals or sham-lesioned control animals. Prior to this, Rhodes and Killcross [13] examined the ability of rats with IL-lesions to acquire conditioned inhibition using a similar simultaneous feature negative design. As Meyer and Bucci also found, IL lesions were without effect in the acquisition of conditioned inhibition in this design, coming, like sham-operated control animals, to respond reliably more to A+ than AX− compounds. However, Rhodes and Killcross subsequently examined the status of the conditioned inhibitor X in both summation and retardation tests. In a summation test in which inhibitor X was paired with novel excitor B+, both lesioned and control animals showed an impact of the inhibitor X on responding, confirming that inhibition had accrued to X during training. In the retardation test, which examined the acquisition of conditioned responding to X (now X+) compared to a neutral cue (Y+) to which animals had had equivalent exposure, only sham-operated control animals showed the expected better acquisition to Y+ than to the inhibitory X+. For IL-lesioned animals, acquisition of conditioned responding was equal to both X+ and Y+. Rhodes and Killcross [13] concluded that the role of the IL cortex here was related specifically to the acquisition of both excitatory and inhibitory associations with the same cue, echoing its role in the inhibitory learning thought to occur in extinction, and more recent evidence suggesting a more general role in inhibitory associations [14].

However, these studies employing discrete-cue feature negative discriminations may not be directly comparable to those examining top-down modulation of behaviour by contextual cues, where the contextual cues are held to act as modulating factors. Whilst feature discriminations such as those described above are laid out as occasion-setting preparations, whereby the feature X can come to modulate the performance to the target A (much like the contextual cues may do in the studies outlined previously), evidence suggests that this is unlikely when simultaneous presentations of the cues in compound are used (as was the case in the above studies). Rather, simultaneous presentation of feature and target cues in compound (AX−) encourages the development of direct (inhibitory) associations between X and the target US or the behaviour engendered by presentation of A [4,15]. By contrast, however, modulatory relationships are favored when the feature and target compounds are presented sequentially or in series (that is, X followed by A). In these preparations, there is evidence that the feature X comes to modulate the relationship between A and the US (see, e.g., Reference [16]).

If sequentially-arranged feature discriminations are underpinned by occasion-setting relationships, the use of such procedures would seem a strong test-bed in which to further examine the role of PL and IL function. In particular, it would permit examination of both the development and execution of modulatory control over ambiguous relationships in discrete-cue Pavlovian conditioning in a manner that can be compared and contrasted with evidence derived from studies examining contextual modulation in both the Stroop analogue and extinction-based procedures. Such an addition would provide a broader base of evidence from which to derive conclusions about PL and IL function, specifically in the context of modulation of performance by top-down processes in which behavioural control must be exerted to regulate responding to cues with an ambiguous or mixed history of reinforcement.

Of course, as the argument above makes clear, simply observing the acquisition of feature discriminations does not, in itself, reveal the underlying associative structure; whilst we might arrange serial feature-target compounds to promote the development of hierarchical occasion setting control, this does not mean this is how the animals learn the tasks (they could, for example, nevertheless produce direct associations between features and the US). Whilst the precise associative structure underpinning occasion setting relationships are still somewhat in debate, in research that does evidence a hierarchical account over a configural one, the failure of complete transfer between occasion-setting cues plays a central role [4,16]. In general, features (X, Y) used in either sequential feature negative (A+, XA−) or feature positive (B−, YB+) discriminations do not show transfer of control over separately trained CSs (e.g., XC, or YD), and whilst there may be some (incomplete) transfer from one feature positive discrimination to another similarly trained feature positive discrimination, transfer does not occur between feature positive and feature negative discriminations under normal occasion setting circumstances [17]. The reason for this is that the modulation of the relationship between CS and US (whereby sometimes the CS predicts the occurrence of the US and sometimes it doesn't) is found to be substantially CS and US specific, emphasizing that the feature modulates the relationship between CS and US, rather than the level of activation of associative representations of CS and/or US directly. Another factor made plain by this account is that the relationship between CS and US must be ambiguous (having a history of reinforcement and non-reinforcement) for occasion setting to play a strong role. Accordingly, a test of transfer provides a clear method by which to explicitly assess the associative structure underpinning feature discrimination.

The purpose of the current study is therefore two-fold. Firstly, we aimed to implement training of serial feature-positive and feature-negative discriminations and assess whether, under normal circumstances, animals acquire these discriminations via hierarchical occasion-setting mechanisms. Secondly, we aimed to examine the role of PL and IL cortices in this process—whether lesions of the PL or IL cortex impact acquisition of feature positive and feature negative discriminations, and/or the manner in which these are acquired. To achieve this, we trained rats (following excitotoxic lesions of PL, IL, or sham control surgery) simultaneously on both Pavlovian serial feature negative (A+ XA−) and Pavlovian serial feature positive (B+, YB−) discrete cue discriminations. Following acquisition of these discriminations, we examined the capacity of the features X and Y to transfer control to their oppositely trained targets (probe tests XB and YA in extinction). It is specifically by the use of the transfer task that one can reveal the specificity of the hierarchical control; if the training had brought the relationships between A and B and the US under hierarchical occasion setting control by X and Y respectively, then we would expect to see little or no transfer of control from X to B or Y to A. In contrast, if the normal processes of occasion setting were disrupted, we might expect this to be revealed in transfer of control from features X and Y to novel targets B and A.

If the PL cortex plays a general role in top-down control of both Pavlovian and instrumental tasks (as we have suggested, see Reference [11]), and the IL cortex plays a role in promoting and acquiring the basic associative relationships that are to be modulated, then the use of feature positive and feature negative occasion setting and transfer tasks should be revealing. It was expected that sham-operated control animals would demonstrate discriminative control of responding in both the feature positive and feature negative tasks, and furthermore would not show transfer of this control in the probe test. This would support the claim that discriminable responding to target cues in serially arranged occasion-setting preparations typically falls under hierarchical control via the feature cues. Given prior work indicating a role for the PL cortex in top-down modulation of performance towards ambiguous cues, one may expect PL-lesioned animals to show an impairment in learning the discriminations (for which there is some evidence in feature-negative preparations [18]). In addition, if they are able to learn the discrimination, it was expected that the transfer test would reveal this not to be a function of hierarchical control over responding (that is, these animals would show significant transfer). It is more difficult to come up with specific predictions as to whether and how lesions of the IL cortex may impact learning of the discriminations, since the main hypotheses regarding IL function are either firmly embedded in the context of extinction procedures [7] or relate to the development of stimulus-response associations [11] which do not have a clear translation in the context of Pavlovian conditioning. However, given the body of literature supporting dissociable functions of PL and IL regions of the cortex, it would be interesting to determine if a similar dissociation is observed in this paradigm.

2. Materials and Methods

2.1. Subjects

Subjects for this experiment comprised twenty-four (N = 24) experimentally naive, adult male Long-Evans rats (Monash Animal Services, Gippsland, Victoria, Australia), weighing between 307–412 g at the start of experimentation. They were housed eight rats per cage, in a temperature- and humidity-controlled environment (22 °C) operating on a 12-h light-dark cycle (lights on at 7:00 a.m.). All experimental procedures took place during the light cycle. Following recovery from surgery, animals were placed on a food restriction schedule on which it was ensured they maintained at least 85% of free-feeding weight. Water was available ad libitum. All procedures were carried out in accordance with the National Institute of Health Guide for the Care and Use of Laboratory Animals (NIH publications No. 80-123, revised 1996) and were approved by the University of New South Wales Animal Care and Ethics Committee (ACE:09/39B).

2.2. Surgery

Prior to behavioral training, animals were randomly assigned to receive bilateral excitotoxic lesions of the infralimbic cortex, prelimbic cortex, or sham surgery (n = 8). Surgery was performed under isoflurane anesthesia in a standard stereotaxic frame (World Precision Instruments Inc., Sarasota, FL, USA), using a flat skull position. To produce lesions, 0.4 µL infusions of 10 µg/µL N-methyl-D-aspartic acid (NMDA; Sigma-Aldrich, Buchs, Switzerland) were administered to either the PL (coordinates from bregma; AP +3.2, L ± 0.7, and DV−4.0) or IL (coordinates from bregma; AP +3.0, L ± 0.7, and DV-5.4) cortex using a 1-µl syringe (Hamilton, NV, USA). Infusions proceeded at a rate of 0.1 µL/min, and once complete the syringe was left in place for a further four minutes to allow the solution to diffuse into the tissue. Animals in the sham group underwent an identical procedure, with the exception that no NMDA was administered. The syringe was entered at the PL site for four of the sham animals and at the IL site for the other four. Post-surgery all animals were allowed to recover over a minimum 10-day period, during which time they received daily post-operative observations, and had ad libitum access to both food and water. Animals were subsequently placed on the food restriction schedule, which was maintained for three days prior to the commencement of behavioural training and was continued for the duration of testing.

2.3. Apparatus

Training was carried out using eight standard operant chambers measuring 25 × 25 × 22 cm and housed in light- and sound-attenuating compartments (Paul Fray, Cambridge, UK). Each chamber was composed of three aluminum walls with a clear Perspex front wall and ceiling. The floors consisted of 18 stainless steel bars, 5 mm in diameter and spaced 1.5 cm apart. A magazine was located at the bottom center of the left-hand wall, where grain pellets (45 mg; Bio-Serv, Flemington, NJ, USA) could be delivered. Magazine entries were registered via the action of a Perspex flap that animals opened in order to access the magazine. Auditory stimuli were provided by a speaker fitted into the back center of the chamber's ceiling, which was linked to an audio signal generator (Med Associates ANL-926, Fairfax, VT, USA). Auditory stimuli consisted of a 2.8 kHz tone and white noise. Visual stimuli consisted of a panel light located immediately above the magazine and an LED light located within the magazine itself. Experimental operations were controlled and recorded by a desktop computer equipped with MED-PC software (Med Associates Inc, Fairfax, VT, USA.).

2.4. Procedures

2.4.1. Pretraining

Prior to discrimination training animals were given three 40-min sessions of magazine training, in which they learned to retrieve food pellets that were delivered to the magazine. Pellets were delivered approximately every 60 s according to a variable time schedule (VT60). For the first of these sessions only, the magazine flaps were fixed open to facilitate access to the rewards.

2.4.2. Discrimination Training

All groups received 32 sessions of discrimination training in which animals were exposed to concurrent serial feature positive and serial feature negative Pavlovian discrimination arrangements. In the feature positive arrangement, a visual 'target' stimulus (Magazine Light or Panel Light; designated cue B) was presented either alone with no reinforcement (B−) or was preceded by an auditory 'feature' stimulus (Noise or Tone; designated cue Y) and was accompanied by the delivery of a food reward (YB+). In the feature negative arrangement, the alternate target stimulus (Magazine Light or Panel light; designated cue A) was either presented alone, in which case the presentation was reinforced (A+), or was preceded by the alternate feature stimulus (noise or Tone; designated cue X) and was not reinforced (XA−). A summary of this experimental design is shown in Table 1. Combinations of auditory and visual stimuli were fully counterbalanced across animals.

Table 1. Summary of experimental design.

	Target Alone	Feature — Target	Probe
Feature Positive	B → No US	Y − B → US	Y − A → No US
Feature Negative	A → US	X − A → No US	X − B → No US

Note. A and B represent target stimuli (magazine light and panel light), while X and Y represent feature stimuli (tone and noise). US represents reinforcement via food pellet, and No US represents no reward. Animals are trained and tested on all combinations.

Each session ran for approximately 64 min and consisted of 10 stimulus presentations of each type (A+, XA−, B−, and YB+). In target-alone presentations, the target stimulus was presented for 10sec and was either followed by a reward or not, depending on trial type (A+ or B−). In feature-target presentations (XA− and YB+), the feature stimulus was presented for 10 s and was immediately followed by the 10 s target stimulus. For reinforced presentations, the termination of the target stimulus coincided with the delivery of a reward. These trials were presented in random order with the restriction of no more than two consecutive trials of the same type and were interspersed with variable inter-trial intervals (ITI; M = 60 s).

2.4.3. Probe Test

Following discrimination training, all groups were given a test session incorporating probe trials in which the original feature-target combinations were reversed. During this session groups received the discrimination procedure in its entirety, immediately followed by an additional 15 min in which animals were presented with six reverse feature-target presentations in the absence of reinforcement (three each of YA− and XB−). This was to assess whether the capacity of features X and Y to control responding would transfer to the opposing targets. These trials were interspersed with four more of the usual target-alone presentations (two each of A+ and B−). Trials were presented in random order and were separated by VT60 ITIs.

2.5. Histological Analysis

At the conclusion of behavioural testing, animals were given a lethal dose of sodium pentobarbitone and were transcardially perfused via the ascending aorta with saline-based pre-wash followed by 4% paraformaldehyde solution. Brains were removed and post-fixed in paraformaldehyde for a period of two days, before being transferred to sucrose solution (20% w/v) for a further 24 h. Forty micrometer coronal sections of the brain were taken using a cryostat and mounted onto gelatine-coated slides. Slides were air-dried overnight under a fume-hood and subsequently stained using cresyl violet. Lesion placement was verified under a light microscope, with the extent and location of neuronal damage for each animal recorded with reference to Paxinos and Watson's atlas [19].

2.6. Statistics Analysis

Entry to the food magazine was the conditioned response measure of interest. Relative rates (per 10 s) of conditioned responding were calculated by subtracting average baseline levels of magazine entry from magazine entries performed during stimulus presentations. Baseline responding was defined as the rate of magazine entry during the ITI period, averaged across all trials of the session. Responding was measured over the full 10 s of feature presentations, and the final 5 s of target presentations (to minimize interference from behavioral competition on trials on which the feature preceded the target). Of primary interest were the rates of conditioned responding to target stimuli (A and B) during acquisition and the probe test. Data were analyzed using mixed analysis of variance (ANOVA) and where relevant, significant interactions were followed up with simple effects analysis and/or pairwise comparisons.

3. Results

3.1. Histology

All animals in the IL group showed substantial bilateral damage to the IL region, extending throughout anterior and posterior regions, while neighboring cortical regions were left largely intact ($n = 8$). Similarly, animals in the PL group showed acceptable levels of neuronal loss to the PL region, which extended fully in the anterior direction but showed some sparing of the posterior region ($n = 8$). Figure 1 illustrates the maximum (grey) and minimum (black) extent of lesion damage for both IL and PL groups. Location and extent of lesions in this study are similar to those in previous work, in which dissociable behavioural effects have been demonstrated [8–10,12,18,20].

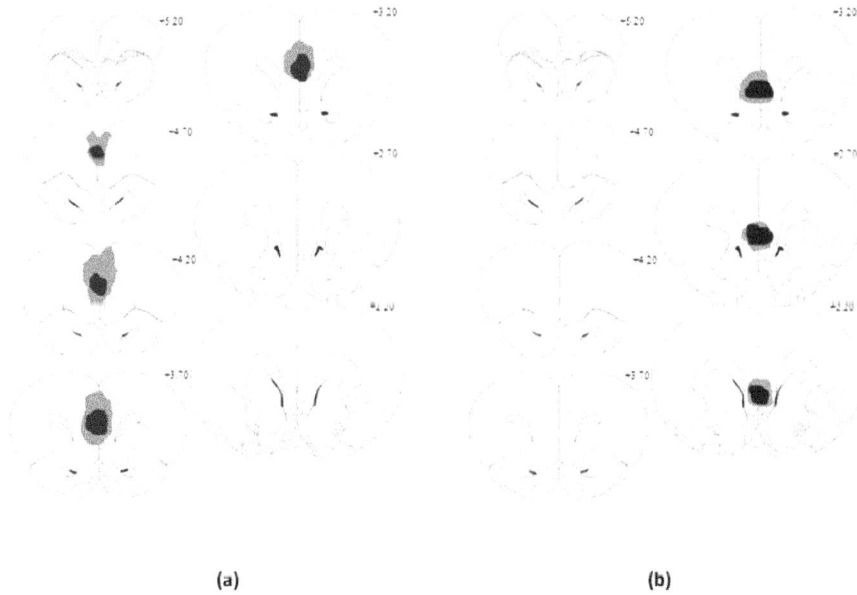

(a)   **(b)**

Figure 1. Schematic representation of location and extent of excitotoxic lesion damage to the prelimbic (PL; **a**) and infralimbic (IL; **b**) cortices. Shaded regions indicate the minimum (black) and maximum (grey) area covered by the lesions. Coronal sections displayed here are +2.20 to +5.20 (in mm from bregma).

3.2. Behaviour

3.2.1. Acquisition

A preliminary analysis of baseline rates magazine entry was performed using a two-way mixed ANOVA in which the between subjects factor was Group (Sham, PL, and IL) and the within subjects factor was Session Block (1–8; blocks of four sessions). Results revealed no significant between-group differences in rates of baseline responding ($F < 1$). Similar ANOVAs (with additional within-subjects factor of Feature; present or absent) were also performed to analyze rates of acquisition of conditioned magazine entry responding to target stimuli in the feature positive (B alone vs. B when preceded by Y) and feature negative (A alone vs. A when preceded by X) discriminations. The data for these analyses are displayed in Figure 2. As illustrated, acquisition of the feature positive association is evidenced by increasing responding on reinforced YB+ trials compared to non-reinforced B- trials, and rate of acquisition did not differ by group. There were significant main effects of Session Block ($F_{7,147} = 21.42$; $p < 0.001$) and Feature ($F_{1,21} = 27.74$; $p < 0.001$) plus a significant Session Block by Feature interaction ($F_{7,147} = 12.19$; $p < 0.001$), but no other effects or interactions were significant (all $F < 1$). Acquisition of the feature negative association is evidenced by increasing responding on reinforced A+ trials, compared to non-reinforced XA− trials. Although it appears that animals in the PL lesion group may have acquired this discrimination more slowly than either the IL lesion or Sham control group (discriminated responding first appears in Block 3 or 4 for IL and Sham groups, but not until Block 6 for the PL lesion group), this was not statistically supported. As for the feature positive discrimination, there were significant main effects of Session Block ($F_{7,147} = 15.13$; $p < 0.001$) and Feature ($F_{1,21} = 9.68$; $p = 0.005$), as well as a Session Block by Feature interaction ($F_{7,147} = 9.35$; $p < 0.001$), but no other effects or interactions were significant (notably no main effect of Group or interaction with Group; all $F < 1$).

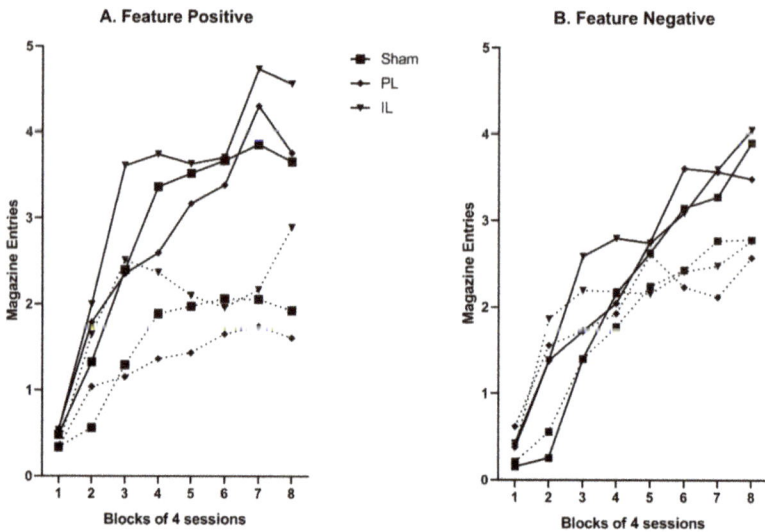

Figure 2. Acquisition of magazine entry responding (rate per 10 s) during target cue presentation in the feature positive (panel **A**) and feature negative (panel **B**) discriminations. Solid line displays responding to the reinforced target (i.e., on (Y)B+ trials for feature positive and A+ trials for feature negative), while dotted line displays responding to the non-reinforced target (i.e., B− trials for the feature positive and (X)A− trials for feature negative).

Responding to target stimuli during the final session of discrimination training is displayed in Figure 3. Rats in all groups showed evidence of having acquired both the feature positive and feature negative discriminations by the end of training, in that conditioned responding was greater on reinforced trials (A+ and (Y)B+) than non-reinforced trials ((X)A− and B−).

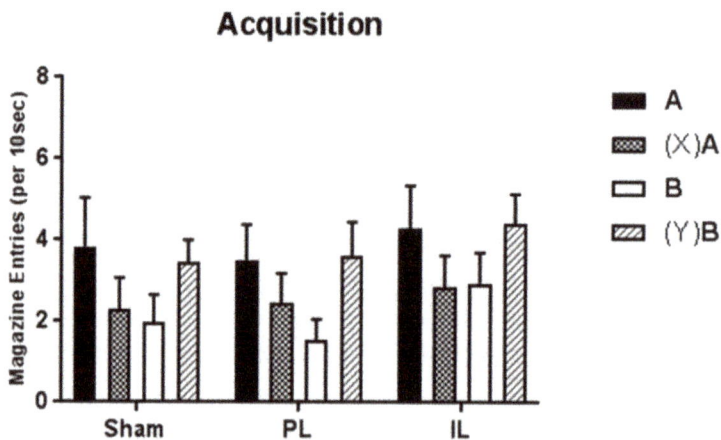

Figure 3. Rate (per 10 s; relative to baseline) of magazine entry during presentation of the target cue on feature-present and feature-absent trials of the feature negative ((X)A and A, respectively) and feature positive ((Y)B and B, respectively) discriminations. Error bars represent +SEM.

Acquisition of conditioned responding to target stimuli in the feature positive (B− and (Y)B+) and feature negative (A+ and (X)A−) discriminations was assessed via a three-way mixed ANOVA. In this analysis, the between subjects factor was Group (Sham, PL, and IL), and within subjects factors were Discrimination (feature negative or feature positive) and Feature (present or absent). Results revealed a significant Discrimination by Feature interaction ($F_{1,21}$ = 29.88; p < 0.001). No other main effects or interactions were significant (all F < 1).

Follow-up simple effects analysis of the interaction term indicate that averaging across groups, conditioned responding during target presentation on the feature negative discrimination was greater on the reinforced feature-absent trials (A+) than the non-reinforced feature-present trials ((X)A−; $F_{1,21}$ = 12.57; p = 0.002). For the feature positive discrimination, conditioned responding during target presentation was greater on the reinforced feature-present trials ((Y)B+) than the non-reinforced feature-absent trials (B−; $F_{1,21}$ = 18.55; p < 0.001). In other words, animals were able to use the feature cue to either inhibit (in the case of the feature negative discrimination) or elevate (in the case of the feature positive discrimination) responding to the target cue, and this did not differ as a function of lesion group.

Analysis of responding during feature presentation was also assessed, using a two-way mixed ANOVA in which the between subjects factor was Group (Sham, PL, and IL) and the within subjects factor was Feature (X or Y; negative and positive discriminations, respectively). Results revealed a significant main effect of Feature ($F_{1,21}$ = 24.86; p < 0.001), whereby conditioned responding during the positive feature Y (which is followed by reinforced target B; M (±SD) for Sham = 3.58 (±2.03), PL = 3.01 (±3.15), and IL = 2.86 (±2.64)) was greater than responding during the negative feature X (which is followed by non-reinforced target A; M (±SD) for Sham = 0.51 (±0.62), PL = 0.64 (±0.26), and IL − 0.54 (±0.49)). No other effect or interaction was significant (both F < 1), indicating that the ability to discriminate between excitatory (Y) and inhibitory (X) features did not differ as a function of lesion group.

3.2.2. Probe Test

Rates of responding to target stimuli during probe trials are displayed in Figure 4. As illustrated, animals in both the PL and IL groups demonstrated differential responding to the target cues according to whether the cues were presented alone (A+ or B−) vs. when they were preceded by the feature opposite to that which they had been paired with in training ((Y)A or (X)B). Specifically, responding to A was increased when preceded by Y, and responding to B was decreased when preceded by X. In contrast, the presence of the reverse features did not appear to have a substantial effect on responding to target stimuli for animals in the Sham group.

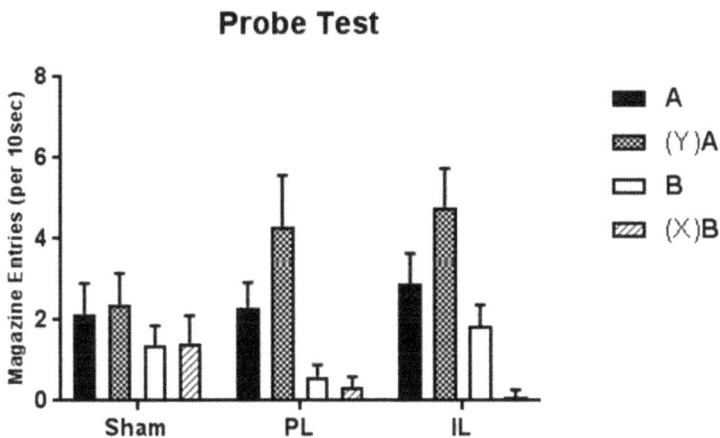

Figure 4. Rate (per 10 s; relative to baseline) of magazine entry during presentation of the target cue on feature-present ((Y)A and (X)B) and feature-absent (A+ and B−) trials of the probe test. Note paired features are the reverse of those in training. Error bars represent +SEM.

These findings are supported by a three-way mixed ANOVA in which the between subjects factor was Group (Sham, PL, and IL) and within subjects factors were Target (responding to A or B) and Feature (present or absent; Y and X, respectively). Results revealed a main effect of Target ($F_{1,21} = 21.35$; $p < 0.001$), whereby responding was greater during presentation of target cue A than target cue B, irrespective of feature presence or absence, and averaged across lesion group. This reflects the history of reinforcement for A and B alone (A+ and B-), and of X and Y as inhibitory and excitatory modulators respectively. Main effects of Feature and Group were not significant ($F_{1,21} = 2.61$; $p = 0.12$ and $F < 1$, respectively).

More informative, however, is a significant three-way interaction between Group, Feature and Target ($F_{2,21} = 4.09$; $p = 0.03$) and two-way interaction between Feature and Target ($F_{1,21} = 16.75$; $p = 0.001$). Neither of the other interactions was significant (Group x Feature, $F_{2,21} = 1.31$; $p = 0.29$; Group × Target, $F_{2,21} = 1.97$; $p = 0.16$). Simple effects analysis clarifies the interaction terms, revealing that responding to target cue A was significantly greater when preceded by feature cue Y than when presented alone for both the PL and IL groups ($F_{1,21} = 9.60$; $p = 0.005$ and $F_{1,21} = 8.59$; $p = 0.008$, respectively), but not for the Sham group ($F < 1$). In addition, responding to target cue B was significantly lower when preceded by cue X than when presented alone for the IL group ($F_{1,21} = 12.05$; $p = 0.002$), though not for the PL or Sham groups (both $F < 1$). In the case of the PL group, however, this is likely to be a floor effect given responding was already minimal to B when presented alone.

Together, these results indicate that both PL- and IL-lesioned animals demonstrate transfer of feature properties to different targets to a greater extent than sham-operated control animals. Specifically, in both these groups there is evidence of additive excitatory stimulus components to both A and Y, and in the IL group there is evidence of additive inhibitory stimulus components to both B and X. While this latter effect is not statistically supported in the PL group, it appears from that this may be a floor effect, in that responding was already minimal to B when presented alone.

4. Discussion

Here we have described a single experiment designed to examine the role of PL and IL regions of the mPFC in the development of hierarchical control in discrete cue Pavlovian feature negative and feature positive discriminations. In sham-operated control animals, simultaneous acquisition of the two discriminations proceeded uneventfully; although training was protracted, performance at the end of training indicated good control of performance in both discriminations, with significantly more responding to the rewarded cues (A+, and B+ following Y) than to non-rewarded cues (A− following X, and B−). A very similar pattern was observed in animals that had received lesions of the PL and IL prior to training, and no significant differences in acquisition were observed.

However, as indicated in the Introduction, performance during acquisition of these discriminations does not necessarily reveal the underpinning associative structure. As such we examined transfer of feature control over targets in separate probe tests. As expected (given the parameters used in the study such as the serial presentations of features and targets [17]), sham-lesioned control animals showed no transfer whatsoever across feature negative and feature positive discriminations. That is, probe presentations of positive feature Y prior to previously rewarded A failed to produce any significant enhancement of performance; similarly probe presentations of negative feature X prior to previously non-rewarded B failed to produce any significant decrement in performance. As such, we would conclude that in these sham-lesioned animals, the performance of the feature positive and feature negative discriminations was very likely to be the product of an underpinning hierarchical relationship in which the features came to modulate conditioned responding to targets with a mixed history of reinforcement.

In contrast, discrete lesions of either the PL or IL resulted in probe test performance that was markedly different. In the case of IL lesions, presentations of the positive feature Y enhanced performance to novel target A, and presentations of the negative feature X attenuated conditioned responding to novel target B. A very similar pattern of responding was observed following PL lesions, although the decrement in conditioned responding to cue B following presentations of negative feature X failed to reach significance in post-hoc analyses. It is possible that this could simply reflect a floor effect as baseline responding to target B (in the absence of X) was especially low in this group of animals.

As such, one would have to argue that the control of performance in the feature positive and feature negative discriminations in groups with lesions of the PL or IL regions, whilst superficially similar to that of the sham-operated control group, was not controlled by the same underpinning occasion setting structure. Rather, the evidence of both positive and negative transfer from features to targets suggests that instead, the features have come to control performance by something other than a hierarchical modulation of the association between targets and rewards. Based on alternative findings from the occasion setting literature investigating the potential associative structures that may control feature positive and feature negative discriminations (see, e.g., References [4,16]), it seems likely that the features X and Y had developed their own associations with the US (inhibitory and excitatory, respectively), and so came to control performance by a process of summation with separate associations formed between targets A and B with the US (excitatory and inhibitory, respectively). Accordingly, acquisition of the discriminations in lesioned groups may be understood in terms of straight-forward error-correction models of associative learning (in particular the Rescorla-Wagner model [21]), whereby excitatory and inhibitory associations of features and targets with the US sum to control performance. Briefly the Rescorla-Wagner model posits that associative learning occurs by a process of error correction whereby the outcome expected to occur following presentation of a stimulus is compared to that which actually occurs and the difference—the prediction error—is then used to adjust the expectancy when the stimulus is next encountered. A key tenet of this model is that associative strength (or in other words, outcome expectancy) accrues separately to all stimuli present on a trial, and is additive; hence the expectancy that is generated when a number of stimuli are presented is equal to the sum of the expectancy for each stimulus (for example inhibition accruing to X can offset excitation accruing to A, leading to lower expectancy on XA trials and hence to lower CRs).

Much previous work has implicated a role for the PL region of the mPFC in the top-down control of behavior. Inactivation of the PL cortex impairs performance in a rodent analogue of the Stroop task [2] and a contextual biconditional discrimination task [3], and PL lesions impair renewal of an extinguished fear response [10] and acquisition of a compound feature negative discrimination [12]. In addition, of particular relevance to this study MacLeod and Bucci [18] found evidence for a modest impairment in the rate of acquisition of a serial feature negative discrimination following lesions targeting the PL region (but not following lesions of the IL region). Whilst there were no statistically significant differences in acquisition between the three groups in the present study, there was some indication that learning of the feature negative discrimination may have been slower in the PL-lesioned group; rats with PL lesions failed to respond differentially to A+ and AX− until about the 6th block of training, compared to about the 3rd or 4th in Sham and IL-lesioned rats. Combined with the data showing transfer of occasion setting control, we would suggest that—as expected—lesions of the PL mPFC lead to a disruption of the ability of feature cues within occasion setting procedures to act as top-down modulators of associations formed between the target and US. Whilst rats with PL lesions (as we have observed in other Pavlovian procedures [3]) appear to remain able to call upon learning processes that conform to a Rescorla-Wagner model of associative learning [21], they cannot use cues or contexts in a hierarchical manner to modulate performance towards ambiguous stimuli with a mixed history of reinforcement. In this way, the data presented here confirm conclusions from previous work, as well as extending those findings to encompass the role of the PL region in the use of discrete stimuli as hierarchical modulators.

By contrast, the impact of lesions on the IL region on the acquisition and transfer tests are somewhat more surprising. Whilst we found no evidence at all for any deficits in acquisition of the two discriminations, both the positive and negative features were shown to be capable of transfer of control to novel targets, closely aligning with the observations following lesions of the PL region.

In previous work, the impact of manipulation of PL and IL regions has tended to produce clearly dissociable results, often described as providing complementary functionality that collectively supports the appropriate implementation of flexible, task-appropriate behaviour. As discussed previously, while the PL cortex has been implicated in expression of Pavlovian conditioned associations, the IL cortex is implicated in the expression of extinction learning [7,22]. Furthermore, while substantial evidence exists to implicate the IL region in inhibitory control [23,24], the PL cortex does not appear to be involved in this operation, being implicated in perseverative rather than premature responding [25]. Marquis et al. [2], Haddon and Killcross [1], and MacLeod and Bucci ([12]; see also Reference [18], also provide explicit evidence of dissociations between PL and IL cortices in the contextual control of instrumental actions, acquisition of occasion-setting modulation of Pavlovian responding, and conditioned inhibition. In addition, similar effects have been found in studies using an optimal set-shifting procedure [26] designed to assess the capacity to form attentional set (as opposed to switching attentional set, cf. Reference [27]), which again found dissociations between PL and IL regions. Other recent work has also highlighted dissociations between PL and IL function (albeit using pharmacogenetic activation of local parvalbumin interneurons as a means to silence local neuronal activity [28]), although these results stand at odds with many previous findings in suggesting deficits in intra-dimensional set shifting following silencing of the PL, but *not* IL, region of the mPFC. Earlier studies found no deficit in intradimensional set shifting following extensive mPFC lesions [27], and clear evidence of set-formation deficits following IL lesions [26].

In seeking to explain the current findings, there are two possible alternatives. The first of these is that the IL and PL cortices do not have separable roles, despite previous suggestions, and instead subserve highly similar functions. However, extant literature such as that described above strongly argues against this possibility. Thus, the present findings do not discount the weight of previous evidence that, in the context of both Pavlovian and instrumental learning, PL and IL cortices subserve differential functions (e.g., References [11,29]). As such, it remains to attempt to reconcile the current results with the notion that IL and PL cortices do operate in different ways. With this in mind, a second alternative explanation is that in the current studies, lesion groups show parallel deficits, but for different reasons.

If we are to assume that the failure of PL-lesioned animals to acquire hierarchical occasion setting control over behavioural responses [11], but that the function of the IL region is complementary (and potentially opposing), then what are the options? The IL region has been implicated in the encoding of inhibition irrespective of motivational value [14], extinction of Pavlovian fear conditioning [30] as well as extinction in appetitive conditioning procedures [8,9], the development of opposing excitatory and inhibitory associations linked to the same CS [13], the ability of training to influence choice performance [1], habitual performance [20,31], and the promotion of well-learned responses over those governed by top-down control [11]. Some researchers have also highlighted the notion that the IL cortex supports behavioural flexibility in the context of extinction, but appears to oppose flexibility in the context of its promotion of extensively trained, habitual responses [32], and have proposed a role for IL in contingency tracking. In all cases, there is a link whereby the IL appears to have a central role in the development of inhibitory relationships. In the broadest context, these might be inhibitory associations between CS and US [33], encoding of CS-No US associations [34] or CS-No Event associations [35], encoding of inhibitory S-R associations [4], or bidirectional encoding of reinforced and unreinforced lever presses on an operant schedule [32]. In all cases, the IL appears to be responsible for the overlay of inhibitory or 'no event' relationships to existing excitatory associations or positive contingencies (see also Reference [36]). Recall also that rats lacking IL fail to show retardation in a test of inhibition that requires excitatory associations to be overlaid on existing inhibitory associations [13], suggesting this role in the encoding of opposing relationships may be bidirectional.

In the context of the current experiment, one of the requirements for the development of a hierarchical occasion setting relationship is that the target cues have a mixed history of reinforcement. It is precisely the representation of this ambiguous relationship that is modulated by the presence of the feature to afford top-down control over responding to the target. Following IL lesions, we propose that animals are no longer able successfully to encode opposing relationships or contingencies around the target cues, and therefore cannot form the type of relationship that attracts (or indeed may necessitate) the development of occasion setting. This, in turn, leaves the animals to solve the task in a manner that appears to make use of more basic associative structures, such that responding to XA− can be reduced by offsetting excitation accruing to A (following A+ trials) with inhibition to X (acquired on AX− trials); similarly inhibition accruing to B will offset excitation to Y, allowing solution of the feature positive B− YB+ discrimination. Note also that previous work has found intact summation in IL-lesioned animals, confirming that they are able to offset excitation and inhibition across separate cues [13]. Further experiments where both excitatory and inhibitory relationships are arranged with single cues would help to further elucidate this potential role of the IL.

5. Conclusions

Overall, the results of the current experiment then lead one to refine further the potential complementary relationship between PL and IL regions of the mPFC. Once again we have demonstrated that the PL region appears critical for the development of top-down control processes, and now further hypothesize that the IL region may be needed to represent those ambiguous relationships in the world that attract this top-down control. Of course, in many situations (and as we have shown here) animals may make use of simpler associative structures to provide behavioural solutions to non linear discriminations, and indeed there are also configural associative structures that can provide a solution in many cases [37]. However, in order to achieve the hierarchical control that is the hallmark of truly flexible decision making, we would argue that the PL and IL must work in concert to produce the necessary template from which genuine rule-based behaviour can emerge. Understanding how rule-based behaviour is supported by these structures has the potential to open up new avenues in the treatment or prevention of human mental disorders where normal decision-making processes are disrupted, such as addiction and obsessive-compulsive disorder.

Author Contributions: Conceptualization, S.R. and S.K.; Data curation, S.K.; Formal analysis, S.R. and S.K.; Funding acquisition, S.R. and S.K.; Investigation, S.R. and S.K.; Methodology, S.R. and S.K.; Project administration, S.K.; Resources, S.K.; Software, S.R.; Supervision, S.K.; Validation, S.R. and S.K.; Visualization, S.R.; Writing—original draft, S.R. and S.K.; Writing—review & editing, S.R. and S.K.

Funding: This research was funded by an Australian Research Council Discovery Grant to Simon Killcross, grant number DP120103564, and by an Australian Postgraduate scholarship to Stephanie Roughley.

Conflicts of Interest: The authors declare no conflict of interest.

References

1. Haddon, J.E.; Killcross, S. Inactivation of the infralimbic prefrontal cortex in rats reduces the influence of inappropriate habitual responding in a response-conflict task. *Neuroscience* **2011**, *199*, 205–212. [CrossRef] [PubMed]

2. Marquis, J.P.; Killcross, S.; Haddon, J.E. Inactivation of the prelimbic, but not infralimbic, prefrontal cortex impairs the contextual control of response conflict in rats. *Eur. J. Neurosci.* **2007**, *25*, 559–566. [CrossRef] [PubMed]

3. Sharpe, M.J.; Killcross, S. The prelimbic cortex uses higher-order cues to modulate both the acquisition and expression of conditioned fear. *Front. Syst. Neurosci.* **2015**, *8*, 235. [CrossRef] [PubMed]

4. Trask, S.; Thrailkill, E.A.; Bouton, M.E. Occasion setting, inhibition, and the contextual control of extinction in Pavlovian and instrumental (operant) learning. *Behav. Process.* **2017**, *137*, 64–72. [CrossRef] [PubMed]

5. Delamater, A.R.; Westbrook, R.F. Psychological and neural mechanisms of experimental extinction: A selective review. *Neurobiol. Learn. Mem.* **2014**, *108*, 38–51. [CrossRef] [PubMed]

6. Bouton, M.E. Context, ambiguity, and unlearning: Sources of relapse after behavioral extinction. *Biol. Psychiatry* **2002**, *52*, 976–986. [CrossRef]

7. Quirk, G.J.; Russo, G.K.; Barron, J.L.; Lebron, K. The role of ventromedial prefrontal cortex in the recovery of extinguished fear. *J. Neurosci.* **2000**, *20*, 6225–6231. [CrossRef] [PubMed]
8. Rhodes, S.E.V.; Killcross, A.S. Lesions of rat infralimbic cortex enhance renewal of extinguished appetitive Pavlovian responding. *Eur. J. Neurosci.* **2007**, *25*, 2498–2503. [CrossRef] [PubMed]
9. Rhodes, S.E.V.; Killcross, S. Lesions of rat infralimbic cortex enhance recovery and reinstatement of an appetitive Pavlovian response. *Learn. Mem.* **2004**, *11*, 611–616. [CrossRef] [PubMed]
10. Sharpe, M.; Killcross, S. The prelimbic cortex uses contextual cues to modulate responding towards predictive stimuli during fear renewal. *Neurobiol. Learn. Mem.* **2015**, *118*, 20–29. [CrossRef] [PubMed]
11. Sharpe, M.J.; Killcross, S. Modulation of attention and action in the medial prefrontal cortex of rats. *Psychol. Rev.* **2018**, *125*, 822–843. [CrossRef] [PubMed]
12. Meyer, H.C.; Bucci, D.J. The contribution of medial prefrontal cortical regions to conditioned inhibition. *Behav. Neurosci.* **2014**, *128*, 644–653. [CrossRef] [PubMed]
13. Rhodes, S.E.V.; Killcross, A.S. Lesions of rat infralimbic cortex result in disrupted retardation but normal summation test performance following training on a Pavlovian conditioned inhibition procedure. *Eur. J. Neurosci.* **2007**, *26*, 2654–2660. [CrossRef] [PubMed]
14. Lingawi, N.W.; Holmes, N.M.; Westbrook, R.F.; Laurent, V. The infralimbic cortex encodes inhibition irrespective of motivational significance. *Neurobiol. Learn. Mem.* **2018**, *150*, 64–74. [CrossRef] [PubMed]
15. Holland, P.C. Conditioned stimulus as a determinant of form of Pavlovian conditioned response. *J. Exp. Psychol. Anim. Behav. Process.* **1977**, *3*, 77–104. [CrossRef] [PubMed]
16. Bonardi, C.; Robinson, J.; Jennings, D. Can existing associative principles explain occasion setting? Some old ideas and some new data. *Behav. Process.* **2017**, *137*, 5–18. [CrossRef] [PubMed]
17. Holland, P.C. Transfer of negative occasion setting and conditioned inhibition across conditioned and unconditioned stimuli. *J. Exp. Psychol. Anim. Behav. Process.* **1989**, *15*, 311–328. [CrossRef] [PubMed]
18. MacLeod, J.E.; Bucci, D.J. Contributions of the subregions of the medial prefrontal cortex to negative occasion setting. *Behav. Neurosci.* **2010**, *124*, 321–328. [CrossRef] [PubMed]
19. Paxinos, G.; Watson, C. *The Rat Brain in Stereotaxic Coordinates*, 6th ed.; Academic Press/Elsevier: Amsterdam, The Netherlands; Boston, MA, USA, 2007.
20. Killcross, S.; Coutureau, E. Coordination of actions and habits in the medial prefrontal cortex of rats. *Cereb. Cortex* **2003**, *13*, 400–408. [CrossRef] [PubMed]
21. Rescorla, R.A.; Wagner, A.R. A theory of Pavlovian conditioning: Variations in the effectiveness of reinforcement and nonreinforcement. In *Classical Conditioning II: Current Theory and Research*; Black, A.H., Prokasy, W.F., Eds.; Appleton-Century-Crofts: New York, NY, USA, 1972; pp. 64–99.
22. Vidal-Gonzalez, I.; Vidal-Gonzalez, B.; Rauch, S.L.; Quirk, G.J. Microstimulation reveals opposing influences of prelimbic and infralimbic cortex on the expression of conditioned fear. *Learn. Mem.* **2006**, *13*, 728–733. [CrossRef] [PubMed]
23. Chudasama, Y.; Passetti, F.; Rhodes, S.E.V.; Lopian, D.; Desai, A.; Robbins, T.W. Dissociable aspects of performance on the 5-choice serial reaction time task following lesions of the dorsal anterior cingulate, infralimbic and orbitofrontal cortex in the rat: Differential effects on selectivity, impulsivity and compulsivity. *Behav. Brain Res.* **2003**, *146*, 105–119. [CrossRef] [PubMed]
24. Murphy, E.R.; Dalley, J.W.; Robbins, T.W. Local glutamate receptor antagonism in the rat prefrontal cortex disrupts response inhibition in a visuospatial attentional task. *Psychopharmacology* **2005**, *179*, 99–107. [CrossRef] [PubMed]
25. Chudasama, Y.; Muir, J.L. Visual attention in the rat: A role for the prelimbic cortex and thalamic nuclei? *Behav. Neurosci.* **2001**, *115*, 417–428. [CrossRef] [PubMed]
26. George, D.N.; Duffaud, A.M.; Killcross, S. Neural correlates of attentional set. In *Attention and Associative Learning: From Brain to Behaviour*; Mitchell, C.J., Le Pelley, M.E., Eds.; Oxford University Press: Oxford, UK, 2010; pp. 351–383.
27. Birrell, J.M.; Brown, V.J. Medial frontal cortex mediates perceptual attentional set shifting in the rat. *J. Neurosci.* **2000**, *20*, 4320–4324. [CrossRef] [PubMed]
28. Mukherjee, A.; Caroni, P. Infralimbic cortex is required for learning alternatives to prelimbic promoted associations through reciprocal connectivity. *Nat. Commun.* **2018**, *9*, 2727. [CrossRef] [PubMed]

29. Sharpe, M.J.; Stalnaker, T.; Schuck, N.W.; Killcross, S.; Schoenbaum, G.; Niv, Y. An Integrated Model of Action Selection: Distinct Modes of Cortical Control of Striatal Decision Making. *Annu. Rev. Psychol.* **2019**, *70*, 53–76. [CrossRef] [PubMed]

30. Rosas-Vidal, L.E.; Do-Monte, F.H.; Sotres-Bayon, F.; Quirk, G.J. Hippocampal–prefrontal BDNF and memory for fear extinction. *Neuropsychopharmacology* **2014**, *39*, 2161–2169. [CrossRef] [PubMed]

31. Coutureau, E.; Killcross, S. Inactivation of the infralimbic prefrontal cortex reinstates goal-directed responding in overtrained rats. *Behav. Brain Res.* **2003**, *146*, 167–174. [CrossRef] [PubMed]

32. Barker, J.M.; Glen, W.B.; Linsenbardt, D.N.; Lapish, C.C.; Chandler, L.J. Habitual Behavior Is Mediated by a Shift in Response-Outcome Encoding by Infralimbic Cortex. *eNeuro* **2017**, *4*. [CrossRef] [PubMed]

33. Delamater, A.R. Experimental extinction in Pavlovian conditioning: Behavioural and neuroscience perspectives. *Q. J. Exp. Psychol.-B* **2004**, *57*, 97–132. [CrossRef] [PubMed]

34. Pearce, J.M.; Hall, G. A model for Pavlovian learning - variations in the effectiveness of conditioned but not of unconditioned stimuli. *Psychol. Rev.* **1980**, *87*, 532–552. [CrossRef] [PubMed]

35. Hall, G.; Rodriguez, G. Associative and nonassociative processes in latent inhibition: An elaboration of the Pearce-Hall model. In *Latent Inhibition: Cognition, Neuroscience and Applications to Schizophrenia*; Lubow, R.E., Weiner, I., Eds.; Cambridge University Press: Cambridge, UK, 2010; pp. 114–136.

36. Barker, J.M.; Taylor, J.R.; Chandler, L.J. A unifying model of the role of the infralimbic cortex in extinction and habits. *Learn. Mem.* **2014**, *21*, 441–448. [CrossRef] [PubMed]

37. Pearce, J.M. Similarity and discrimination: A selective review and a connectionist model. *Psychol. Rev.* **1994**, *101*, 587–607. [CrossRef] [PubMed]

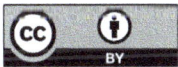

brain
sciences

MDPI

Review

Loss of Prefrontal Cortical Higher Cognition with Uncontrollable Stress: Molecular Mechanisms, Changes with Age, and Relevance to Treatment

Dibyadeep Datta and Amy F. T. Arnsten *

Department Neuroscience, Yale Medical School, New Haven, CT 06510, USA; Dibyadeep.datta@yale.edu
* Correspondence: amy.arnsten@yale.edu; Tel.: +1-203-785-4431; Fax: +1-203-785-5263

Received: 17 April 2019; Accepted: 13 May 2019; Published: 17 May 2019

Abstract: The newly evolved prefrontal cortex (PFC) generates goals for "top-down" control of behavior, thought, and emotion. However, these circuits are especially vulnerable to uncontrollable stress, with powerful, intracellular mechanisms that rapidly take the PFC "off-line." High levels of norepinephrine and dopamine released during stress engage α1-AR and D1R, which activate feedforward calcium-cAMP signaling pathways that open nearby potassium channels to weaken connectivity and reduce PFC cell firing. Sustained weakening with chronic stress leads to atrophy of dendrites and spines. Understanding these signaling events helps to explain the increased susceptibility of the PFC to stress pathology during adolescence, when dopamine expression is increased in the PFC, and with advanced age, when the molecular "brakes" on stress signaling are diminished by loss of phosphodiesterases. These mechanisms have also led to pharmacological treatments for stress-related disorders, including guanfacine treatment of childhood trauma, and prazosin treatment of veterans and civilians with post-traumatic stress disorder.

Keywords: prefrontal cortex; stress adolescence; aging; calcium; cAMP; dopamine; norepinephrine

1. Introduction

The prefrontal cortex (PFC) provides "top-down" control of behavior, thought, and emotion. However, these newly evolved circuits are especially vulnerable to uncontrollable stress, with built-in mechanisms to rapidly take the PFC "off-line" and switch the brain from a reflective to reflexive state. The current review summarizes the role of PFC circuits in top-down control, the unique molecular mechanisms governing PFC synapses that induce this rapid loss of function during stress exposure, and, with repeated stress, the atrophy of dendrites and spines. Understanding the molecular events that drive these powerful changes in brain state has direct relevance to the etiology of stress-related disorders such as depression, post-traumatic stress disorder (PTSD), substance abuse, schizophrenia, and late onset Alzheimer's disease (LOAD). These molecular mechanisms also help to explain why the PFC is so susceptible to stress pathology during adolescence (when catecholamine expression is increased in the PFC), and with advanced age (when the molecular "brakes" on stress signaling are diminished). Finally, understanding the molecular basis of the stress response in PFC has led to pharmacological treatments that are in widespread clinical use, a rare instance of successful translation from animals to humans.

2. The PFC Circuitry in Primates Serving Top-Down Control

The PFC provides top-down regulation of thought, action, and emotion [1], and has extensive connections to either promote or inhibit these neural events [2–6]. The PFC expands greatly in primate evolution, with the ventral and medial PFC (vmPFC) specialized for the regulation of emotion (internal states), while the more dorsal and lateral regions of the PFC (dlPFC) mediate cognition (external states) [2–4,7]. The most rostral, frontal pole serves metacognition, e.g., insight about oneself and others [8]. These regions all interconnect to provide a holistic mental state, where more newly evolved rostral and dorsolateral regions can provide top-down regulation of more ancient, caudal structures.

Evidence of "top-down" regulation by rostral and dlPFC–physiological recordings from monkeys have provided extensive evidence of "top-down" regulation by the dlPFC and rostral PFC circuits. Early studies found that these areas have the ability to generate neural activity in the absence of sensory stimulation, e.g., during a working memory task, the foundation of abstract thought [9,10]. This persistent firing during working memory could also be used to guide behavior, e.g., inhibiting an inappropriate response [11], and to suppress responding to distractors [12]. More recent studies have shown extensive roles in categorization and abstract rules, top-down control of attention, and strategic decision making, e.g., References [13–17]. Recordings from rostral medial PFC circuits have revealed signatures of high order cognitive capabilities, including social aspects of decision-making such as "theory of mind," i.e., understanding the minds of others [18], as well as metacognitive self-evaluation, i.e., insights about one's own decisions, in the frontal pole (area 10) [19,20]. These physiological recordings are consonant with studies of monkeys and patients with lesions to these regions, which demonstrate deficits in the top-down control of social and emotional behavior (reviewed in Reference [21]).

Ventral and medial PFC circuits regulate emotion. The ventral (orbital) and medial PFC provide flexible evaluation of affective information such as reward and punishment [18,22–25]. Although these regions are often referred to in a unitary fashion as simply "vmPFC," a more careful examination of the human imaging data, coupled with the known anatomical connections of this region in nonhuman primates, indicates important differentiations which likely mediate distinct functional contributions. The medial PFC includes the cingulate cortices: the anterior cingulate cortex, also known as Brodmann Area (BA)24, and the cingulate cortex under the genu of the corpus callosum, often called the subgenual cingulate, or BA25 (Figure 1; numbering scheme of Reference [26]). BA24 and BA25 as well as the insular cortex are all key parts of a medial circuit that processes the emotional aspects of pain [27,28]. These structures are overactive in neuropathic pain [29], and have been surgically removed to treat intractable pain [30]. The anterior cingulate also activates with cognitive conflict, e.g., mental errors [31], emphasizing the mental nature of its function. The anterior cingulate projects to nearby premotor areas, e.g., BA6d, to influence motor responses such as eye or hand movements (Figure 1). Information also flows from BA24 and the insular cortex to BA25, which serves as the major visceromotor output for the PFC (Figure 1). BA25 is of particular interest given its overactivity in depression, and is thus a focus of deep brain stimulation treatment [32]. This area has extensive projections to limbic areas such as the amygdala, ventral striatum, and hypothalamus to control emotion and visceral responses [3,33]. This includes projections to hypothalamus and brainstem centers that coordinate the stress response [34], consistent with its activity correlating with increased cortisol release in stressed human subjects (see Table S2 in the Supplement of Reference [35]). BA25 also interconnects with the medial subthalamic nucleus [36], which, if playing a role similar to that in motor circuits, may provide pervasive inhibition relevant to symptoms of "mental paralysis," a hypothesis supported by the antidepressant effects of subthalamic deep brain stimulation [37].

Anatomical tracing studies in monkeys [38] indicate that dlPFC may be able to regulate BA25 through indirect connections via areas BA10m and BA32 (Figure 1A). Human imaging studies suggest these connections may be important in regulating stress and depression, as dlPFC functional connectivity correlates with that of vmPFC BA32 as subjects overcome their response to stress [35], and as activity in this "medial corridor" is related to a sustained anti-depressant response to deep brain stimulation [39]. Furthermore, the antidepressant effects of TMS to strengthen the left dlPFC have been related to its ability to reduce the activity of BA25 [40], supporting the circuit model shown in Figure 1. Conversely, dlPFC and medial PFC deactivate during uncontrollable stress (Figure 1B), as described below. The loss of top-down control by the dlPFC and rostral circuits with stress has been of special interest, as these newly evolved circuits are especially vulnerable in neuropsychiatric disorders. Thus, they have been a focus of neurobiological research.

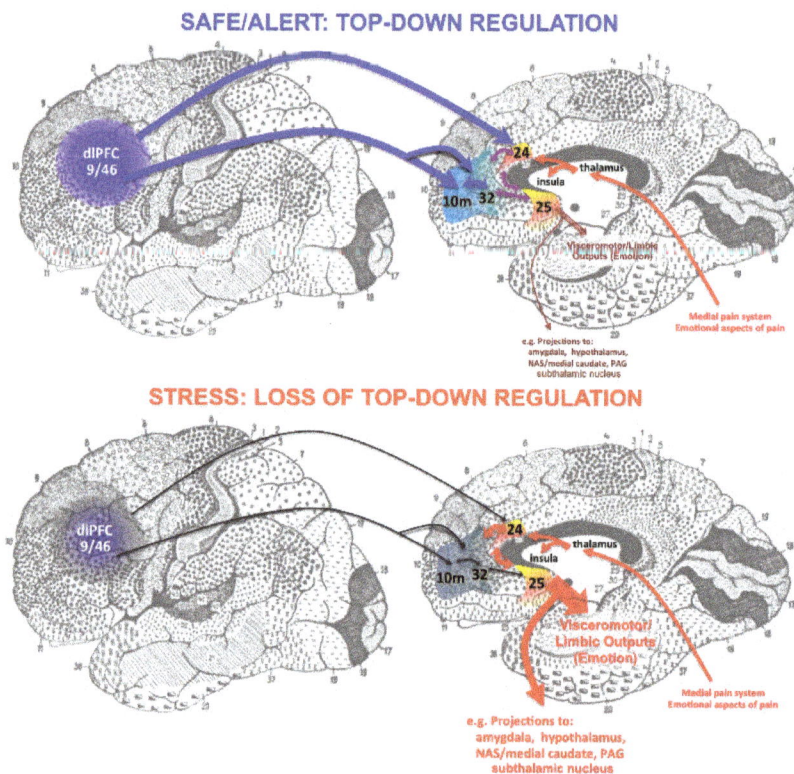

Figure 1. Schematic diagram of prefrontal cortex (PFC) circuits providing top-down regulation of emotion, and the effects of arousal state on connectivity. (**Top**): Under non-stress conditions, newly evolved dorsolateral PFC (dlPFC) and rostral areas (e.g., BA10) project back to anterior (BA24) and subgenual (BA25) cingulate via BA32 to regulate visceromotor output and emotional response. Note that these cingulate areas are part of the pathway that mediates the emotional aspects of the pain response. (**Bottom**): Under conditions of uncontrollable stress, the connectivity of dlPFC and the rostral aspect of medial PFC are weakened, and the top-down suppression of BA25 is diminished, promoting activation of subcortical structures such as the amygdala. Anatomical projections are based on tracing studies in monkeys [38], but are portrayed on a Brodmann drawing of the human brain to facilitate translation to human brain imaging results.

3. The Microcircuitry for Generating Top-Down Goals for Regulating Thought, Action, and Emotion

The work of Goldman-Rakic [41] and of González-Burgos [42,43] has uncovered the microcircuitry in deep layer III of dlPFC that allows the persistent representation of information in the absence of sensory stimulation, the neural basis for top-down control. Tract tracing studies of primate dlPFC in vivo [41] and in slices [42] have shown extensive horizontal connections in deep layer III, the anatomical basis for extensive recurrent excitation. This research showed that the persistent firing of neurons across the delay period in a working memory task arises from the recurrent excitation of pyramidal cells with shared characteristics (Figure 2A). For example, a group of pyramidal cells will continue to fire across the delay epoch after a spatial cue is presented at a location 90° from the fixation point, but not other locations. These neurons are able to continue firing without sensory stimulation due to their recurrent excitatory network connections, as illustrated in Figure 2A. These pyramidal cells excite each other through glutamatergic NMDAR synapses even after the cue has been extinguished, thus maintaining the memory of 90° across the delay period. Conversely, the spatial tuning of neuronal firing is refined by lateral inhibition from parvalbumin-containing GABA interneurons, reducing firing for nonpreferred information [41]. This contrasts with classic circuits in the sensory cortex, where feedforward inhibition rather than lateral inhibition is the rule. Studies of dlPFC slices were able to identify GABAergic basket and chandelier cells inhibiting pyramidal cells to produce lateral inhibition, consistent with the in vivo recordings [43]. These layer III microcircuits have expanded greatly in primate brain evolution [44], and are the neurons most afflicted in schizophrenia, with loss of dendrites and spines from pyramidal cells, and compensatory weakening of GABA interneurons [45]. These pyramidal cells also fill with neurofibrillary tangles and degenerate in Alzheimer's Disease [46]. It is not known whether medial and rostral PFC regions also contain recurrent microcircuits, which would be an important area for future research.

4. The Unique Neurotransmission and Neuromodulation of dlPFC Synapses

The recurrent excitatory synapses on pyramidal cell spines in deep layer III of dlPFC have characteristics that render them especially vulnerable to stress and atrophy, including important roles of calcium signaling (Figure 2B). These characteristics include unusual glutamate neurotransmission and neuromodulatory actions, where cAMP-calcium signaling weakens rather than strengthens network connectivity, e.g., during uncontrollable stress exposure.

Neurotransmission classic glutamatergic circuits, e.g., in V1, rely heavily on AMPA receptor (AMPAR) stimulation, which provides the permissive excitation for NMDA receptor (NMDAR actions during neuroplasticity [47]. These circuits have few NMDAR with NR2B subunits in the adult, although they predominate early in development [48]. In contrast, dlPFC delay cells have only a minor reliance on AMPAR, and are greatly reliant on NMDAR-NR2B, which are found exclusively in the post-synaptic density and not at extra-synaptic locations [49], and are concentrated in pyramidal cell synapses [50]. Layer III reliance on NMDAR is also seen in human dlPFC, where pyramidal cells express a greater NMDAR than AMPAR message, while the converse is true in layer V [51]. Layer III delay cells also do not rely on AMPAR to permit NMDAR actions. Instead this permissive role is played by cholinergic stimulation [52], which occurs during waking but not deep sleep, contributing to conscious cortical activity. The reliance of layer III dlPFC circuits on NMDAR-NR2B is particularly interesting, as these receptors close slowly and allow a large amount of calcium into the post-synaptic spine (schematically shown in Figure 2B), and calcium plays a major neuromodulatory role in determining the strength of these network connections through powerful neuromodulatory actions.

Neuromodulation layer III dlPFC pyramidal cells also have unique neuromodulatory influences, where calcium-cAMP signaling weakens connections by opening potassium (K^+) channels on spines. We have proposed that calcium plays a critical, negative feedback role in these recurrent excitatory circuits where there is little feedback inhibition, and thus may prevent excessive neuronal firing [6]. We see evidence of feedforward calcium-cAMP signaling in spines near K^+ channels that are regulated by calcium itself (e.g., SK channels [53]), or by cAMP-PKA signaling (HCN and KCNQ channels) [6,54,55]. As schematized in Figure 2B, layer III dlPFC spines have extensive smooth endoplasmic reticulum (SER), which stores and releases calcium into the cytosol (the SER is called the spine apparatus where it extends and elaborates in the spine). In layer III of dlPFC, the spine apparatus is the focus of extensive cAMP-signaling machinery [54,56–58], consistent with feedforward calcium-cAMP signaling. Thus, calcium release can drive the production of cAMP, which activates PKA, which drives further calcium release [55]. Feedforward signaling promotes a rapid build-up of calcium-cAMP-PKA activity to open K^+ channels and reduce firing. These detrimental actions are prevented under optimal arousal conditions by NE stimulation of α2A-AR [54] and NAAG/glutamate stimulation of mGluR3 [59]. These receptors are concentrated on layer III dlPFC post-synaptic spines where they inhibit cAMP signaling, close K$^+$ channels, and enhance firing. Under healthy conditions, PKA also activates the phosphodiesterases (e.g., PDE4A) to catabolize cAMP and thus provide brakes on cAMP-calcium signaling after it has been activated. However, this negative feedback is lost with age and with inflammation, as described below.

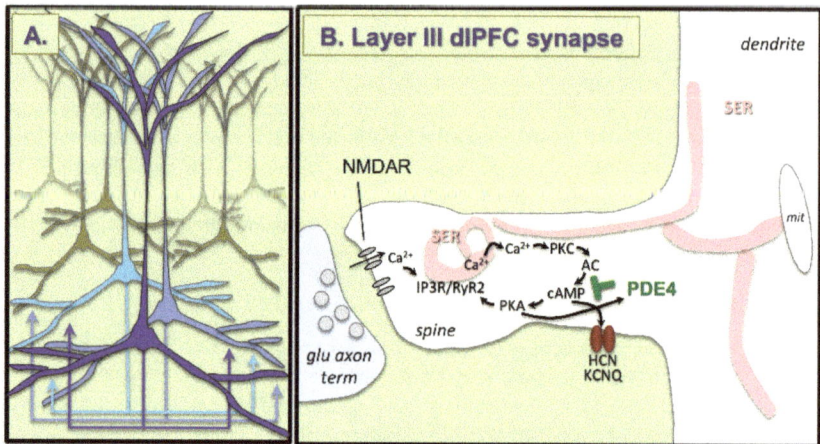

Figure 2. Recurrent excitation in deep layer III of the dlPFC. (**A**) Schematic drawing of clusters of pyramidal cells in deep layer III of dlPFC with shared characteristics that excite each other through extensive recurrent excitatory glutamatergic connections to keep information "in mind" in the absence of sensory stimulation. (**B**) A glutamate synapse on a pyramidal cell spine in deep layer III of dlPFC. These synapses depend on NMDAR stimulation, and have extensive elaboration of the calcium-containing smooth endoplasmic reticulum (SER) "spine apparatus" in the spine, where there is evidence of feedforward calcium-cAMP signaling, which can open HCN and KCNQ channels to reduce firing. This process is held in check by the phosphodiesterases (PDE4), which catabolize cAMP and are anchored to the spine apparatus by DISC1 [56].

5. Stress Rapidly Takes PFC Circuits "Offline"

Even mild uncontrollable stress increases catecholamine release in the PFC to drive feedforward calcium-cAMP-K$^+$ signaling and rapidly take the PFC "off-line." These effects were initially observed in rodent medial PFC, but similar mechanisms have been documented in the primate dlPFC. Due to the early work of Steven Maier, it has long been appreciated that it is the uncontrollable aspect of the stressor that initiates the stress response and leads to cognitive deficits, e.g., Reference [60], and an acute, uncontrollable stress can induce a distracted behavior profile [61]. In contrast, a controllable stressor does not induce dopamine release in the PFC [62]. Biochemical studies documented increased catecholamine release in the rat medial PFC in response to mild uncontrollable stress [63–65]. High levels of dopamine (DA) D1R and norepinephrine (NE) α1-AR stimulation in the PFC impair working memory performance by driving feedforward calcium-cAMP-K$^+$ signaling [66–69], as schematically illustrated in Figure 3. Both α1R (Figure 3A; [70]) and D1R [57,71] have been localized on dendritic spines in layer III of primate dlPFC, and their activation drives feedforward calcium-cAMP signaling (Figure 3B). Thus, stimulation of α1R or D1R reduces the task-related firing of dlPFC neurons in monkeys performing a working memory task, while blockade or closure of HCN channels rescues firing [68–70,72]. These stress signaling pathways may interact with neuroinflammation, which may remove the brakes on the stress response by inhibiting PDE4s, as illustrated in Figure 3B. Specifically, in vitro studies have shown that MK2 inflammatory signaling can inhibit PDE4 regulation of the stress response by un-anchoring PDE4s from their correct location and preventing PKA activation of PDE4 negative feedback on the cAMP-PKA response [73,74]. Similar actions in PFC pyramidal cells would accelerate and prolong the response to uncontrollable stress.

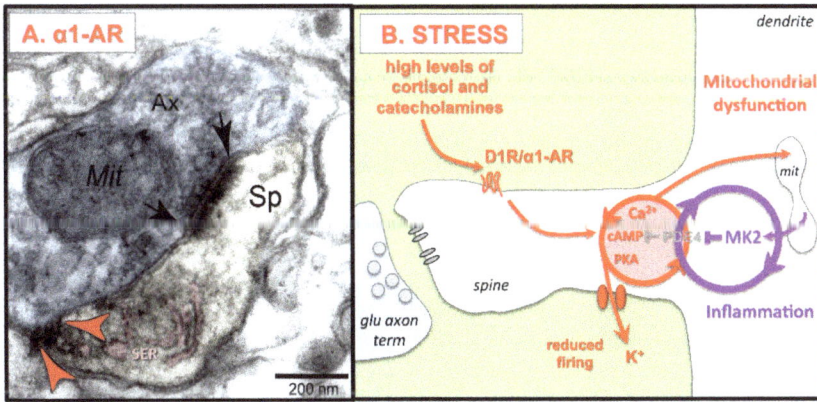

Figure 3. Uncontrollable stress weakens PFC synaptic connectivity through α1-AR and D1R drive of calcium-cAMP-K$^+$ signaling. (**A**) DAB immunolabeling shows that α1-AR (red arrowheads) are localized on dendritic spines in layer III dlPFC near the calcium-containing SER spine apparatus, pseudocolored in pink. The synapse is indicated by black arrows. Sp = spine, Ax = axon terminal, Mit = mitochondrion. Figure 3A adapted from Reference [70]. (**B**) Schematic drawing showing that uncontrollable stress induces cortisol and catecholamine release; high levels of NE and DA activate α1-AR and D1R, which drive feedforward, calcium-cAMP opening of HCN and KCNQ channels to reduce cell firing. With sustained stress exposure, calcium overload of mitochondria may induce inflammatory responses such as MK2 signaling, which inhibits PDE4 and thus removes the "brakes" on stress signaling pathways, ultimately leading to spine loss.

In contrast to the PFC, high levels of catecholamine strengthen the emotional responses of the amygdala and the habitual responding of the striatum [75–77], and can enhance the functioning of the primary sensory cortex [78]. Thus, high levels of catecholamine released during uncontrollable stress switch the brain from a slow, thoughtful, reflective PFC-regulated state to a more reactive, reflexive state that may be advantageous during danger, but would be detrimental when more thoughtful solutions are needed [79].

The detrimental effects of stress-induced catecholamine release are exacerbated by glucocorticoids (cortisol in primates, corticosterone in rodents). Cortisol blocks extraneuronal catecholamine transporters, and thus expands the effects of catecholamines [80]. Corticosterone has been shown to exacerbate the catecholamine response in rat brain, both in impairing PFC working memory [81] and in fortifying the amygdala's enhanced consolidation of emotional memories [82].

Stress-induced PFC dysfunction has now been documented in rats, monkeys, and humans, indicating that this is a highly conserved response. For example, exposure to violent images impairs performance of a working memory task and reduces the activity of the dlPFC in humans [83], and the degree of impairment is related to COMT genotype, with greater catecholamines associated with greater dlPFC dysfunction [84]. Functional brain imaging has also been used to assess the dynamic changes in PFC and cortisol release in response to viewing violent images. This study showed that cortisol release correlated with activation of a caudal region that included BA25, while the suppression of the cortisol response was related to activity in the vmPFC (e.g., BA32), which initially deactivated with stress but reactivated in correlation with coping [35]. Importantly, the reactivation of BA32 correlated with its connectivity with dlPFC, indicating a network of PFC subregions regulating the stress response in humans. It would be helpful to extend this approach to the nonhuman primate, for example to determine the molecular mechanisms governing medial PFC (BA32, BA24, BA25) connectivity and neuronal firing.

6. Architectural Changes with Chronic Stress

Chronic stress exposure leads to additional architectural changes, including spine loss and dendritic atrophy from the medial PFC in rodents, and PFC gray matter loss seen with structural imaging in humans. Dendritic atrophy induced by chronic stress was originally observed in the rat hippocampus [85], but has been found to be even more sensitive in the rat medial PFC [86–90]. Dendritic changes are circuit-specific, where PFC pyramidal cells projecting to entorhinal cortex atrophy with chronic stress, while those projecting to and activating the basolateral amygdala show dendritic expansion [89]. The dendrites of amygdala neurons also expand [91], thus strengthening more primitive emotional circuits in concert with the loss of PFC cortical–cortical connections. Importantly, the loss of spines and dendrites in medial PFC correlates with impaired PFC cognitive functioning on working memory [92,93] and attention-shifting [87] tasks, demonstrating that these architectural changes have great functional relevance. Dendritic integrity is restored with a prolonged period of non-stress following the chronic stress, at least in young animals [94]. Antidepressant treatments also induce spinogenesis in medial PFC [90], and longitudinal in vivo imaging has revealed the retraction and subsequent recovery of spines with antidepressant treatment, (although the return of PFC spines was needed for the long-term maintenance of antidepressant effects on motivated escape behavior but not for their initial induction [95]).

Parallel findings have been seen in human subjects with brain imaging, where exposure to repeated stressors is associated with reduced gray matter in the rostral PFC areas that provide top-down control [96]. Sustained stress also has been shown to induce weaker functional connectivity with the dlPFC that correlates with impaired set-shifting attentional regulation that returns to normal after the stress is over [97]. Reduced functional connectivity with PFC is also seen in human subjects with severe childhood abuse [98]. Thus, there are strong parallels between animal and human studies.

It is important to understand the molecular signaling events that cause loss of PFC connections so that we can develop informed strategies for treatment. The loss of dendritic spines with chronic stress can be prevented by daily treatment with agents such as guanfacine that inhibit PKA signaling [93], or chelerythrine, which inhibits PKC signaling [92]. Sustained high levels of feedforward, calcium-PKC cAMP-PKA signaling may cause dendritic atrophy through a variety of downstream mechanisms. For example, excessive calcium leak from the SER can cause calcium overload of mitochondria, initiating inflammatory cascades, and sustained high levels of PKC activity. High levels of PKC activity can phosphorylate MARCKS (myristoylated alanine-rich C-kinase substrate), which detaches the actin cytoskeleton from the plasma membrane, causing spine collapse [99]. It is also noteworthy that PKC activates GSK3β signaling, and both PKC and GSK3β are inhibited by anti-manic medications that rescue PFC gray matter in patients [100,101]. Interestingly, the rapidly-acting antidepressant, ketamine, induces spine formation through activation of mTOR and inhibition of GSK3β signaling [102]. Thus, this is an exciting arena of current research with immediate clinical relevance.

7. Females Have a Greater Stress Response Than Males

Understanding the molecular basis of the stress response in PFC may help to explain the prominent sex differences in the stress response in animals and humans. Female rats with circulating estrogen have a greater stress response, e.g., due to greater promotion of noradrenergic [103], and dopaminergic [104] actions. A parallel relationship can be seen in humans, where women have reduced expression of COMT [105], and thus less catabolism of catecholamines. Female rats with circulating estrogen have greater stress-induced PFC dysfunction than males (but outperform males when they are ovariectomized) [106,107]. Female rats with circulating estrogen also have a greater architectural response to chronic stress, with increased dendritic expansion in PFC neurons projecting to amygdala [108].

These neurobiological findings may help to explain the increased prevalence of depression and PTSD in women [109–112]. However, cultural factors also likely play an important role, as women are often given less control in society, and are even encouraged to be helpless, factors that would increase the stress response.

8. Increased Susceptibility to Stress-Induced PFC Dysfunction During Adolescence

The neurobiology of stress can also help to explain differences in top-down control over the lifespan. Adolescence is a time of biological susceptibility, for example due to hormonal changes and to pruning of dendritic spines in cortex [113]. Adolescents are especially vulnerable to emotional stress [114,115], with an increased risk of issues such as addiction [116]. Adolescence is also a time of increased DA signaling in the PFC. There is an increased DA innervation of layer III in the macaque dlPFC during adolescence [117,118], and increased expression of D1R on rat prelimbic PFC neurons that project to the nucleus accumbens [119]. Thus, the stress response in PFC may be magnified during adolescence, and may lower the threshold for high-risk behaviors and poor decision-making under emotionally stressful conditions.

9. Increased Vulnerability During Aging Loss of Brakes on Stress Signaling Pathways

The stress response is also magnified with advanced age, due, at least in part, to the loss of regulation at the intracellular and circuit levels. The PFC atrophies with advancing age, with loss of spines from the layer III microcircuits that generate working memory [120]. For example, cortisol levels are higher in elderly individuals, especially in older women [121], and this may involve weaker PFC inhibition of the HPA axis with age. Aging may also alter the stress response through molecular changes. Although there is a decline in PFC DA with advancing age [122], there is also a loss of PDE4 expression from spines, the enzymes that normally catabolize cAMP and hold stress signaling events in check [58]. These data suggest that there may be a higher threshold to activate the stress response in aged individuals, but that once stress signaling is initiated, it would be more prolonged. Increased stress calcium-cAMP signaling in the association cortex may have many consequences that would increase risk of pathology, including mitochondrial abnormalities [123,124], spine loss [120], and phosphorylation of tau [58,125], all of which are seen in layer III of aged monkey dlPFC. Stress is now recognized as a risk factor for late onset AD, with stressful events linked to higher disease onset decades later [126–128]. Indeed, recent evidence shows that increased cortisol is a risk factor for disease [129]. The more prominent stress response in women may also help to explain the increased prevalence of late onset AD in women compared to men [130,131], especially as AD pathology begins decades before disease onset, at a time when estrogen mechanisms could exacerbate the biological response to stress.

10. Successful Translation to Clinical Treatments

Pharmacological manipulations can protect dlPFC connectivity by inhibiting stress-induced calcium-cAMP-K^+ signaling and maintaining synaptic efficacy. It is possible that treatments such as GCPII inhibitors that enhance stimulation of mGluR3 may be helpful in the future. However, two treatments that have been helpful in animals—the α2A-AR agonist guanfacine, and the α1-AR antagonist prazosin—are now in widespread clinical use for treating stress-related disorders.

The α2A-AR agonist, guanfacine, prevents PFC dysfunction caused by either acute [132] or chronic [93] stress, including rescuing spine loss from PFC neurons (Figure 4A). Studies in monkeys have shown that guanfacine acts by inhibiting cAMP-opening of HCN channels on spines (Figure 4B), strengthening connectivity, persistent firing, and working memory abilities [54]. α2A-AR stimulation also has anti-inflammatory actions, e.g., deactivation of microglia [133]. Based on research in animals, extended release guanfacine (Intuniv®, Shire Takada Pharmaceuticals) is now in widespread use for treating ADHD, but is also being used to treat traumatized children [134], including those with oppositional behaviors often arising from maltreatment [135].

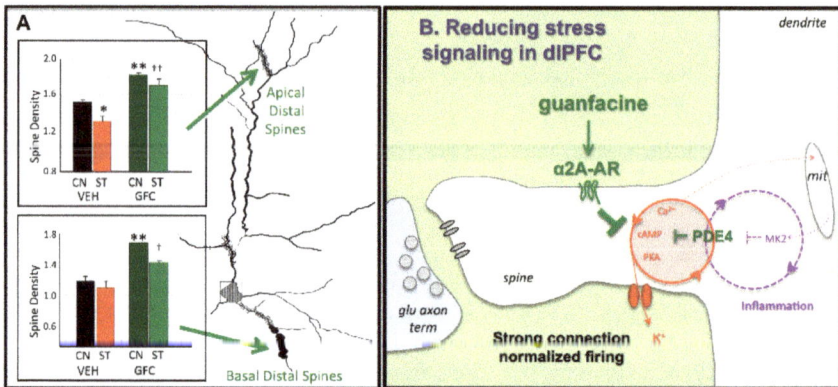

Figure 4. The α2A-AR agonist guanfacine can strengthen PFC connectivity and protect the PFC from stress. (**A**) Chronic restraint stress causes loss of apical distal spines from layer II/III prelimbic PFC pyramidal cells in rats. Daily pre-treatment with guanfacine prevents spine loss and protects working memory function. CN = control, ST = chronic restraint stress, VEH = vehicle, GFC = guanfacine. * or ** significantly different from vehicle control; † or †† significantly different from vehicle stress at $p < 0.05$ or 0.01 levels, respectively. Figure 4A adapted from [93]. (**B**) Schematic diagram showing that guanfacine stimulation of α2A-AR on spines strengthens connectivity and protects PFC from stress by inhibiting cAMP-calcium-K$^+$ channel signaling.

The α1-AR antagonist prazosin is in widespread use for treating PTSD in adults [136]. As described above, stimulation of α1-AR is a key part of stress-induced PFC dysfunction, and also contributes to the strengthening of amygdala during conditions of high NE release. Prazosin has been found to be helpful in treating combat-related PTSD, including daytime hyperarousal symptoms and improving global clinical status [137]. It is noteworthy that the hyperarousal subscale used to rate PTSD symptoms includes many PFC-related deficits (e.g., impaired concentration, impaired regulation of mood and aggression), in addition to alterations in sleep–wakefulness. Another double-blind placebo-controlled study of civilians addressed whether daytime-only prazosin treatment reduced PTSD symptoms during a trauma-relevant stress paradigm that measured PFC-related executive function through use of an emotional version of the Stroop interference task [138]. Prazosin simultaneously reduced subjective stress and improved cognitive performance [138]. High doses of prazosin may also be helpful in the treatment of daytime PTSD symptoms, when levels of NE release are higher [139]. Prazosin may also be helpful in reducing substance abuse, which is common in PTSD. Initial trials suggest that prazosin can reduce cravings for and use of alcohol in patients with PTSD [140], as well as reducing stress-induced craving for alcohol in subjects without PTSD [141].

11. Outstanding Questions and Future Directions

Although there has been remarkable progress in this field, with many similarities bridging across rodent and both nonhuman and human primate species, there are still many outstanding questions. Greater understanding of circuit specific changes with stress exposure is an important arena for future research, but challenging to extend from rodent to primate. The rodent medial PFC represents many primordial features of the PFC, and projections are organized in gradients rather than in discrete subregions [142]. The great expansion of the PFC in primates suggests that these processes elaborate and differentiate in brain evolution, and yet we know very little about the molecular regulation of the primate medial PFC, including the subgenual cingulate BA25 that is powerfully positioned to activate the stress response. Future research may find distinct molecular regulation of PFC subcircuits that may help us target therapies more effectively.

Funding: This work was funded in part by PHS grant AG061190-01 to AFTA, and by an Alzheimer's Association Research Fellowship AARF-17-533294 to DD.

Conflicts of Interest: A.F.T.A. and Yale University receive royalties from the USA sales of nongeneric Intuniv. They do not receive royalties from generic or international sales.

References

1. Goldman-Rakic, P.S. The prefrontal landscape: Implications of functional architecture for understanding human mentation and the central executive. *Phil. Trans. R. Soc. London* **1996**, *351*, 1445–1453.
2. Goldman-Rakic, P.S. Circuitry of the primate prefrontal cortex and the regulation of behavior by representational memory. In *Handbook of Physiology, The Nervous System, Higher Functions of the Brain*; Plum, F., Ed.; American Physiological Society: Bethesda, MD, USA, 1987; pp. 373–417.
3. Ongür, D.; Price, J.L. The organization of networks within the orbital and medial prefrontal cortex of rats, monkeys and humans. *Cereb. Cortex* **2000**, *10*, 206–219. [CrossRef]
4. Ghashghaei, H.T.; Barbas, H. Pathways for emotion: Interactions of prefrontal and anterior temporal pathways in the amygdala of the rhesus monkey. *Neuroscience* **2002**, *115*, 1261–1279. [CrossRef]
5. Barbas, H.; Medalla, M.; Alade, O.; Suski, J.; Zikopoulos, B.; Lera, P. Relationship of prefrontal connections to inhibitory systems in superior temporal areas in the rhesus monkey. *Cereb. Cortex* **2005**, *15*, 1356–1370. [CrossRef]
6. Arnsten, A.F.T.; Wang, M.; Paspalas, C.D. Neuromodulation of thought: Flexibilities and vulnerabilities in prefrontal cortical network synapses. *Neuron* **2012**, *76*, 223–239. [CrossRef] [PubMed]
7. Barbas, H.; Saha, S.; Rempel Clower, N.; Ghashghaei, T. Serial pathways from primate prefrontal cortex to autonomic areas may influence emotional expression. *BMC Neurosci.* **2003**, *4*, 25. [CrossRef] [PubMed]
8. Amodio, D.M.; Frith, C.D. Meeting of minds: The medial frontal cortex and social cognition. *Nat. Rev. Neurosci.* **2006**, *7*, 268–277. [CrossRef] [PubMed]
9. Fuster, J.M.; Alexander, G.E. Neuron activity related to short-term memory. *Science* **1971**, *173*, 652–654. [CrossRef]
10. Funahashi, S.; Bruce, C.J.; Goldman-Rakic, P.S. Mnemonic coding of visual space in the monkey's dorsolateral prefrontal cortex. *J. Neurophysiol.* **1989**, *61*, 331–349. [CrossRef]
11. Funahashi, S.; Chafee, M.V.; Goldman-Rakic, P.S. Prefrontal neuronal activity in rhesus monkeys performing a delayed anti-saccade task. *Nature* **1993**, *365*, 753–756. [CrossRef]
12. Suzuki, M.; Gottlieb, J. Distinct neural mechanisms of distractor suppression in the frontal and parietal lobe. *Nat. Neurosci.* **2013**, *16*, 98–104. [CrossRef]
13. Wallis, J.D.; Anderson, K.C.; Miller, E.K. Single neurons in prefrontal cortex encode abstract rules. *Nature* **2001**, *411*, 953–956. [CrossRef]
14. Kim, S.; Hwang, J.; Lee, D. Prefrontal coding of temporally discounted values during intertemporal choice. *Neuron* **2008**, *59*, 161–172. [CrossRef]
15. Miller, E.K. The prefrontal cortex and cognitive control. *Nat. Rev. Neurosci.* **2000**, *1*, 59–65. [CrossRef] [PubMed]
16. Buschman, T.J.; Miller, E.K. Top-down versus bottom-up control of attention in the prefrontal and posterior parietal cortices. *Science* **2007**, *315*, 1860–1862. [CrossRef]
17. Sun, Y.; Yang, Y.; Galvin, V.C.; Yang, S.; Arnsten, A.F.; Wang, M. Nicotinic α4β2 cholinergic receptor influences on dorsolateral prefrontal cortical neuronal firing during a working memory task. *J. Neurosci.* **2017**, *37*, 5366–5377. [CrossRef]
18. Lee, D.; Seo, H. Neural Basis of Strategic Decision Making. *Trends Neurosci.* **2016**, *39*, 40–48. [CrossRef]
19. Tsujimoto, S.; Genovesio, A.; Wise, S.P. Evaluating self-generated decisions in frontal pole cortex of monkeys. *Nat. Neurosci.* **2010**, *13*, 120–126. [CrossRef] [PubMed]
20. Tsujimoto, S.; Genovesio, A.; Wise, S.P. Frontal pole cortex: Encoding ends at the end of the endbrain. *Trends Cogn. Sci.* **2011**, *15*, 169–176. [CrossRef]
21. Szczepanski, S.M.; Knight, R.T. Insights into human behavior from lesions to the prefrontal cortex. *Neuron* **2014**, *83*, 1002–1018. [CrossRef]
22. Rolls, E.T. The orbitofrontal cortex and reward. *Cereb. Cortex* **2000**, *10*, 284–294. [CrossRef]

23. Wallis, J.D.; Miller, E.K. Neuronal activity in primate dorsolateral and orbital prefrontal cortex during performance of a reward preference task. *Eur. J. Neurosci.* **2003**, *18*, 2069–2081. [CrossRef] [PubMed]

24. Bouret, S.; Richmond, B.J. Ventromedial and orbital prefrontal neurons differentially encode internally and externally driven motivational values in monkeys. *J. Neurosci.* **2010**, *30*, 8591–8601. [CrossRef]

25. Rudebeck, P.H.; Saunders, R.C.; Lundgren, D.A.; Murray, E.A. Specialized Representations of Value in the Orbital and Ventrolateral Prefrontal Cortex: Desirability versus Availability of Outcomes. *Neuron* **2017**, *95*, 1208–1220. [CrossRef]

26. Ongür, D.; Ferry, A.; Price, J.L. Architectonic subdivision of the human orbital and medial prefrontal cortex. *J. Comp. Neurol.* **2003**, *460*, 425–449. [CrossRef] [PubMed]

27. Vogt, B.A.; Sikes, R.W. The medial pain system, cingulate cortex, and parallel processing of nociceptive information. *Prog. Brain Res.* **2000**, *22*, 223–235.

28. Bushnell, M.C.; Ceko, M.; Low, L.A. Cognitive and emotional control of pain and its disruption in chronic pain. *Nat. Rev. Neurosci.* **2013**, *14*, 502–511. [CrossRef]

29. Jaggi, A.S.; Singh, N. Role of different brain areas in peripheral nerve injury-induced neuropathic pain. *Brain Res.* **2011**, *1381*, 187–201. [CrossRef] [PubMed]

30. Viswanathan, A.; Harsh, V.; Pereira, E.A.; Aziz, T.Z. Cingulotomy for medically refractory cancer pain. *Neurosurg. Focus.* **2013**, *35*, E1. [CrossRef] [PubMed]

31. Van Veen, V.; Carter, C.S. The anterior cingulate as a conflict monitor: fMRI and ERP studies. *Physiol. Behav.* **2002**, *77*, 477–482. [CrossRef]

32. Mayberg, H.S.; Lozano, A.M.; Voon, V.; McNeely, H.E.; Seminowicz, D.; Hamani, C.; Schwalb, J.M.; Kennedy, S.H. Deep brain stimulation for treatment-resistant depression. *Neuron* **2005**, *45*, 651–660. [CrossRef] [PubMed]

33. Neafsey, E.J. Prefrontal control of the autonomic nervous system: Anatomical and physiological observations. *Prog. Brain Res.* **1990**, *85*, 147–165.

34. An, X.; Bandler, R.; Ongür, D.; Price, J.L. Prefrontal cortical projections to longitudinal columns in the midbrain periaqueductal gray in macaque monkeys. *J. Comp. Neurol.* **1998**, *401*, 455–479. [CrossRef]

35. Sinha, R.; Lacadie, C.M.; Constable, R.T.; Seo, D. Dynamic neural activity during stress signals resilient coping. *Proc. Natl. Acad. Sci. USA* **2016**, *113*, 8837–8842. [CrossRef] [PubMed]

36. Haynes, W.I.; Haber, S.N. The organization of prefrontal-subthalamic inputs in primates provides an anatomical substrate for both functional specificity and integration: Implications for Basal Ganglia models and deep brain stimulation. *J. Neurosci.* **2013**, *33*, 4804–4814. [CrossRef]

37. Birchall, E.L.; Walker, H.C.; Cutter, G.; Guthrie, S.; Joop, A.; Memon, R.A.; Watts, R.L.; Standaert, D.G.; Amara, A.W. The effect of unilateral subthalamic nucleus deep brain stimulation on depression in Parkinson's disease. *Brain Stimul.* **2017**, *10*, 651–656. [CrossRef]

38. Barbas, H.; Pandya, D.N. Architecture and intrinsic connections of the prefrontal cortex in the rhesus monkey. *J. Comp. Neurol.* **1989**, *286*, 353–375. [CrossRef]

39. Riva-Posse, P.; Choi, K.S.; Holtzheimer, P.E.; McIntyre, C.C.; Gross, R.E.; Chaturvedi, A.; Crowell, A.L.; Garlow, S.J.; Rajendra, J.K.; Mayberg, H.S. Defining Critical White Matter Pathways Mediating Successful Subcallosal Cingulate Deep Brain Stimulation for Treatment-Resistant Depression. *Biol. Psychiatry* **2014**, *76*, 963–969. [CrossRef]

40. Fox, M.D.; Buckner, R.L.; White, M.P.; Greicius, M.D.; Pascual-Leone, A. Efficacy of transcranial magnetic stimulation targets for depression is related to intrinsic functional connectivity with the subgenual cingulate. *Biol. Psychiatry* **2012**, *72*, 595–603. [CrossRef]

41. Goldman-Rakic, P.S. Cellular basis of working memory. *Neuron* **1995**, *14*, 477–485. [CrossRef]

42. González-Burgos, G.; Barrionuevo, G.; Lewis, D.A. Horizontal synaptic connections in monkey prefrontal cortex: An in vitro electrophysiological study. *Cereb. Cortex* **2000**, *10*, 82–92. [CrossRef] [PubMed]

43. González-Burgos, G.; Krimer, L.S.; Povysheva, N.V.; Barrionuevo, G.; Lewis, D.A. Functional properties of fast spiking interneurons and their synaptic connections with pyramidal cells in primate dorsolateral prefrontal cortex. *J. Neurophysiol.* **2005**, *93*, 942–953. [CrossRef]

44. Elston, G.N.; Benavides-Piccione, R.; Elston, A.; Zietsch, B.; Defelipe, J.; Manger, P.; Casagrande, V.; Kaas, J.H. Specializations of the granular prefrontal cortex of primates: Implications for cognitive processing. *Anat Rec. A Discov. Mol. Cell Evol. Biol.* **2006**, *288*, 26–35. [CrossRef] [PubMed]

45. Glausier, J.R.; Lewis, D.A. Mapping pathologic circuitry in schizophrenia. *Handb. Clin. Neurol.* **2018**, *150*, 389–417.

46. Bussière, T.; Giannakopoulos, P.; Bouras, C.; Perl, D.P.; Morrison, J.H.; Hof, P.R. Progressive degeneration of nonphosphorylated neurofilament protein-enriched pyramidal neurons predicts cognitive impairment in Alzheimer's disease: Stereologic analysis of prefrontal cortex area 9. *J. Comp. Neurol.* **2003**, *463*, 281–302. [CrossRef]

47. Yang, S.T.; Wang, M.; Paspalas, C.P.; Crimins, J.L.; Altman, M.T.; Mazer, J.A.; Arnsten, A.F. Core differences in synaptic signaling between primary visual and dorsolateral prefrontal cortex. *Cereb. Cortex* **2018**, *28*, 1458–1471. [CrossRef]

48. Liu, X.B.; Murray, K.D.; Jones, E.G. Switching of NMDA receptor 2A and 2B subunits at thalamic and cortical synapses during early postnatal development. *J. Neurosci.* **2004**, *24*, 8885–8895. [CrossRef]

49. Wang, M.; Yang, Y.; Wang, C.J.; Gamo, N.J.; Jin, L.E.; Mazer, J.A.; Morrison, J.H.; Wang, X.-J.; Arnsten, A.F. NMDA receptors subserve working memory persistent neuronal firing In dorsolateral prefrontal cortex. *Neuron* **2013**, *77*, 736–749. [CrossRef]

50. Rotaru, D.C.; Yoshino, H.; Lewis, D.A.; Ermentrout, G.B.; Gonzalez-Burgos, G. Glutamate receptor subtypes mediating synaptic activation of prefrontal cortex neurons: Relevance for schizophrenia. *J. Neurosci.* **2011**, *31*, 142–156. [CrossRef] [PubMed]

51. Datta, D.; Arion, D.; Lewis, D.A. Developmental Expression Patterns of GABAA Receptor Subunits in Layer 3 and 5 Pyramidal Cells of Monkey Prefrontal Cortex. *Cereb. Cortex* **2014**, *25*, 2295–2305. [CrossRef]

52. Yang, Y.; Paspalas, C.D.; Jin, L.E.; Picciotto, M.R.; Arnsten, A.F.T.; Wang, M. Nicotinic α7 receptors enhance NMDA cognitive circuits in dorsolateral prefrontal cortex. *Proc. Nat. Acad. Sci. USA* **2013**, *110*, 12078–12083. [CrossRef] [PubMed]

53. Brennan, A.R.; Dolinsky, B.; Vu, M.A.; Stanley, M.; Yeckel, M.F.; Arnsten, A.F. Blockade of IP3-mediated SK channel signaling in the rat medial prefrontal cortex improves spatial working memory. *Learn. Mem.* **2008**, *15*, 93–96. [CrossRef]

54. Wang, M.; Ramos, B.; Paspalas, C.; Shu, Y.; Simen, A.; Duque, A.; Vijayraghavan, S.; Brennan, A.; Dudley, A.G.; Nou, E.; et al. Alpha2A-adrenoceptor stimulation strengthens working memory networks by inhibiting cAMP-HCN channel signaling in prefrontal cortex. *Cell* **2007**, *129*, 397–410. [CrossRef]

55. Arnsten, A.F. Stress weakens prefrontal networks: Molecular insults to higher cognition. *Nat. Neurosci.* **2015**, *18*, 1376–1385. [CrossRef]

56. Paspalas, C.D.; Min Wang, M.; Arnsten, A.F.T. Constellation of HCN Channels and cAMP regulating proteins in dendritic spines of the primate prefrontal cortex–Potential substrate for working memory deficits in schizophrenia. *Cereb. Cortex* **2013**, *23*, 1643–1654. [CrossRef]

57. Arnsten, A.F.T.; Wang, M.; Paspalas, C.D. Dopamine's actions in primate prefrontal cortex: Challenges for treating cognitive disorders. *Pharmacological Rev.* **2015**, *67*, 681–696. [CrossRef]

58. Carlyle, B.C.; Nairn, A.C.; Wang, M.; Yang, Y.; Jin, L.E.; Simen, A.A.; Ramos, B.P.; Bordner, K.A.; Craft, G.E.; Davies, P.; et al. cAMP-PKA phosphorylation of tau confers risk for degeneration in aging association cortex. *Proc. Natl. Acad. Sci. USA* **2014**, *111*, 5036–5041. [CrossRef] [PubMed]

59. Jin, L.E.; Wang, M.; Galvin, V.C.; Lightbourne, T.C.; Conn, P.J.; Arnsten, A.F.T.; Paspalas, C.D. mGluR2 vs. mGluR3 in Primate Prefrontal Cortex: Postsynaptic mGluR3 Strengthen Cognitive Networks. *Cereb. Cortex* **2018**, *28*, 974–987. [CrossRef]

60. Minor, T.R.; Jackson, R.L.; Maier, S.F. Effects of task-irrelevant cues and reinforcement delay on choice-escape learning following inescapable shock: Evidence for a deficit in selective attention. *J. Exp. Psychol. Anim. Behav. Process.* **1984**, *10*, 543–556. [CrossRef] [PubMed]

61. Arnsten, A.F.; Berridge, C.W.; Segal, D.S. Stress produces opioid-like effects on investigatory behavior. *Pharmacol Biochem Behav.* **1985**, *22*, 803–809. [CrossRef]

62. Bland, S.T.; Hargrave, D.; Pepin, J.L.; Amat, J.; Watkins, L.R.; Maier, S.F. Stressor controllability modulates stress-induced dopamine and serotonin efflux and morphine-induced serotonin efflux in the medial prefrontal cortex. *Neuropsychopharmacology* **2003**, *28*, 1589–1596. [CrossRef] [PubMed]

63. Deutch, A.Y.; Roth, R.H. The determinants of stress-induced activation of the prefrontal cortical dopamine system. *Prog. Brain Res.* **1990**, *85*, 367–403.

64. Finlay, J.M.; Zigmond, M.J.; Abercrombie, E.D. Increased dopamine and norepinephrine release in medial prefrontal cortex induced by acute and chronic stress: Effects of diazepam. *Neuroscience* **1995**, *64*, 619–628. [CrossRef]

65. Goldstein, L.E.; Rasmusson, A.M.; Bunney, S.B.; Roth, R.H. Role of the amygdala in the coordination of behavioral, neuroendocrine and prefrontal cortical monoamine responses to psychological stress in the rat. *J. Neurosci.* **1996**, *16*, 4787–4798. [CrossRef] [PubMed]

66. Murphy, B.L.; Arnsten, A.F.T.; Goldman-Rakic, P.S.; Roth, R.H. Increased dopamine turnover in the prefrontal cortex impairs spatial working memory performance in rats and monkeys. *Proc. Nat. Acad. Sci. U.S.A.* **1996**, *93*, 1325–1329. [CrossRef]

67. Birnbaum, S.G.; Gobeske, K.T.; Auerbach, J.; Taylor, J.R.; Arnsten, A.F.T. A role for norepinephrine in stress-induced cognitive deficits: Alpha-1-adrenoceptor mediation in prefrontal cortex. *Biol. Psychiatry* **1999**, *46*, 1266–1274. [CrossRef]

68. Birnbaum, S.B.; Yuan, P.; Wang, M.; Vijayraghavan, S.; Bloom, A.; Davis, D.; Gobeske, K.; Sweatt, D.; Manji, H.K.; Arnsten, A.F.T. Protein kinase C overactivity impairs prefrontal cortical regulation of working memory. *Science* **2004**, *306*, 882–884. [CrossRef]

69. Gamo, N.J.; Lur, G.; Higley, M.J.; Wang, M.; Paspalas, C.D.; Vijayraghavan, S.; Yang, Y.; Ramos, B.P.; Peng, K.; Kata, A.; et al. Stress impairs prefrontal cortical function via D1 dopamine receptor interactions with HCN channels. *Biol. Psychiatry* **2015**, *78*, 860–870. [CrossRef]

70. Datta, D.; Yang, S.T.; Galvin, V.C.; Solder, J.; Luo, F.; Morozov, Y.M.; Arellano, J.; Duque, A.; Rakic, P.; Arnsten, A.F.T.; et al. Noradrenergic α1-Adrenoceptor Actions in the Primate Dorsolateral Prefrontal Cortex. *J. Neurosci.* **2019**, *39*, 2722–2734. [CrossRef] [PubMed]

71. Smiley, J.F.; Levey, A.I.; Ciliax, B.J.; Goldman-Rakic, P.S. D1 dopamine receptor immunoreactivity in human and monkey cerebral cortex: Predominant and extrasynaptic localization in dendritic spines. *Proc. Natl. Acad. Sci. USA* **1994**, *91*, 5720–5724. [CrossRef]

72. Vijayraghavan, S.; Wang, M.; Birnbaum, S.G.; Bruce, C.J.; Williams, G.V.; Arnsten, A.F.T. Inverted-U dopamine D1 receptor actions on prefrontal neurons engaged in working memory. *Nat. Neurosci.* **2007**, *10*, 376–384. [CrossRef]

73. MacKenzie, K.F.; Wallace, D.A.; Hill, E.V.; Anthony, D.F.; Henderson, D.J.; Houslay, D.M.; Arthur, J.S.; Baillie, G.S.; Houslay, M.D. Phosphorylation of cAMP-specific PDE4A5 (phosphodiesterase-4A5) by MK2 (MAPKAPK2) attenuates its activation through protein kinase A phosphorylation. *Biochem. J.* **2011**, *435*, 755–769. [CrossRef]

74. Houslay, K.F.; Christian, F.; MacLeod, R.; Adams, D.R.; Houslay, M.D.; Baillie, G.S. Identification of a multifunctional docking site on the catalytic unit of phosphodiesterase-4 (PDE4) that is utilised by multiple interaction partners. *Biochem. J.* **2017**, *474*, 597–609. [CrossRef]

75. Cahill, L.; McGaugh, J.L. Modulation of memory storage. *Curr. Opin. Neurobiol.* **1996**, *6*, 237–242. [CrossRef]

76. Packard, M.G.; Teather, L.A. Amygdala modulation of multiple memory systems: Hippocampus and caudate-putamen. *Neurobiol. Learning Mem.* **1998**, *69*, 163–203. [CrossRef]

77. Ferry, B.; Roozendaal, B.; McGaugh, J.L. Basolateral amygdala noradrenergic influences on memory storage are mediated by an interaction between beta- and alpha-1-adrenoceptors. *J. Neurosci.* **1999**, *19*, 5119–5123. [CrossRef]

78. Waterhouse, B.D.; Moises, H.C.; Woodward, D.J. Alpha-receptor-mediated facilitation of somatosensory cortical neuronal responses to excitatory synaptic inputs and iontophoretically applied acetylcholine. *Neuropharmacology* **1981**, *20*, 907–920. [CrossRef]

79. Arnsten, A.F.T. Stress signaling pathways that impair prefrontal cortex structure and function. *Nature Reviews Neuroscience* **2009**, *10*, 410–422. [CrossRef]

80. Grundemann, D.; Schechinger, B.; Rappold, G.A.; Schomig, E. Molecular identification of the cortisone-sensitive extraneuronal catecholamine transporter. *Nat. Neurosci.* **1998**, *1*, 349–351. [CrossRef]

81. Barsegyan, A.; Mackenzie, S.M.; Kurose, B.D.; McGaugh, J.L.; Roozendaal, B. Glucocorticoids in the prefrontal cortex enhance memory consolidation and impair working memory by a common neural mechanism. *Proc. Natl. Acad. Sci. USA* **2010**, *107*, 16655–16660. [CrossRef]

82. Roozendaal, B.; Quirarte, G.L.; McGaugh, J.L. Glucocorticoids interact with the basolateral amygdala beta-adrenoceptor-cAMP/cAMP/PKA system in influencing memory consolidation. *Eur. J. Neurosci.* **2002**, *15*, 553–560. [CrossRef]

83. Qin, S.; Hermans, E.J.; Van Marle, H.J.F.; Lou, J.; Fernandez, G. Acute psychological stress reduces working memory-related activity in the dorsolateral prefrontal cortex. *Biol. Psychiatry* **2009**, *66*, 25–32. [CrossRef] [PubMed]

84. Qin, S.; Cousijn, H.; Rijpkema, M.; Luo, J.; Franke, B.; Hermans, E.J.; Fernández, G. The effect of moderate acute psychological stress on working memory-related neural activity is modulated by a genetic variation in catecholaminergic function in humans. *Front. Integr. Neurosci.* **2012**, *6*, 16. [CrossRef] [PubMed]

85. Magariños, A.M.; McEwen, B.S. Stress-induced atrophy of apical dendrites of hippocampal CA3c neurons: Comparison of stressors. *Neuroscience* **1995**, *69*, 83–88. [CrossRef]

86. Izquierdo, A.; Wellman, C.L.; Holmes, A. Brief uncontrollable stress causes dendritic retraction in infralimbic cortex and resistance to fear extinction in mice. *J. Neurosci.* **2006**, *26*, 5733–5738. [CrossRef]

87. Liston, C.; Miller, M.M.; Goldwater, D.S.; Radley, J.J.; Rocher, A.B.; Hof, P.R.; Morrison, J.H.; McEwen, B.S. Stress-induced alterations in prefrontal cortical dendritic morphology predict selective impairments in perceptual attentional set-shifting. *J. Neurosci.* **2006**, *26*, 7870–7874. [CrossRef]

88. Radley, J.J.; Rocher, A.B.; Miller, M.; Janssen, W.G.; Liston, C.; Hof, P.R.; McEwen, B.S.; Morrison, J.H. Repeated stress induces dendritic spine loss in the rat medial prefrontal cortex. *Cereb. Cortex* **2006**, *16*, 313–320. [CrossRef] [PubMed]

89. Shansky, R.M.; Hamo, C.; Hof, P.R.; McEwen, B.S.; Morrison, J.H. Stress-induced dendritic remodeling in the prefrontal cortex is circuit specific. *Cereb. Cortex* **2009**, *106*, 17957–17962. [CrossRef]

90. Licznerski, P.; Duman, R.S. Remodeling of axo-spinous synapses in the pathophysiology and treatment of depression. *Neuroscience* **2013**, *251*, 33–50. [CrossRef]

91. Vyas, A.; Mitra, R.; Shankaranarayana Rao, B.S.; Chattarji, S. Chronic stress induces contrasting patterns of dendritic remodeling in hippocampal and amygdaloid neurons. *J. Neurosci.* **2002**, *22*, 6810–6818. [CrossRef]

92. Hains, A.B.; Vu, M.A.; Maciejewski, P.K.; Van Dyck, C.H.; Gottron, M.; Arnsten, A.F. Inhibition of protein kinase C signaling protects prefrontal cortex dendritic spines and cognition from the effects of chronic stress. *Proc. Natl. Acad. Sci. USA* **2009**, *106*, 17957–17962. [CrossRef]

93. Hains, A.B.; Yabe, Y.; Arnsten, A.F.T. Chronic stimulation of alpha-2A-adrenoceptors with guanfacine protects rodent prefrontal cortex dendritic spines and cognition from the effects of chronic stress. *Neurobiol. Stress* **2015**, *2*, 1–9. [CrossRef]

94. Bloss, E.B.; Janssen, W.G.; Ohm, D.T.; Yuk, F.J.; Wadsworth, S.; Saardi, K.M.; McEwen, B.S.; Morrison, J.H. Evidence for reduced experience-dependent dendritic spine plasticity in the aging prefrontal cortex. *J. Neurosci.* **2011**, *31*, 7831–7839. [CrossRef]

95. Moda-Sava, R.N.; Murdock, M.H.; Parekh, P.K.; Fetcho, R.N.; Huang, B.S.; Huynh, T.N.; Witztum, J.; Shaver, D.C.; Rosenthal, D.L.; Always, E.J.; et al. Sustained rescue of prefrontal circuit dysfunction by antidepressant-induced spine formation. *Science* **2019**, *364*. [CrossRef]

96. Ansell, E.B.; Rando, K.; Tuit, K.; Guarnaccia, J.; Sinha, R. Cumulative adversity and smaller gray matter volume in medial prefrontal, anterior cingulate, and insula regions. *Biol. Psychiatry* **2012**, *72*, 57–64. [CrossRef] [PubMed]

97. Liston, C.; McEwen, B.S.; Casey, B.J. Psychosocial stress reversibly disrupts prefrontal processing and attentional control. *Proc. Nat. Acad. Sci. USA* **2009**, *106*, 912–917. [CrossRef] [PubMed]

98. Hart, H.; Lim, L.; Mehta, M.A.; Chatzieffraimidou, A.; Curtis, C.; Xu, X.; Breen, G.; Simmons, A.; Mirza, K.; Rubia, K. Reduced functional connectivity of fronto-parietal sustained attention networks in severe childhood abuse. *PLoS ONE* **2017**, *12*, e0188744. [CrossRef]

99. Calabrese, B.; Halpain, S. Essential role for the PKC target MARCKS in maintaining dendritic spine morphology. *Neuron* **2005**, *48*, 77–90. [CrossRef] [PubMed]

100. Manji, H.K.; Lenox, R.H. Signaling: Cellular insights into the pathophysiology of bipolar disorder. *Biol. Psychiatry* **2000**, *48*, 518–530. [CrossRef]

101. Moore, G.J.; Bebchuk, J.M.; Wilds, I.B.; Chen, G.; Manji, H.K. Lithium-induced increase in human brain gray matter. *The Lancet* **2000**, *356*, 1241–1242. [CrossRef]

102. Liu, R.J.; Fuchikami, M.; Dwyer, J.M.; Lepack, A.E.; Duman, R.S.; Aghajanian, G.K. GSK-3 inhibition potentiates the synaptogenic and antidepressant-like effects of subthreshold doses of ketamine. *Neuropsychopharmacology.* **2013**, *38*, 2268–2277. [CrossRef]

103. Bangasser, D.A.; Valentino, R.J. Sex differences in molecular and cellular substrates of stress. *Cell Mol. Neurobiol.* **2012**, *32*, 709–723. [CrossRef]

104. Küppers, E.; Ivanova, T.; Karolczak, M.; Beyer, C. Estrogen: A multifunctional messenger to nigrostriatal dopaminergic neurons. *J. Neurocytol.* **2000**, *29*, 375–385. [CrossRef]
105. Tunbridge, E.M. The catechol-O-methyltransferase gene: Its regulation and polymorphisms. *Int. Rev. Neurobiol.* **2010**, *95*, 7–27.
106. Shansky, R.M.; Glavis-Bloom, C.; Lerman, D.; McRae, P.; Benson, C.; Miller, K.; Cosand, L.; Horvath, T.L.; Arnsten, A.F.T. Estrogen mediates sex differences in stress-induced prefrontal cortex dysfunction. *Mol. Psychiatry* **2004**, *9*, 531–538. [CrossRef]
107. Shansky, R.M.; Rubinow, K.; Brennan, A.; Arnsten, A.F. The effects of sex and hormonal status on restraint-stress-induced working memory impairment. *Behav. Brain Funct.* **2006**, *2*, 8. [CrossRef]
108. Shansky, R.M.; Hamo, C.; Hof, P.R.; Lou, W.; McEwen, B.S.; Morrison, J.H. Estrogen promotes stress sensitivity in a prefrontal cortex-amygdala pathway. *Cereb. Cortex* **2010**, *20*, 2560–2567. [CrossRef]
109. Weiss, E.L.; Longhurst, J.G.; Mazure, C.M. Childhood sexual abuse as a risk factor for depression in women: Psychosocial and neurobiological correlates. *Am. J. Psychiatry* **1999**, *156*, 816–828. [CrossRef]
110. Bebbington, P.; Dunn, G.; Jenkins, R.; Lewis, G.; Brugha, T.; Farrell, M.; Meltzer, H. The influence of age and sex on the prevalence of depressive conditions: Report from the National Survey of Psychiatric Morbidity. *Int. Rev. Psychiatry.* **2003**, *15*, 74–83. [CrossRef]
111. Breslau, N. The epidemiology of trauma, PTSD, and other posttrauma disorders. *Trauma Violence Abuse* **2009**, *10*, 198–210. [CrossRef]
112. Johnson, D.P.; Whisman, M.A. Gender differences in rumination: A meta-analysis. *Pers. Individ. Dif.* **2013**, *55*, 367–374. [CrossRef]
113. Arnsten, A.F.; Shansky, R.M. Adolescence: Vulnerable period for stress-induced prefrontal cortical function? Introduction to part IV. *Ann. N.Y. Acad. Sci.* **2004**, *1021*, 143–147. [CrossRef]
114. Duckworth, A.L.; Kim, B.; Tsukayama, E. Life stress impairs self-control in early adolescence. *Front. Psychol.* **2012**, *3*, 608. [CrossRef]
115. Hanson, J.L.; Chung, M.K.; Avants, B.B.; Rudolph, K.D.; Shirtcliff, E.A.; Gee, J.C.; Davidson, R.J.; Pollak, S.D. Structural variations in prefrontal cortex mediate the relationship between early childhood stress and spatial working memory. *J. Neurosci.* **2012**, *32*, 7917–7925. [CrossRef]
116. Hammond, C.J.; Mayes, L.C.; Potenza, M.N. Neurobiology of Adolescent Substance Use and Addictive Behaviors: Prevention and Treatment Implications. *Adolesc. Med. State Art Rev.* **2014**, *25*, 15–32.
117. Rosenberg, D.R.; Lewis, D.A. Changes in the dopaminergic innervation of monkey prefrontal cortex during late postnatal development: A tyosine hydroxylase immunohistochemical study. *Biol. Psychiat.* **1994**, *36*, 272–277. [CrossRef]
118. Rosenberg, D.R.; Lewis, D.A. Postnatal maturation of the dopaminergic innervation of monkey prefrontal cortices: A tyrosine hydroxylase immunohistochemical analysis. *J. Comp. Neurol.* **1995**, *358*, 383–400. [CrossRef]
119. Brenhouse, H.C.; Sonntag, K.C.; Andersen, S.L. Transient D1 dopamine receptor expression on prefrontal cortex projection neurons: Relationship to enhanced motivational salience of drug cues in adolescence. *J. Neurosci.* **2008**, *28*, 2375–2382. [CrossRef]
120. Morrison, J.H.; Baxter, M.G. The ageing cortical synapse: Hallmarks and implications for cognitive decline. *Nat. Rev. Neurosci.* **2012**, *13*, 240–250. [CrossRef]
121. Otte, C.; Hart, S.; Neylan, T.C.; Marmar, C.R.; Yaffe, K.; Mohr, D.C. A meta-analysis of cortisol response to challenge in human aging: Importance of gender. *Psychoneuroendocrinology* **2005**, *30*, 80–91. [CrossRef]
122. Goldman-Rakic, P.S.; Brown, R.M. Regional changes of monoamines in cerebral cortex and subcortical structures of aging rhesus monkeys. *Neuroscience* **1981**, *6*, 177–187. [CrossRef]
123. Hara, Y.; Yuk, F.; Puri, R.; Janssen, W.G.; Rapp, P.R.; Morrison, J.H. Presynaptic mitochondrial morphology in monkey prefrontal cortex correlates with working memory and is improved with estrogen treatment. *Proc. Natl. Acad. Sci. USA* **2014**, *111*, 486–491. [CrossRef]
124. Morozov, Y.M.; Datta, D.; Paspalas, C.D.; Arnsten, A.F. Ultrastructural evidence for impaired mitochondrial fission in the aged rhesus monkey dorsolateral prefrontal cortex. *Neurobiol. Aging* **2017**, *51*, 9–18. [CrossRef]
125. Paspalas, C.D.; Carlyle, B.; Leslie, S.; Preuss, T.M.; Crimins, J.L.; Huttner, A.J.; Van Dyck, C.H.; Rosene, D.L.; Nairn, A.C.; Arnsten, A.F.T. The aged rhesus macaque manifests Braak-stage III/IV Alzheimer's-like pathology. *Alzheimer's Dementia* **2018**, *14*, 680–691. [CrossRef]

126. Johansson, L.; Guo, X.; Hällström, T.; Norton, M.C.; Waern, M.; Ostling, S.; Bengtsson, C.; Skoog, I. Common psychosocial stressors in middle-aged women related to longstanding distress and increased risk of Alzheimer's disease: A 38-year longitudinal population study. *BMJ Open* **2013**, *3*, e003142. [CrossRef]

127. Johansson, L.; Guo, X.; Duberstein, P.R.; Hällström, T.; Waern, M.; Ostling, S.; Skoog, I. Midlife personality and risk of Alzheimer disease and distress: A 38-year follow-up. *Neurology* **2014**, *83*, 1538–1544. [CrossRef]

128. Flatt, J.D.; Gilsanz, P.; Quesenberry, C.P.J.; Albers, K.B.; Whitmer, R.A. Post-traumatic stress disorder and risk of dementia among members of a health care delivery system. *Alzheimers Dement.* **2018**, *14*, 28–34. [CrossRef]

129. Ennis, G.E.; An, Y.; Resnick, S.M.; Ferrucci, L.; O'Brien, R.J.; Moffat, S.D. Long-term cortisol measures predict Alzheimer disease risk. *Neurology* **2017**, *88*, 371–378. [CrossRef]

130. Altmann, A.; Tian, L.; Henderson, V.W.; Greicius, M.D.; Alzheimer's Disease Neuroimaging Initiative Investigators. Sex modifies the APOE-related risk of developing Alzheimer disease. *Ann. Neurol.* **2014**, *75*, 563–573. [CrossRef]

131. Alzheimer's Association. 2014 Alzheimer's disease facts and figures. *Alzheimers Dement.* **2014**, *10*, e47–e92. [CrossRef]

132. Birnbaum, S.G.; Podell, D.M.; Arnsten, A.F.T. Noradrenergic alpha-2 receptor agonists reverse working memory deficits induced by the anxiogenic drug, FG7142, in rats. *Pharmacol. Biochem. Behav.* **2000**, *67*, 397–403. [CrossRef]

133. Gyoneva, S.; Traynelis, S.F. Norepinephrine modulates the motility of resting and activated microglia via different adrenergic receptors. *J. Biol. Chem.* **2013**, *288*, 15291–15302. [CrossRef]

134. Connor, D.F.; Grasso, D.J.; Slivinsky, M.D.; Pearson, G.S.; Banga, A. An open-label study of guanfacine extended release for traumatic stress related symptoms in children and adolescents. *J. Child. Adolesc. Psychopharmacol.* **2013**, *23*, 244–251. [CrossRef]

135. Connor, D.F.; Findling, R.L.; Kollins, S.H.; Sallee, F.; López, F.A.; Lyne, A.; Tremblay, G. Effects of guanfacine extended release on oppositional symptoms in children aged 6–12 years with attention-deficit hyperactivity disorder and oppositional symptoms: A randomized, double-blind, placebo-controlled trial. *CNS Drugs* **2010**, *24*, 755–768. [CrossRef]

136. Arnsten, A.F.T.; Raskind, M.; Taylor, F.B.; Connor, D.F. The effects of stress exposure on prefrontal cortex: Translating basic research into successful treatments for Post-Traumatic Stress Disorder. *Neurobiol. Stress* **2015**, *1*, 89–99. [CrossRef]

137. Raskind, M.A.; Peterson, K.; Williams, T.; Hoff, D.J.; Hart, K.; Holmes, H.; Homas, D.; Hill, J.; Daniels, C.; Calohan, J.; et al. A trial of prazosin for combat trauma PTSD with nightmares in active-duty soldiers returned from Iraq and Afghanistan. *Am. J. Psychiatry.* **2013**, *170*, 1003–1010. [CrossRef]

138. Taylor, F.B.; Lowe, K.; Thompson, C.; McFall, M.M.; Peskind, E.R.; Kanter, E.D.; Allison, N.; Williams, J.A.; Martin, P.; Raskind, M.A. Daytime prazosin reduces psychological distress to trauma specific cues in civilian trauma posttraumatic stress disorder. *Biol Psychiatry* **2006**, *59*, 577–581. [CrossRef]

139. Koola, M.M.; Varghese, S.P.; Fawcett, J.A. High-dose prazosin for the treatment of post-traumatic stress disorder. *Ther. Adv. Psychopharmacol.* **2014**, *4*, 43–47. [CrossRef]

140. Simpson, T.L.; Saxon, A.J.; Meredith, C.W.; Malte, C.A.; McBride, B.; Ferguson, L.C.; Gross, C.A.; Hart, K.L.; Raskind, M. A pilot trial of the alpha-1 adrenergic antagonist, prazosin, for alcohol dependence. *Alcohol Clin. Exp. Res.* **2009**, *33*, 255–263. [CrossRef]

141. Fox, H.C.; Anderson, G.M.; Tuit, K.; Hansen, J.; Kimmerling, A.; Siedlarz, K.M.; Morgan, P.T.; Sinha, R. Prazosin effects on stress- and cue-induced craving and stress response in alcohol-dependent individuals: Preliminary findings. *Alcohol Clin. Exp. Res.* **2012**, *36*, 351–360. [CrossRef]

142. Gabbott, P.L.; Warner, T.A.; Jays, P.R.; Salway, P.; Busby, S.J. Prefrontal cortex in the rat: Projections to subcortical autonomic, motor, and limbic centers. *J. Comp. Neurol* **2005**, *492*, 145–177. [CrossRef]

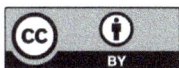

Article

Reliability of Fronto–Amygdala Coupling during Emotional Face Processing

Camilla L Nord [1,2], Alan Gray [2], Oliver J Robinson [2] and Jonathan P Roiser [2,*]

[1] MRC Cognition and Brain Sciences Unit, University of Cambridge, Cambridge CB2 7EF, UK
[2] Institute of Cognitive Neuroscience, University College London, London WC1N 3AZ, UK
* Correspondence: j.roiser@ucl.ac.uk; Tel.: +44-020-7679-1170

Received: 28 March 2019; Accepted: 9 April 2019; Published: 19 April 2019

Abstract: One of the most exciting translational prospects for brain imaging research is the potential use of functional magnetic resonance imaging (fMRI) 'biomarkers' to predict an individual's risk of developing a neuropsychiatric disorder or the likelihood of responding to a particular intervention. This proposal depends critically on reliable measurements at the level of the individual. Several previous studies have reported relatively poor reliability of amygdala activation during emotional face processing, a key putative fMRI 'biomarker'. However, the reliability of amygdala connectivity measures is much less well understood. Here, we assessed the reliability of task-modulated coupling between three seed regions (left and right amygdala and the subgenual anterior cingulate cortex) and the dorsomedial frontal/cingulate cortex (DMFC), measured using a psychophysiological interaction analysis in 29 healthy individuals scanned approximately two weeks apart. We performed two runs on each day of three different emotional face-processing tasks: emotion identification, emotion matching, and gender classification. We tested both between-day reliability and within-day (between-run) reliability. We found good-to-excellent within-subject reliability of amygdala–DMFC coupling, both between days (in two tasks), and within day (in one task). This suggests that disorder-relevant regional coupling may be sufficiently reliable to be used as a predictor of treatment response or clinical risk in future clinical studies.

Keywords: reliability; functional magnetic resonance imaging (fMRI); connectivity; emotion processing; amygdala; prefrontal cortex

1. Introduction

Measurement reliability is essential when translating research findings to clinical practice. Any study that describes brain function associated with risk or resilience to developing a neuropsychiatric disorder or with good or poor treatment outcome following treatment, rests on the assumption that the measurement has adequate reliability. For example, if a study finds that depressed patients who respond to fluoxetine have higher subgenual anterior cingulate cortex (sgACC) activation than non-responders, assessed with functional magnetic resonance imaging (fMRI), this could only be of clinical use if the measurement of each patient's sgACC activation were reliable, such that the clinical prognosis derived from the scan of an individual patient was consistent over time. Only then could brain activation (in the sgACC in this example) be tested as a putative fMRI 'biomarker' to predict clinical response.

Recently, we conducted a test–retest reliability analysis of activation for three commonly proposed biomarkers for depression, the left and right amygdala and the sgACC, measuring fMRI activation during three different emotional face paradigms [1]. Discouragingly, we found consistently poor reliability across all three tasks, both across days (two weeks apart) and within the scan session (two runs 15 minutes apart). This replicated some previous poor reliability findings in the amygdala [2], although others have produced more optimistic estimates [3,4].

Several recent studies have suggested various measures of functional connectivity—i.e., the covariation of fMRI signal between two or more brain regions over time—as putative 'biomarkers'. For example, studies have reported a relationship between functional connectivity and ketamine response in depression [5], antipsychotic response in schizophrenia [6], response to brain stimulation (repetitive transcranial magnetic stimulation, rTMS) in depression [7], and cognitive behavioural therapy (CBT) response in anxiety [8]. However, the reliability of these connectivity measures has not been comprehensively tested. In this paper, we therefore explore the reliability of a specific connectivity measure in the same dataset we analysed previously.

The example we focus on in this manuscript is a cortical–subcortical circuit that may play an important role in threat processing [9], a behaviour with transdiagnostic relevance across affective and anxiety disorders [10]. This circuit involves a region that encompasses areas of the dorsomedial frontal/cingulate (DMFC) cortex, which shows increased connectivity with the amygdala during both induced and pathological anxiety [9,11]. A large body of evidence in humans and rodents implicates the extended amygdala in aversive processing [12–15], a key cognitive mechanism in anxiety disorders [16]. However, the amygdala functions in concert with more frontal ('higher-order') neural regions. There is substantial evidence suggesting that anxiety-related processes, in fact, reflect a bidirectional modulation between amygdala and medial prefrontal circuitry, in particular the DMFC [16,17], which itself has been shown to be overactive in pathological anxiety [18]. Nonhuman primate research has found that amygdala–DMFC coupling is involved in fear learning and other anxiety-related behaviours [16,19,20]. Moreover, this coupling can be down-regulated by attentional instruction, suggesting that psychological therapy might function via similar neural mechanisms [21]. Therefore, DMFC–amygdala coupling is a crucial potential biomarker of anxiety and, potentially, also of therapeutic response [16,22].

We built on our previous work by examining the test–retest reliability of task-modulated covariation of fMRI signal between our initial 'biomarker' regions (the left and right amygdala and the sgACC) and the DMFC target region derived from a circuit implicated in anxiety [9]. Specifically, we tested whether the psychophysiological interaction (PPI, i.e., the modulation of coupling by a psychological factor, in this case, processing emotional faces) between the amygdalae and sgACC seed regions and the DMFC target was reliable within an individual. We examined reliability across scan days two weeks apart, as well as within the same scanning session across two runs of the task.

2. Materials and Methods

This re-analysis was performed on a previously acquired dataset; the initial fMRI analysis was described in more detail in our earlier publication [1]. In summary, we extended the initial task-related *activation* analysis to encompass *connectivity*. The key details are re-stated below for completeness.

2.1. Participants

We recruited healthy controls (N = 29, age range 18–40, mean age 26 (SD = 6.24), 10 male) through the UCL Institute of Cognitive Neuroscience and Department of Psychology subject databases. We included only right-handed fluent English speakers (meeting standard MRI safety criteria) without a recent (six-week) history of illegal substance use or any history of neurological or psychiatric disorders (the latter was screened by using the Mini International Neuropsychiatric Interview, version 5.0.0 [23]). We initially recruited 35 participants: 4 of them did not attend their follow-up fMRI scan, and data loss occurred for 2 of them.

The study was approved by the UCL Departmental Research Ethics Committee (ID: fMRI/2013/005). The participants provided informed consent in accordance with the Helsinki Declaration and were compensated £30 for taking part.

2.2. Protocol

Our experimental protocol involved three separate testing days. The participants first attended a screening session at the UCL Institute of Cognitive Neuroscience to determine eligibility and complete practice versions of the fMRI tasks. The second and third sessions took place at the Birkbeck-UCL Centre for Neuroimaging 9–21 days later (mean 14.33, *SD* = 2.10). On each of these scan sessions, the participants performed three tasks twice in the scanner (order counterbalanced between participants, with order kept constant within each participant), using an MR-compatible button box.

The tasks have been described in detail previously [1] (see Table 1 for summary). Briefly, the emotional identification (EI) task involved explicitly judging the emotion (happy, fearful, or neutral) of sixty face stimuli (task adapted from a separate study [11]). Two participants were excluded from this task analysis because of a high proportion of non-responses (>20 trials). The face matching (FM) task [24] consisted of 30 trials (split into five blocks) of either shape matching (18 trials, 3 blocks) or face matching (12 trials, 2 blocks). In both cases, the participants were instructed to match a centrally presented emotional face or centrally presented shape (both displayed for 5 s) with one of two alternatives displayed at the bottom (two test faces or two test shapes). No participants were excluded because of poor task performance. In the gender classification (GC) task [25], the participants were instructed to classify the gender of emotional faces (displayed for 2 seconds, happy, fearful, or neutral faces, separated into blocks; equal proportion of male and female faces, displayed in a random order). Each emotion block occurred 4 times per run (12 blocks total, 8 stimuli per block). One participant (with performance worse than chance) was excluded from this analysis.

Table 1. Task characteristics.

Characteristic	Emotion Identification (EI)	Face Matching (FM)	Gender Classification (GC)
Task duration	4:03	5:55	6:24
Task design	Event-related	Blocked	Blocked
Regressors of interest	Happy; fearful; neutral	Faces; shapes	Happy; fearful; neutral
Instruction	Explicit (match emotion)	Implicit (match face or shape to test stimuli)	Implicit (classify gender of face)
Regressors of no interest	6 movement parameters	6 movement parameters	6 movement parameters + errors
Contrast	Faces > fixation	Faces > shapes	Faces > fixation

Design and analysis characteristics of the three emotional processing tasks used.

2.3. Image Acquisition and Analysis

fMRI image acquisition has been described in detail previously [1]. Briefly, gradient-echo T2*-weighted images were acquired using a Siemens Avanto 1.5 Tesla MRI scanner employing a 32-channel head coil (this head coil improves signal-to-noise ratio up to 3.5 times compared to standard 8- or 12-channel coils [26]). We collected 36 slices per volume, slice gap 1 mm (2 mm slices; 50% distance factor) (see Table 1). The echo planar imaging (EPI) sequence was highly optimised to minimise ventral prefrontal cortex dropout (for extensive sequence details, see previous work [1,25,27]): echo time = 50 ms, repetition time/slice = 87 ms, slice thickness = 2 mm, in-plane resolution = 2 × 2 mm. One fieldmap per participant per day was acquired using identical parameters to the EPI scans; for each participant, we also acquired one magnetization-prepared rapid gradient-echo T1-weighted 1 mm isotropic anatomical scan.

We used Statistical Parametric Mapping (SPM12; Wellcome Trust Centre for Neuroimaging, London, UK, www.fil.ion.ucl.ac.uk/spm) in Matlab R2015a (for the initial region-of-interest (ROI)-based analyses and Matlab R2018a (for the PPI analyses). All data were slice-time corrected to account for the long repetition time (TR) (3.132 seconds). Preprocessing was identical to that described previously [1].

2.4. Psychophysiological Interaction Analysis

We used these data to conduct a PPI analysis, a functional connectivity method commonly applied to task-based fMRI data. This analysis reveals how experimental task conditions modulate the covariation in signal between a 'seed' region and the rest of the brain [28]. This is in contrast to the so-called "resting-state" functional connectivity, which examines such covariation independent of any specific cognitive demands. Therefore, PPI analysis can reveal which voxels in the brain exhibit different covariation with the seed region as a function of task condition [28] (in our study: for GC and EI, faces > fixation cross; for FM, faces > shapes). Note that PPI analyses do not provide any inferences about the directionality of this relationship or whether any connections are direct or indirect.

We followed the steps of a PPI analysis outlined by O'Reilly and colleagues [28]. We first defined anatomical masks for our three seed regions (PickAtlas left and right amygdala masks and a custom-made sgACC mask described previously [1]; note the sgACC mask was bilateral, to adhere with typical practice in the field and maintain comparability between these and our previous results [1]) and extracted representative time courses for each seed region. One subject did not show any suprathreshold activation in the left amygdala seed on any of the tasks; for this subject, we analysed only the right amygdala and the sgACC. Next, we computed the PPI time course (a single regressor describing the interaction between the time course of each region and the time course of each task). Finally, we entered this interaction regressor into a general linear model which included the physiological and psychological time courses as covariates. All models also included six movement regressors of no interest, and for the gender classification task, an error regressor only in those participants who made errors. For each task, we constructed parameter estimate images for the primary contrast of interest (for gender classification and emotion identification, faces > fixation cross, the implicit baseline; for emotion matching, faces > shapes). The results (voxels where activation was significantly explained by the interaction between seed and task time course) therefore describe only those voxels where the variance explained was over and above (1) the physiological covariation between each voxel and the seed region, and (2) the haemodynamic response function (HRF)-convolved time course of the task [28].

We performed a PPI analysis for each region ($N = 3$) and each task ($N = 3$). We took an a priori ROI approach to the analysis. Our a priori ROI was defined as the more rostral of two functionally defined ROIs created from clusters emerging from a whole-brain threat-by-valence interaction during a threat of shock task [11] and included, primarily, areas of DMFC (see Figure 1A; see Figure 1B,C for amygdala and sgACC masks, respectively). Our ROI analysis approach proceeded in much the same way as the ROI analyses in our previous paper, but now the extracted betas represented the modulation of covariance between the ROI and the seed by the task, rather than activation within the ROI.

Across an average of all four runs of each task (two on each day), we conducted one-way t-tests to verify there was a significant PPI effect between these regions. We then selected the regions showing a significant effect to perform reliability testing. We also tested for effects of day, run, and the interaction between day and run, using an analysis of variance on each ROI for each task.

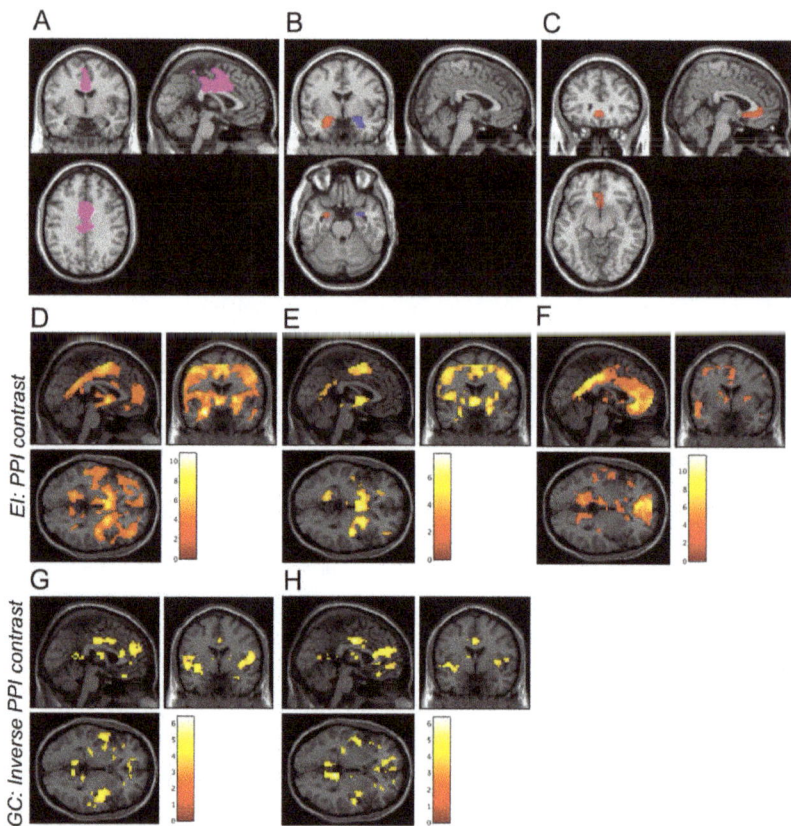

Figure 1. A priori ROIs and whole-brain PPI connectivity averaged across all runs and scan days. Figure A depicts the DMFC ROI used as a target region in the PPI analysis (**A**). Figure B,C depict the three seed regions: the left and right amygdala (**B**) and the subgenual anterior cingulate cortex (**C**). D,H depict results from seed regions showing significant PPI effects in the DMFC cortex ROI. Increases in whole-brain connectivity (positive PPI contrast) were observed during the EI task for the left amygdala (**D**), right amygdala (**E**), and subgenual anterior cingulate cortex (**F**) seeds. Decreases in whole-brain PPI connectivity (negative PPI contrast) were observed during the GC task for the left amygdala (**G**) and right amygdala (**H**) seeds. For illustrative purposes only, images were thresholded at $p < 0.001$ (uncorrected), and the colour bars indicate t-values. The inverse PPI contrast is displayed for the GC task (G,H) because mean PPI connectivity with the DMFC ROI was significantly negative (see Figure 2).

2.5. Reliability Testing

To quantify within-subject reliability, we performed intraclass correlation coefficient (ICC) analyses on the PPI results, using the Statistical Package for the Social Sciences 22 (http://www.ibm.com/analytics/us/en/technology/spss/). The ICC enabled us to quantify the stability of measurement across each fMRI session [29] and is usually interpreted as a ratio of between-subjects to within-subjects variance [30] (an ICC = 1.0 would indicate perfect agreement between test and retest fMRI sessions). For each seed region (left and right amygdala; sgACC), we calculated five ICCs: three between-day ICCs (averaged across both runs, as well as separately for the first and second runs) and two within-day ICCs (between the two runs, separately for each day).

We employed a two-way mixed effects ICC [31], defined as:

$$ICC(3,1) = BMS - EMS/BMS + (k - 1)*EMS$$

This form of the ICC has three important characteristics: it assumes the effect of measure (scanner) to be fixed, the effect of participant to be random, and tests for "consistency" (rather than "absolute" agreement) between sessions. We report average measures (rather than single measures) ICCs.

We adhered to a conventional interpretation of ICCs: ICC < 0.4 was interpreted as poor reliability; ICC = 0.4–0.75 as moderate-to-good reliability; ICC > 0.75 as excellent reliability [2,32]. We also report p-values and 95% confidence intervals obtained from an F-test against the null hypothesis.

2.6. Power Analysis

Our power analysis was computed for the original reliability dataset. To achieve 80% power to detect a moderate-to-large effect size (correlation r = 0.5, which we chose as a clinically meaningful degree of reliability) at our specified alpha (0.05, two-tailed), we required 26 participants [1].

3. Results

3.1. PPI Analysis

We first analysed the overall PPI effects (collapsing across day and run); we report average PPI effect size (Cohen's d, or standardised mean difference, averaged across all voxels within the DMFC ROI) for each task and region. For the FM task [24], there was no significant (p < 0.05) PPI effect between any of our seed regions and the DMFC ROI (all p > 0.2, Figure 2B; left amygdala: d = −0.233; right amygdala: d = −0.088; sgACC: d = 0.162). Therefore, the FM task was not analysed further.

For the EI task, the average PPI effect for all three seed regions was significant (all p < 0.002, Figure 2A; left amygdala: d = 0.966; right amygdala: d = 0.726; sgACC: d = 1.09). For the GC task, the average PPI effect for the sgACC was non-significant (p > 0.1), and, therefore, this seed was not analysed further. The GC task PPI effect for both left and right amygdala was significant (both p < 0.003) (Figure 2C; left amygdala: d = −0.657; right amygdala: d = −0.624; sgACC: d = −0.162). It is notable that one of the tasks (EI) evoked considerably more robust PPI effects, both within the DMFC ROI (Figure 2) and across the entire brain (see Figure 1).

The participants showed very high accuracy in both of the tasks analysed: for the EI task, over 91% of button presses were accurate (SD = 8.06); for the GC task, over 94% of button presses were accurate (SD = 6.33). There was no association between PPI activation and accuracy on the EI (sgACC: r = 0.194, p = 0.332; left amygdala: r = 0.247, p = 0.225; right amygdala: r = 0.249, p = 0.210) or GC task (left amygdala: r = 0.172, p = 0.382; right amygdala: r = 0.291, p = 0.126).

For the seed regions resulting in a significant DMFC PPI effect, we conducted ANOVAs, testing for effects of day, run, and the interaction between day and run. There were no significant main effects of day or run for either task, nor any significant interaction between day and run in the EI task, for either the amygdala or the sgACC. However, both regions tested for the GC task (left and right amygdala) showed a day-by-run interaction (left amygdala: F(1,27) = 7.12, p = 0.013; right amygdala: F(1,28) = 6.63, p = 0.016), such that activation decreased from run 1 to run 2 on day 1, but *increased* from run 1 to run 2 on day 2 (see Figure 2C).

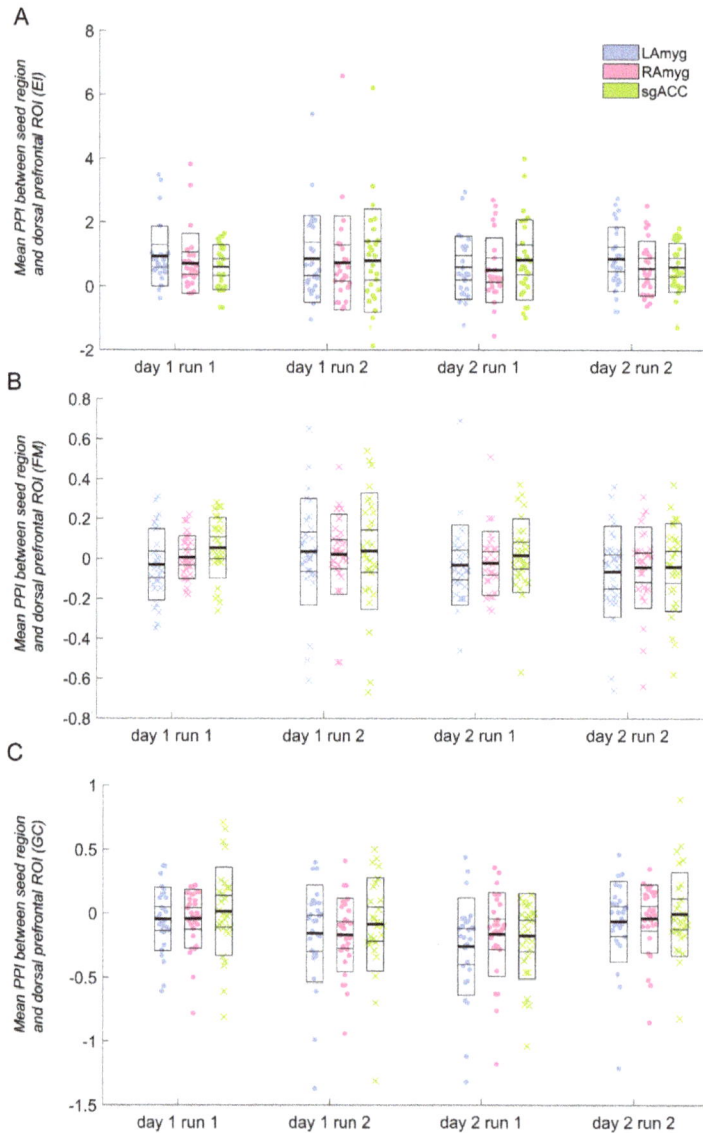

Figure 2. Psychophysiological interaction (PPI) parameter estimates for each task between the seed regions and the dorsomedial frontal/cingulate (DMFC) cortex region of interest. Data marked with "x" (as opposed to those marked with a filled circle) indicate runs that were not significantly different from zero (and therefore were not analysed further). Horizontal lines in the box plots indicate the mean (darkest line), standard deviation, and 95% confidence interval. A: Emotion identification (EI) task; B: Face matching (FM) task (not analysed further, as the average PPI parameter estimates were not significantly different from zero); C: Gender classification (GC) task (the subgenual anterior cingulate cortex (sgACC) seed was not analysed further, as the average PPI parameter estimate was not significantly different from zero). ROI: region of interest; LAmyg: left amygdala; RAmyg: right amygdala.

3.2. Reliability

We performed ICC analyses to test the within-subject reliability of the PPI effect, across days and runs (two-way fixed effects mixed ICCs; testing for consistency rather than absolute agreement). Table 2 details all reliability statistics computed; scatter plots illustrating the average between-day reliability for the amygdala seed regions are presented in Figure 3.

Table 2. Results from intraclass correlation coefficient (ICC) analysis of PPI for the EI and GC tasks, extracted from the DMFC region of interest.

Task	Reliability	LAmyg ICC (95% CI)	p-value	RAmyg ICC (95% CI)	p-value	sgACC ICC (95% CI)	p-value
FI	Between-day (both runs)	**0.704** (0.340 to 0.867)*	0.002	**0.738** (0.427 to 0.881)*	0.001	0.121 (−0.928 to 0.600)	0.372
	Between-day (run 1)	**0.585** (0.074 to 0.814)*	0.010	**0.708** (0.405 to 0.902)*	<0.001	0.167 (−0.828 to 0.620)	0.323
	Between-day (run 2)	**0.573** (0.047 to 0.808)*	0.019	**0.555** (0.008 to 0.801)*	0.024	0.017 (−1.158 to 0.552)	0.483
	Within-day (day 1)	**0.652** (0.224 to 0.844)*	0.005	**0.832** (0.626 to 0.925)*	<0.001	0.314 (−0.504 to 0.688)	0.171
	Within-day (day 2)	**0.768** (0.482 to 0.896)*	<0.001	**0.699** (0.339 to 0.863)*	0.002	**0.408** (0.299 to 0.730)*	0.094
GC	Between-day (both runs)	**0.442** (−0.206 to 0.742)*	0.068	**0.627** (0.206 to 0.825)*	0.006	Not analysed	
	Between-day (run 1)	0.071 (−1.01 to 0.570)	0.425	**0.579** (0.103 to 0.802)*	0.013	Not analysed	
	Between-day (run 2)	**0.493** (−0.095 to 0.765)*	0.042	0.326 (−0.435 to 0.684)	0.151	Not analysed	
	Within-day (day 1)	0.143 (−0.852 to 0.603)	0.346	0.146 (−0.818 to 0.599)	0.339	Not analysed	
	Within-day (day 2)	0.171 (−0.792 to 0.616)	0.315	−0.319 (−1.810 to 0.381)	0.766	Not analysed	

ICCs, their 95% confidence intervals (CI) and associated *p*-values are presented for each seed region analysed, for each task; * indicates ICCs exceeding 0.4 (these ICCs are depicted in bold), the lower bound for moderate reliability. EI=emotion identification; GC=gender classification; LAmyg=left amygdala; RAmyg=right amygdala; sgACC=subgenual anterior cingulate cortex; DMFC=dorsomedial frontal cortex; CI=confidence interval.

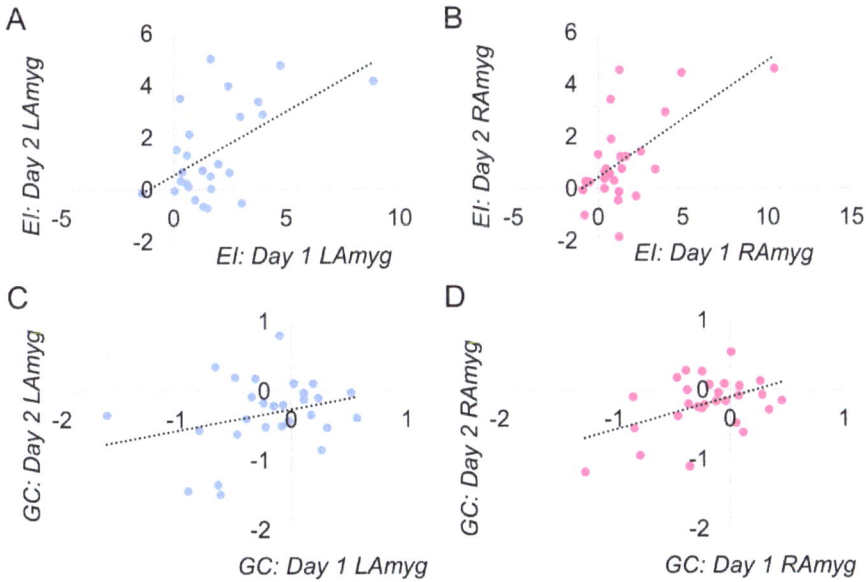

Figure 3. Distribution of PPI effect averaged across days. The regions displayed exceeded our threshold for reliability (ICC > 0.4, see Table 1 for full statistics). The sgACC in the EI task did not exceed our threshold for reliability and is not displayed. EI=emotion identification; GC=gender classification; LAmyg=left amygdala; RAmyg=right amygdala.

3.3. Emotion Identification

For the EI task, we found good-to-excellent reliability (all ICCs between 0.5 and 0.9) in all between-day and within-day ICC analyses (see Table 1). Note the high between-day reliability averaging across both runs in both left and right amygdala (left: ICC = 0.704 (95%CI = 0.340 to 0.867), *p* = 0.002; right: ICC = 0.738 (95%CI = 0.427 to 0.881), *p* = 0.001), as well as excellent reliability between runs on day 1 for the right amygdala (ICC = 0.832 (95%CI = 0.626 to 0.925), $p < 0.001$) (the same analysis for the left amygdala showed good reliability: ICC = 0.652 (95%CI = 0.224 to 0.844), $p = 0.005$; similarly good reliability was obtained for both amygdalae on day 2). In contrast, the sgACC had only one instance of moderate reliability across all analyses: the within-day reliability on the second day (ICC = 0.408 (95%CI = 0.299 to 0.730), $p = 0.094$). See Figure 3 for average between-day reliability.

3.4. Gender Classification

For the GC task, reliability was more variable. There were two instances of moderate between-day reliability, for the left amygdala (overall, between days, averaging across both runs: ICC = 0.442 (95%CI = 0.206 to 0.742), $p = 0.068$; and between the second runs of both days (ICC = 0.493 (95%CI = 0.095 to 0.765), $p = 0.042$) and for the right amygdala (overall, between days, averaging across both runs: ICC = 0.627 (95%CI = 0.206 to 0.825), $p = 0.006$; and between the first runs of both days (ICC = 0.579 (95%CI = 0.103 to 0.802), $p = 0.013$). However, there were no instances of moderate (or higher) within-day reliability (see Table 2).

4. Discussion

We tested the reliability of amygdala–DMFC and sgACC–DMFC connectivity using a ROI-guided PPI analysis of three emotion-processing tasks. Following initial analyses, only two tasks were analysed for reliability, as one task (face matching) did not show a significant PPI effect using our specific analytic approach. In contrast to our previous results, which showed poor within-subject reliability across these tasks for evoked hemodynamic responses [1], we found good-to-excellent reliability in every amygdala reliability analysis for the emotion identification task. We generally found poorer reliability for sgACC–DMFC task-modulated coupling and mixed reliability for the amygdala–DMFC PPI effect during the gender classification task.

These findings have particular implications for translational neuroimaging work in anxiety and related disorders. Converging human and animal data have implicated coupling between the DMFC and amygdala in both normal and pathological anxiety [9,16–20]. There are well-known contributions of the amygdala to fear and aversive processing [12–15] and of the DMFC region in fear appraisal, expression, and pathological anxiety [17,18]. However, there is substantial and bidirectional coupling between the DMFC and the amygdala [19,20]; anxiety behaviours may emerge from changes in the balance of (reciprocal) fronto–amygdala information flow [16]. This coupling has been suggested to represent a common neurobiological phenotype underpinning affective and anxiety disorders (within the 'negative valence systems' construct of the Research Domain Criteria) [16], making its investigation as a putative biomarker essential.

Our target ROI was taken directly from the anxiety literature [11] (ROI available at https://figshare.com/authors/Oliver_Robinson/568652). This enabled us to test whether task-related amygdala–DMFC coupling was sufficiently reliable to justify its exploration as a biomarker of treatment response, as previously suggested [9]. We provide support for the use of one of our tasks (emotion identification) in this endeavour and weaker support for another (gender classification).

It is notable that one of the tasks (emotion identification) evoked very robust PPI effects, both in the ROI (see Figure 2) and the brain as a whole (see Figure 1). One of the tasks (face matching) showed no significant PPI effect in the DMFC ROI, and for the other (gender classification), the PPI effect was more modest. The tasks differed in several key aspects which could have contributed to these differences: the emotion identification task was the only one that required explicit emotional labelling; one possibility is that such labelling evokes greater prefrontal–subcortical coupling than the incidental processing of emotional faces. Indeed, somewhat surprisingly, while we identified a significant increase in amygdala–DMFC covariation during the emotion identification task (relative to fixation baseline), this covariation was significantly decreased during the gender classification task.

Limitations and Future Directions

There are a number of important limitations to our findings. First, we conducted a very specific type of connectivity analysis (PPI), so our cautiously optimistic finding of good within-subject reliability for PPI with the amygdala, particularly in the emotion identification task, may not apply to data analysed using a different method. Others have reported similarly high reliability estimates of so-called "resting-state" connectivity measures, ranging from moderate to large [33–35], though these differ widely depending on the methodology used and the measure tested [35]. It is also worth noting that at least some resting-state reliability estimates may be artificially inflated because of the extremely high reliability of physiological noise (cardiac and respiratory) [36], while this is much less of a concern for our PPI analyses (as such, physiological noise is presumably similar between the task conditions). Second, it will be essential to test the reliability of activation and PPI effects in clinical samples, who may differ in relevant aspects from our sample of healthy controls. Finally, in larger samples than ours, it will also be important to perform more exploratory analyses of PPI between these seed regions and the rest of the brain. In this study, we restricted ourselves to a single DMFC ROI (and a single fMRI contrast for each task, as in our previous work [1]). This allowed us to constrain our hypotheses to avoid false positives, which could arise from a combination of multiple testing and low statistical power (common in PPI) [28]; however, this approach precludes inference about other regions.

5. Conclusions

We report good within-subject reliability of amygdala–DMFC PPI using emotion processing tasks, both between days (in two tasks) and within-day (between runs, in one task). This suggests that PPI may have more utility as a 'biomarker' to predict treatment outcome than task-related hemodynamic responses, which (in this dataset at least), showed very poor within-subject reliability [1]. Functional connectivity has been implicated as a possible 'biomarker' across a number of studies and treatment modalities, including pharmacological [5,6,37], psychological [8,37], and brain stimulation [38]. It is certainly a compelling suggestion that regional coupling implicated in a disorder could be tested as a predictor of treatment response. Our finding of relatively good within-subject reliability tentatively supports testing this ambitious proposal in future translational work.

Author Contributions: Conceptualization, C.L.N., O.J.R. and J.P.R.; Data curation, C.L.N., A.G. and J.P.R.; Formal analysis, C.L.N., O.J.R. and J.P.R.; Funding acquisition, J.P.R.; Investigation, C.L.N., A.G., O.J.R. and J.P.R.; Methodology, O.J.R. and J.P.R.; Project administration, A.G.; Resources, J.P.R.; Supervision, O.J.R. and J.P.R.; Visualization, C.L.N.; Writing – original draft, C.L.N.; Writing – review & editing, C.L.N., O.J.R. and J.P.R.

Funding: This work was supported by a Wellcome Trust Senior Investigator Award (to J.P.R.: 101798/Z/13/Z). O.J.R. is funded by a Medical Research Council Senior Fellowship MR/R020817/1. C.L.N. is funded by the Medical Research Council and the NIHR Cambridge Biomedical Research Centre.

Acknowledgments: The authors would like to thank Dr Rebecca Lawson and Dr Caroline Charpentier for imaging analysis scripts, and Oris Shenyan for additional help with the PPI analysis. The authors also thank Prof Karl Friston and Dr Peter Zeidman for their helpful discussions about PPI analyses.

Conflicts of Interest: J.P.R. consults for Cambridge Cognition, Takeda Ltd and GE. The other authors report no conflict of interest.

References

1. Nord, C.L.; Gray, A.; Charpentier, C.J.; Robinson, O.J.; Roiser, J.P. Unreliability of putative fMRI biomarkers during emotional face processing. *Neuroimage* **2017**, *156*, 119–127. [CrossRef]
2. Plichta, M.M.; Schwarz, A.J.; Grimm, O.; Morgen, K.; Mier, D.; Haddad, L.; Gerdes, A.B.; Sauer, C.; Tost, H.; Esslinger, C.; et al. Test–retest reliability of evoked BOLD signals from a cognitive–emotive fMRI test battery. *Neuroimage* **2012**, *60*, 1746–1758. [CrossRef]
3. Johnstone, T.; Somerville, L.H.; Alexander, A.L.; Oakes, T.R.; Davidson, R.J.; Kalin, N.H.; Whalen, P.J. Stability of amygdala BOLD response to fearful faces over multiple scan sessions. *Neuroimage* **2005**, *25*, 1112–1123. [CrossRef] [PubMed]

4. Manuck, S.B.; Brown, S.M.; Forbes, E.E.; Hariri, A.R. Temporal stability of individual differences in amygdala reactivity. *Am. J. Psychiat.* **2007**, *164*, 1613–1614. [CrossRef] [PubMed]
5. Salvadore, G.; Cornwell, B.R.; Sambataro, F.; Latov, D.; Colon-Rosario, V.; Carver, F.; Holroyd, T.; DiazGranados, N.; Machado-Vieira, R.; Grillon, C.; et al. Anterior cingulate desynchronization and functional connectivity with the amygdala during a working memory task predict rapid antidepressant response to ketamine. *Neuropsychopharmacology* **2010**, *35*, 1415. [CrossRef] [PubMed]
6. Sarpal, D.K.; Argyelan, M.; Robinson, D.G.; Szeszko, P.R.; Karlsgodt, K.H.; John, M.; Weissman, N.; Gallego, J.A.; Kane, J.M.; Lencz, T.; et al. Baseline striatal functional connectivity as a predictor of response to antipsychotic drug treatment. *Am. J. Psychiat.* **2015**, *173*, 69–77. [CrossRef] [PubMed]
7. Hanson, J.L.; Knodt, A.R.; Brigidi, B.D.; Hariri, A.R. Heightened connectivity between the ventral striatum and medial prefrontal cortex as a biomarker for stress-related psychopathology: understanding interactive effects of early and more recent stress. *Psychol. Med.* **2018**, *48*, 1835–1843. [CrossRef]
8. Klumpp, H.; Keutmann, M.K.; Fitzgerald, D.A.; Shankman, S.A.; Phan, K.L. Resting state amygdala-prefrontal connectivity predicts symptom change after cognitive behavioral therapy in generalized social anxiety disorder. *Biol. Mood Anxiety Disord.* **2014**, *4*, 14. [CrossRef]
9. Robinson, O.J.; Krimsky, M.; Lieberman, L.; Allen, P.; Vytal, K.; Grillon, C. The dorsal medial prefrontal (anterior cingulate) cortex–amygdala aversive amplification circuit in unmedicated generalised and social anxiety disorders: an observational study. *Lancet Psychiatry* **2014**, *1*, 294–302. [CrossRef]
10. Feldker, K.; Heitmann, C.; Neumeister, P.; Tupak, S.; Schrammen, E.; Moeck, R.; Zwitserlood, P.; Bruchmann, M.; Straube, T. Transdiagnostic brain responses to disorder-related threat across four psychiatric disorders. *Psychol. Med.* **2017**, *47*, 730–743. [CrossRef] [PubMed]
11. Robinson, O.J.; Charney, D.R.; Overstreet, C.; Vytal, K.; Grillon, C. The adaptive threat bias in anxiety: amygdala–dorsomedial prefrontal cortex coupling and aversive amplification. *Neuroimage* **2012**, *60*, 523–529. [CrossRef] [PubMed]
12. Boeke, E.A.; Moscarello, J.M.; LeDoux, J.E.; Phelps, E.A.; Hartley, C.A. Active avoidance: neural mechanisms and attenuation of Pavlovian conditioned responding. *J. Neurosci.* **2017**, *37*, 4808–4818. [CrossRef] [PubMed]
13. Campese, V.D.; Gonzaga, R.; Moscarello, J.M.; LeDoux, J.E. Modulation of instrumental responding by a conditioned threat stimulus requires lateral and central amygdala. *Front. Behav. Neurosci.* **2015**, *9*, 293. [CrossRef]
14. Sengupta, A.; Yau, J.O.; Jean-Richard-Dit-Bressel, P.; Liu, Y.; Millan, E.Z.; Power, J.M.; McNally, G.P. Basolateral amygdala neurons maintain aversive emotional salience. *J. Neurosci.* **2018**, *38*, 3001–3012. [CrossRef]
15. Terburg, D.; Morgan, B.; Montoya, E.; Hooge, I.; Thornton, H.; Hariri, A.; Panksepp, J.; Stein, D.; Van Honk, J. Hypervigilance for fear after basolateral amygdala damage in humans. *Transl. Psychiatr.* **2012**, *2*, e115. [CrossRef]
16. Carlisi, C.O.; Robinson, O.J. The role of prefrontal–subcortical circuitry in negative bias in anxiety: Translational, developmental and treatment perspectives. *Brain Neurosci Adv.* **2018**, *2*, 2398212818774223. [CrossRef] [PubMed]
17. Etkin, A.; Egner, T.; Kalisch, R. Emotional processing in anterior cingulate and medial prefrontal cortex. *Trends. Cogn. Sci.* **2011**, *15*, 85–93. [CrossRef] [PubMed]
18. Kalisch, R.; Gerlicher, A.M. Making a mountain out of a molehill: On the role of the rostral dorsal anterior cingulate and dorsomedial prefrontal cortex in conscious threat appraisal, catastrophizing, and worrying. *Neurosci. Biobehav. Rev.* **2014**, *42*, 1–8. [CrossRef]
19. Klavir, O.; Genud-Gabai, R.; Paz, R. Functional connectivity between amygdala and cingulate cortex for adaptive aversive learning. *Neuron* **2013**, *80*, 1290–1300. [CrossRef]
20. Livneh, U.; Paz, R. Amygdala-prefrontal synchronization underlies resistance to extinction of aversive memories. *Neuron* **2012**, *75*, 133–142. [CrossRef] [PubMed]
21. Robinson, O.; Krimsky, M.; Lieberman, L.; Vytal, K.; Ernst, M.; Grillon, C. Anxiety-potentiated amygdala–medial frontal coupling and attentional control. *Transl. Psychiatr.* **2016**, *6*, e833. [CrossRef]
22. Klumpp, H.; Fitzgerald, J.M.; Kinney, K.L.; Kennedy, A.E.; Shankman, S.A.; Langenecker, S.A.; Phan, K.L. Predicting cognitive behavioral therapy response in social anxiety disorder with anterior cingulate cortex and amygdala during emotion regulation. *NeuroImage-Clin.* **2017**, *15*, 25–34. [CrossRef] [PubMed]

23. Sheehan, D.V.; Lecrubier, Y.; Sheehan, K.H.; Amorim, P.; Janavs, J.; Weiller, E.; Hergueta, T.; Baker, R.; Dunbar, G.C. The Mini-International Neuropsychiatric Interview (MINI): the development and validation of a structured diagnostic psychiatric interview for DSM-IV and ICD-10. *J. Clin. Psychiatry* **1998**.

24. Hariri, A.R.; Mattay, V.S.; Tessitore, A.; Kolachana, B.; Fera, F.; Goldman, D.; Egan, M.F.; Weinberger, D.R. Serotonin transporter genetic variation and the response of the human amygdala. *Science* **2002**, *297*, 400–403. [CrossRef] [PubMed]

25. O'Nions, E.J.; Dolan, R.J.; Roiser, J.P. Serotonin transporter genotype modulates subgenual response to fearful faces using an incidental task. *J. Cogn. Neurosci.* **2011**, *23*, 3681–3693. [CrossRef]

26. Wiggins, G.; Triantafyllou, C.; Potthast, A.; Reykowski, A.; Nittka, M.; Wald, L. 32-channel 3 tesla receive-only phased-array head coil with soccer-ball element geometry. *Magn. Reson. Med.* **2006**, *56*, 216–223. [CrossRef] [PubMed]

27. Weiskopf, N.; Hutton, C.; Josephs, O.; Deichmann, R. Optimal EPI parameters for reduction of susceptibility-induced BOLD sensitivity losses: a whole-brain analysis at 3 T and 1.5 T. *Neuroimage* **2006**, *33*, 493–504. [CrossRef] [PubMed]

28. O'Reilly, J.X.; Woolrich, M.W.; Behrens, T.E.; Smith, S.M.; Johansen-Berg, H. Tools of the trade: psychophysiological interactions and functional connectivity. *Soc. Cogn. Affect. Neurosci.* **2012**, *7*, 604–609. [CrossRef] [PubMed]

29. Bennett, C.M.; Miller, M.B. How reliable are the results from functional magnetic resonance imaging? *Ann. N. Y. Acad. Sci.* **2010**, *1191*, 133–155.

30. Bartko, J.J. The intraclass correlation coefficient as a measure of reliability. *Psychol. Rep.* **1966**, *19*, 3–11. [CrossRef] [PubMed]

31. Shrout, P.E.; Fleiss, J.L. Intraclass Correlations: Uses in Assessing Rater Reliability. *Psychol. Bull.* **1979**, *86*, 420–428. [CrossRef] [PubMed]

32. Fleiss, J.L. Reliability of measurement. In *The Design and Analysis of Clinical Experiments*; John Wiley & Sons: Hoboken, NJ, USA, 1986; pp. 1–32.

33. Shehzad, Z.; Kelly, A.C.; Reiss, P.T.; Gee, D.G.; Gotimer, K.; Uddin, L.Q.; Lee, S.H.; Margulies, D.S.; Roy, A.K.; Biswal, B.B.; et al. The resting brain: unconstrained yet reliable. *Cereb. Cortex* **2009**, *19*, 2209–2229. [CrossRef] [PubMed]

34. Schwarz, A.J.; McGonigle, J. Negative edges and soft thresholding in complex network analysis of resting state functional connectivity data. *Neuroimage* **2011**, *55*, 1132–1146. [CrossRef] [PubMed]

35. Braun, U.; Plichta, M.M.; Esslinger, C.; Sauer, C.; Haddad, L.; Grimm, O.; Mier, D.; Mohnke, S.; Heinz, A.; Erk, S.; et al. Test–retest reliability of resting-state connectivity network characteristics using fMRI and graph theoretical measures. *Neuroimage* **2012**, *59*, 1404–1412. [CrossRef] [PubMed]

36. Guijt, A.M.; Sluiter, J.K.; Frings-Dresen, M.H. Test-retest reliability of heart rate variability and respiration rate at rest and during light physical activity in normal subjects. *Arch. Med. Res.* **2007**, *38*, 113–120. [CrossRef] [PubMed]

37. Dunlop, B.W.; Rajendra, J.K.; Craighead, W.E.; Kelley, M.E.; McGrath, C.L.; Choi, K.S.; Kinkead, B.; Nemeroff, C.B.; Mayberg, H.S.; et al. Functional connectivity of the subcallosal cingulate cortex and differential outcomes to treatment with cognitive-behavioral therapy or antidepressant medication for major depressive disorder. *Am. J. Psychiat.* **2017**, *174*, 533–545. [CrossRef]

38. Salomons, T.V.; Dunlop, K.; Kennedy, S.H.; Flint, A.; Geraci, J.; Giacobbe, P.; Downar, J. Resting-state cortico-thalamic-striatal connectivity predicts response to dorsomedial prefrontal rTMS in major depressive disorder. *Neuropsychopharmacology* **2014**, *39*, 488–498. [CrossRef] [PubMed]

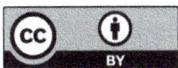

brain sciences

MDPI

Review

Sketching the Power of Machine Learning to Decrypt a Neural Systems Model of Behavior

Monique Ernst [1,*], Joshua L. Gowin [2], Claudie Gaillard [3], Ryan T. Philips [1] and Christian Grillon [1]

[1] Section on Neurobiology of Fear and Anxiety (NFA), National Institute of Mental Health/NIMH, 15K North Drive, Bethesda, MD 20892, USA; ryan.philips@nih.gov (R.T.P.); grillonc@mail.nih.gov (C.G.)
[2] Departments of Radiology and Psychiatry, University of Colorado School of Medicine, Aurora, CO 80045, USA; joshua.gowin@ucdenver.edu
[3] IReach Lab, Unit of Clinical & Health Psychology, Department of Psychology, University of Fribourg, 1700 Fribourg, Switzerland; claudie.gaillard@unifr.ch
[*] Correspondence: ernstm@mail.nih.gov; Tel.: +1-301-402-9355 or +1-301-675-4525; Fax: +1-301-402-2010

Received: 30 January 2019; Accepted: 14 March 2019; Published: 20 March 2019

Abstract: Uncovering brain-behavior mechanisms is the ultimate goal of neuroscience. A formidable amount of discoveries has been made in the past 50 years, but the very essence of brain-behavior mechanisms still escapes us. The recent exploitation of machine learning (ML) tools in neuroscience opens new avenues for illuminating these mechanisms. A key advantage of ML is to enable the treatment of large data, combing highly complex processes. This essay provides a glimpse of how ML tools could test a heuristic neural systems model of motivated behavior, the triadic neural systems model, which was designed to understand behavioral transitions in adolescence. This essay previews analytic strategies, using fictitious examples, to demonstrate the potential power of ML to decrypt the neural networks of motivated behavior, generically and across development. Of note, our intent is not to provide a tutorial for these analyses nor a pipeline. The ultimate objective is to relate, as simply as possible, how complex neuroscience constructs can benefit from ML methods for validation and further discovery. By extension, the present work provides a guide that can serve to query the mechanisms underlying the contributions of prefrontal circuits to emotion regulation. The target audience concerns mainly clinical neuroscientists. As a caveat, this broad approach leaves gaps, for which references to comprehensive publications are provided.

Keywords: triadic neural systems model; development; adolescence; machine learning; networks

---

1. Introduction

Adolescence is a period during which individuals undergo irreversible transformations in multiple physical, biological, cognitive, emotional, social, and behavioral domains. This implies immense complexity in trying to capture the overall landscape of these mutations. This review presents how the use of machine learning (ML) tools could test neural systems theories of motivated behaviors, particularly across the developmental period of adolescence. This is not a tutorial nor a pipeline, but rather an introduction to the growing possibilities that the combination of powerful ML tools with large datasets opens up to probe brain-behavior questions. An effort was made to keep this complex topic as straightforward as possible, at the expense of discussions of limitations and constraints. However, readers are referred to publications that begin to address these gaps.

At present, only simple heuristic models of the ontogeny of neural systems have been proposed to account for the behavioral changes occurring in adolescence (e.g., [1–3]). Among these models, the triadic model [2] figures as the broadest theory that provides functional mechanisms underlying motivated behaviors in general, and specifically across development. The triadic model is based on a functional balance across three neural systems dedicated to (1) approach behavior, (2) avoidance behavior, and (3) control processing (Figure 1). The triadic model, as a whole, has not yet been tested, although individual components have been validated, such as the developmental pattern of the approach system across adolescence [4–6]. We believe that the introduction of machine learning (ML) tools to brain-behavior analyses and the emerging availability of big developmental data can test the entirety of the model. This review will illustrate how this could be achieved.

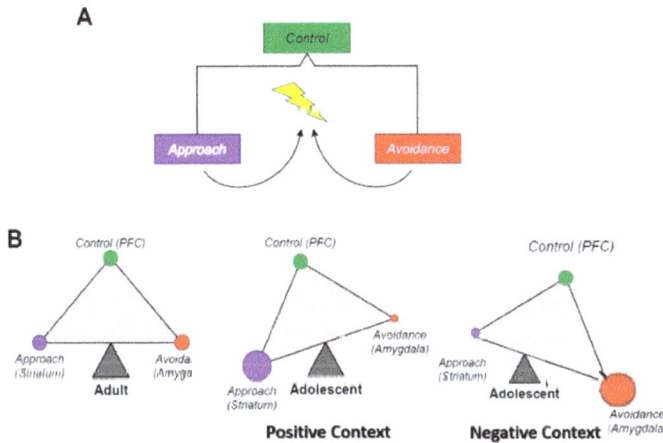

Figure 1. The triadic model. (**A**) This figure shows that at the most elementary level, behavioral responses to a stimulus can take only two forms: approach or avoidance. The selection of the behavioral response is monitored or adjudicated by a supervisory controller (control system). In yellow is the stimulus (i.e., object, situation), purple is the approach response, red is the other possible avoidance response, and green is the controller. (**B**) This represents the neural translation (nodes of the triadic model) of the three behavioral entities described in (**A**). The term node is used here to refer to a neural system whose core structure is unique. The ventral striatum is specific to the approach system, the amygdala to the avoidance system, and the prefrontal cortex (PFC) to the control system. In addition, these three systems establish a balance that is represented as a triangle in equilibrium. The adult balance is used as the yardstick, to which the adolescent is being compared. In an approach context, the adolescent balance is tilted towards the approach system, and away from the avoidance system, in a way that translates the proclivity of adolescent behavior towards approach, including risk-taking. In an avoidance context, the adolescent balance is tilted towards the avoidance system, and away from the approach system, in a way that translates the proclivity of adolescent behavior towards emotional intensity and lability, perhaps reflecting the peak onset of internalizing disorders in adolescence.

This chapter is divided in two main sections. The first section reviews the triadic neural systems model [2,7]. The second section focuses on the ways to test this model, using a hypothetical study of two large community samples, one of adults and the other of children tested repeatedly from childhood into emerging adulthood. Of note, only functional magnetic resonance imaging (fMRI) data were used to identify neural predictors. In addition, we will not provide details on how to acquire, preprocess, and process the fMRI data. All the neural data used for the analyses were scalar variables of intrinsic functional connectivity (iFC) of regions of interest extracted from resting state scans and regional activations in task-related fMRI scans. The iFC values corresponded to Fisher-transformed Pearson correlations.

2. The Triadic Neural Systems Model

The three neural systems of the triadic model consist of an approach, avoidance, and control module. At the most elementary level, motivated behaviors can be reduced to the generation of two possible actions, approach or avoidance, and the decision to adopt one or the other action is ultimately regulated by the control system (Figure 1). The triadic model is a generic heuristic explanation of how input information is processed at the brain neural–systems level to generate a motivated action output.

2.1. Conceptual Definition

We first address the approach and avoidance systems and then the control system.

A fundamental assumption of the model is that the approach and avoidance responses are encoded by two separate, although overlapping, neural systems. The "approach system" is classically associated with positive-value encoding, which underlies reward and motivation functions. The "avoidance system" maps to negative-value encoding, which captures punishment and negative emotion processing. These two "approach" and "avoidance" systems are not just the mirror of one another. They have different properties and behave according to distinct rules. For example, punishments weigh more than rewards. Indeed, economic tasks reveal that the subjective value of a $5.00 loss equates to the subjective value of a $10.00 gain [8]. Another example of these loss/gain differences is the impact of uncertainty onto behavior. Uncertainty, which carries a negative cost, increases avoidance but decreases approach. However, this functional separation of the approach and avoidance systems is far from absolute. Overlaps exist at both behavioral and neural levels.

Accordingly, motivation processing is common to both approach and avoidance systems. In other words, motivation fuels approach and avoidance responses. In fact, "motivated avoidance" is another conceptualization of "active avoidance", a construct currently under investigation in the field of defensive responses (e.g., anxiety, fear) [9–11]. Similarly, emotion takes both negative and positive flavors. Taken together, the approach and avoidance systems bleed into one another, which is reflected at the neural level.

The third component of the triadic model is the control system, which adjudicates courses of action between the approach and avoidance systems. In the context of this chapter, "control" refers to the formation of preference that is transferred to effector sites. Generally, control processes belong to the cognitive domain. Theories on preference formation are still debated, with two main contenders: (1) a feedforward competition of the representation of options and a resolution favoring the strongest signal [12–15], and (2) an inhibitory feedback of one representation, leaving the other option to prevail [16–19]. At this point, these potential mechanisms mediating control have not been considered in the triadic model.

The triadic model is typically represented as a triangle whose angles denote each system, and the sides denote the connections among the systems (Figure 1). Importantly, the triangle can be tilted in various directions, as a function of the weight (i.e., activity) attached to each system. Theoretically, the tilt could be measured by the location of the center of gravity of the triangle.

2.2. Neural Substrates

2.2.1. Approach System

The approach system is centered on the striatum, a relatively large multiplex structure, whose components include the caudate nucleus, nucleus accumbens, putamen, and pallidum. Broadly, the striatum is an essential contributor to the implementation of goals into actions and plays this critical role through the processing of information along parallel striatal–thalamocortical–striatal loops [20]. Although the bulk of research on the striatum has focused on reward function and motivation [21–23], much work in the last two decades has been dedicated to the role of striatal networks in aversive processes [24–28]. While both animal and human data clearly indicate involvement of the striatal circuitry in the processing of aversive stimuli, for instance in active avoidance, the exact mechanism is still unclear. However, it is also well-demonstrated that the recruitment of the striatal circuitry predominates and is more consistent in the processing of appetitive than aversive information [29–31].

2.2.2. Avoidance System

This system is centered on the amygdala. The amygdala is composed of multiple nuclei with distinct functions, which can be grouped into three compartments: (1) an input compartment, carrying multimodal sensory information; (2) a processing compartment, which integrates and broadly interprets the sensory information coming from the cortex and hippocampus; and finally (3) an output compartment, which dispatches the processed signals to effector agents that code physiological and motor responses. The amygdala input receiver is allocated to the lateral nucleus, and the output dispatcher to the extended amygdala (central nucleus of the amygdala and the bed nucleus of the stria terminalis). The information processing takes place in the basal/accessory basal nuclei. This information processing center has not typically been considered an "output region", but it does have an important one-way projection to the striatum to inform complex motor programs. The amygdala has raised considerable research aimed at understanding its function in the processing of aversive stimuli, including aversive learning [32–34]. Similarly, its implication in reward learning has been well established [33,35–39]. However, it is also important to point out that, like the biased responsivity of the striatum towards appetitive stimuli, the amygdala responds prominently and more consistently to aversive than appetitive stimuli [40,41].

2.2.3. Control System

The control system is centered in the prefrontal cortex (PFC). It falls under the umbrella term of cognitive executive function, which is essential to self-directed behavior. Multiple models have been proposed to describe the various components of executive function (e.g., working memory, inhibition, set shifting), and to map these different components onto brain regions (e.g., [42]). The common denominator across these models is the PFC. Regional specialization of the PFC has been parsed out in various ways, depending on theoretical frameworks, such as, to cite just a few, inferior-lateral versus mid-lateral PFC [43], anterior versus posterior PFC [44], or medial versus left lateral versus right lateral PFC [45]. The triadic model does not specify the putative PFC organization to adjudicate on courses of action. However, the framework most fit to accommodate the control of the direction of action (i.e., the decision proper) consists of a combination of regions that integrate the value and salience tagged to the possible options to decide on, and regions that modulate the weight of these value options. The former set of regions receives information (bottom-up process) and the latter apply the information to direct the course of action (top-down). In other words, the first set of regions receives information from the approach (striatum) and avoidance (amygdala) systems, which is sent then to the second set. The second set of regions modulates the activity of the avoidance and/or approach systems, which provides the signal that is dispatched to effectors which implement the action. This framework has been applied to the pattern of the neural mechanisms involved in the expression of defensive responses [46,47], which we generalize to motivated behaviors at large.

2.3. Triadic Model in Adolescence

The foundation of the triadic model is to explain how brain maturational changes underlie the prototypical behavioral changes in adolescence.

At the behavior level, adolescence is characterized by unique patterns in three domains: peak lifetime period of risk-taking, amplified and labile emotions, and highly context-dependent executive control [48–50]. In addition, the adolescent world undergoes a dramatic social reorganization. Accordingly, social processes should be considered as a fourth domain, but it is not yet integrated to the triadic model. Finally, adolescence is a time of vulnerability for psychopathology, as evidenced by a peak rise in the incidence of internalizing, addictive, and psychotic disorders.

The behavioral shifts across adolescence are modeled as a facilitation of approach behaviors, serving an "exploratory purpose." Indeed, adolescence refers to the transition period from childhood into adulthood, when the individual moves away from the protective family nest and learns to independently navigate the world, which requires risk-taking and exploration. This behavioral pattern can also reflect blindness or increased tolerance for possible failures.

According to the triadic neural systems model, the proclivity for exploratory behavior would be supported by an increased reactivity of the approach neural system, which would peak in mid-adolescence and taper down into adulthood. An opposite progression is described for the avoidance neural system in the context of responses to reward, i.e., hypo-responsivity of the avoidance system supposedly to protect exploration. Finally, the adjudication by the control neural system between approach and avoidance is becoming progressively more refined and efficient with age. This elementary description of the developmental dynamics of each unit of the triadic system accounts for the most commonly described changes in the adolescent motivated behavior, i.e., risk-taking and improved cognition [7,51].

Although generally less emphasized, the model also supports exacerbated emotions, positive as well as negative. The avoidance neural system, which contributes most significantly to emotional expression, has been shown to be hyper-responsive to aversive stimuli in adolescents compared to adults (e.g., [52–54]). This finding suggests that, in a negative context, the adolescent may react more emotionally than the adult. Therefore, the direction of the developmental trajectory depends on the context in which these systems are called into play.

This cursory description of how the triadic model is instantiated in adolescence, in a way that can explain typical adolescent behaviors, reveals obvious gaps. For example, it is unclear how the approach (appetitive) system is uniquely affected in aversive contexts in adolescence. The neural delineation of the circuits of each system is only partial. The amount and nature of overlaps among the systems is also unclear, and how these overlaps change with age and with context (appetitive versus aversive) has hardly been addressed. The next section explores how these limitations can be leveraged by the combined use of large datasets and machine learning tools.

3. Testing the Triadic Neural Systems Model

3.1. Introduction to Machine Learning Tools

The potential benefits of machine learning (ML) tools to facilitate discoveries in neuroscience research have generated huge hope and excitement (e.g., [55–58]). Indeed, these tools have gained enormous popularity among neuroscientists, particularly clinical neuroimagers, at a time when large datasets are becoming publicly available (e.g., [59–64]). Historically, ML tools have been developed to pursue artificial intelligence. As a growing field, ML has diversified into branches within statistics, computer science, and mathematics. The interdisciplinary nature of this field presents challenges when applying ML tools to neuroscience questions, especially in the neuroimaging domain, as it requires substantial expertise in a wide range of domains. For example, engineering, neuroscience, advanced physics, and psychology are each deep and well-developed fields. Achieving mastery of each of them is a daunting task. For this reason, collaborative approaches are highly recommended when applying ML tools to neuroscience research, since it behooves a team to have expertise in each of the domains involved in solving a problem.

Machine learning consists of algorithms that train computers to learn patterns from arrays of variables. Computer science, statistics, and engineering research have been instrumental to the development of these mathematical tools. Typically, nuanced solutions require large pools of data. As the neuroscience concepts addressed by the triadic model are complex, large datasets will be needed to apply ML tools to its testing. Machine learning consists of automated and iterative computations that promote computer learning of patterns (i.e., models). These patterns can serve to classify data and to provide predictive models. For example, ML is a critical tool in artificial intelligence, the science that trains computers to reproduce human behavior. Deep learning is a sub-specialized area of ML that uses multiple layers of learning, with successive layers using the output from previous layers as the input (e.g., [65]). Deep-learning algorithms have reached new limits in accuracy compared to other methods, and they permit to learn more precise rules when other ML approaches reach a plateau [66,67]. Deep learning typically requires substantially more data than simpler machine learning models, and this presents a limitation of its use in neuroscience, since large neuroscience datasets are rare for psychiatric disorders.

Finally, ML is divided into "supervised" and "unsupervised" algorithms (e.g., [68]). Supervised ML assumes a ground truth (e.g., patient versus healthy groups; faces versus houses) and trains the computer to use data that will best predict the ground truth. The power of these algorithms lies in the fact that the patterns learned are generalizable to testing datasets (not used to train the model). Some examples of supervised algorithms include multilayer perceptrons (MLP), decision trees, and support vector machines (SVMs). In this manuscript we use decision trees. A more detailed description of this algorithm is included later.

Unsupervised ML is not predicated on a ground truth. It provides training to find reliable patterns in data that can inform the constituents of models. In other words, it attempts to group objects (e.g., brain activation maps) according to their intrinsic properties, as opposed to similarity with some ground truth. These algorithms could also be used to identify important dimensions or components of a dataset. Popular unsupervised algorithms including clustering algorithms such as k-means clustering, hierarchical clustering, Gaussian mixture models (GMMs), and dimensionality reduction tools such as principal component analysis (PCA), and independent component analysis (ICA).

Deep learning is particularly well-suited for these applications. In all cases, ML's initial solutions, computed in a first sample (training sample), must be tested in a new independent sample (test sample) [69,70].

3.2. Overall Strategy for Testing the Triadic Neural Systems Model

The triadic neural–systems model can be tested in three sequential stages to address three main aims (questions) that seek to delineate: (1) the functional architecture of each system: describe and validate the brain mapping of each system (the approach, avoidance, and control system); (2) the dynamic interaction among the three systems: describe and validate how these systems work together to generate adaptive motivated actions; (3) the maturation of the triadic model: model how these three systems and their interactions develop with age. The strategy to test the first two questions is illustrated in Figure 2.

To accomplish these three aims, three types of data need to be collected in healthy individuals. These types of data include measures of (1) functional neural architecture, (2) behavioral characteristics, and (3) changes of neural and behavioral measures with maturation. Furthermore, each of these sets of data should be acquired in three different contexts, an appetitive context for approach responses, an aversive context for avoidance responses, and a cognitive context for control responses.

The first two questions do not require pediatric samples. Although it would be optimal for the samples of Question 1 and Question 2 to be independent, it is not a requirement. The samples should be large enough to apply machine learning analysis, allowing for a larger subsample of >150 subjects to be used as a training sample to define the model, and a smaller subsample of >50 subjects to be used as the testing sample to validate the model. For Question 3, an optimal design would be that of a longitudinal study of a large community sample of children (e.g., $n > 300$). Research consortia such as ABCD, NCANDA, IMAGEN, and connectome [59–62] are currently collecting longitudinal behavioral and neuroimaging measures in large pediatric samples. Since these data are made available to the public, the present discussion is highly propitious.

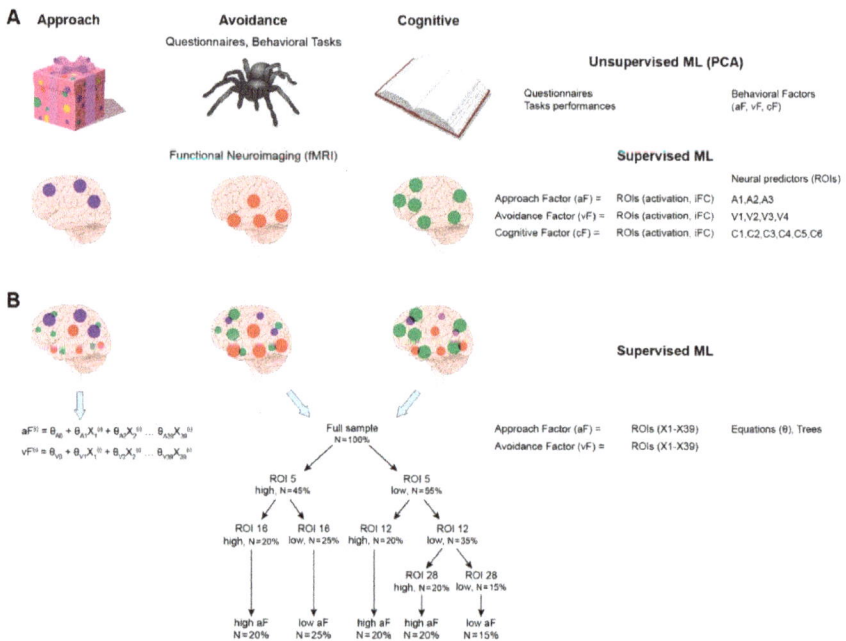

Figure 2. Strategy for Questions 1 and 2 to test the triadic neural systems model. All the data presented in this figure are totally fictitious. They only serve as concrete illustrations. The upper-panel addresses Question 1. Two sequential analyses are presented. (**A**) The first analysis is a principal component analysis (PCA is considered an unsupervised algorithm), which reduces and groups all behavioral data (from questionnaires, physiological, task performance) into latent factors. These factors map to the approach (aF), avoidance (vF), and cognitive (cF) domains. The second analysis applies a supervised ML algorithm. This algorithm uses the latent behavioral factors (aF, vF, cF) provided by the PCA as the predicted (output) data. The input data are all the significant regions of interest identified in the neuroimaging scans (task-related activation: regions of interest (ROIs), and resting state connectivity: intrinsic functional connectivity (iFCs)). In the present example, the input variables are scalar variables. The solution of this algorithm reveals the brain regions (ROIs, iFCs) that best predict the behavioral factors (aF, vF, cF). We consider these brain regions to represent the networks underlying the coding for aF, vF, and cF. These networks consist of three regions for aF, A1–A3, four regions for vF, V1–V4 for vF, and six regions for cF. These networks are drawn on the brain illustrations for concrete illustration. However, their location is not to be interpreted, since they are arbitrary. (**B**) The lower-panel delineates the analytic path to identify the relative contributions of the three neural networks of approach, avoidance, and cognitive (provided by the solution of Question 1) to individual behavioral propensity. This path rests on a supervised ML algorithm. The input variables consist of all neural predictors isolated in Question 1, but extracted from the three task-related fMRI scans, i.e., in the three behavioral contexts of interest. Therefore, 13 brain regions are extracted from each of the reward, aversive, cognitive task-related scans, making up 39 input variables. X1 is the extracted value of ROI1. There are 39 ROIs, and thus 39 X's. The superscript ^{i} corresponds to the subject i. The predicted variables (output variables) are the latent behavioral factors (aF, vF) calculated in Question 1. The cognitive factor is not examined because, presently, the triadic model is specifically focused on modeling approach and avoidance behaviors, and their relative dominance in the behavioral patterns of individuals. The solution of the ML algorithm provides equations and trees. The equations assign weight to each predictor (parameters that are unique to the equation predicting aF and those predicting vF). The trees permit to assess how the different variables interact to predict the behavioral factors (aF, vF).

3.3. Question 1: Functional Architecture of Each System

Question 1 aims at defining the networks that are associated with the generation of three domains of behavior: approach, avoidance, and cognitive control. Two types of data were used for this goal: behavioral and neural measures. The strategy to test Question 1 progressed in two steps for data organization and for the computation of the predictive model (Figure 2).

3.3.1. Data Organization/Reduction

The behavioral measures were expected to be numerous, including paper and pencil measures (self-report, interviews), task performance in both clinic and MRI (cognitive, motivation, emotion tasks), and physiological data (e.g., skin conductance, heart rate, EMG) (Figure 3). Therefore, a first step was to organize and reduce these measures to isolate latent factors most representative of the three domains of approach, avoidance, and control. In other words, rather than dictating which behaviors and questionnaires are associated with any one of the triadic systems, a data-driven approach can yield more objective and valid categorization of behavioral data. Principal component analysis (PCA) [71] is a reasonable approach to map existing behavioral data to distinct functional domains. This way, many metrics (e.g., questionnaire ratings, task performance, stress physiological responses) can be employed to reveal clusters (factors) of behavioral items that best describe the three behavioral domains of approach, avoidance, and control. Principal component analysis identifies the factors (eigen vectors) that best capture the variance in the existing dataset. These factors can be arranged in the order of their importance as defined by their corresponding eigen values. Ideally, a PCA approach would identify three principal factors that account for almost all of the variance of the behavior-based dataset, and which would map to the approach (aF), avoidance (vF), and cognitive control (cF) behavioral domains.

The results of the PCA might be more complex. This analysis could provide more than one factor score for each of the three behavioral domains. In addition, other factors, not related to the triadic domains, could emerge. Finally, the possibility for not being able to clearly identify an approach, avoidance or cognitive factor also exists, although the nature of the inputted items, all related to the behaviors of interest, make this possibility unlikely. For simplicity, only one behavioral factor for each domain will be used as illustration, and each factor score can be used to define two groups, one with individuals scoring low on the given behavioral factor, and the other group scoring high. Finally, additional unrelated factors, which can also emerge from the PCA results, will not be discussed here. The next step was to identify which and how neural measures predict each behavioral domain, respectively.

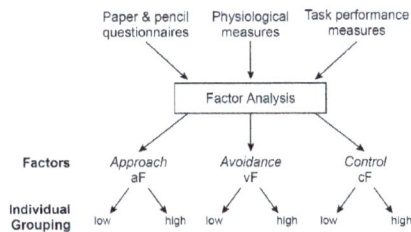

Figure 3. Principal component analysis (PCA) for behavioral data organization and reduction and for addressing Question 1, step 1. This step pools together all behavioral variables that are entered into a PCA. The PCA is aimed at grouping the behavioral variables into components (factors) based on their intrinsic properties. Based on the nature of the input variables, it is most likely that the variables will be groups into at least 3 factors, one capturing approach, another avoidance, and a third cognitive control. Other factors may also emerge. But, for simplicity, we only consider the three factors of interest, aF, vF, and cF for the approach, avoidant, and cognitive factors, respectively. Subjects can then be divided by their score level, e.g., high-score group versus the low-score group. Of note, the number of groups is arbitrary, since subjects could as well be separated into three groups, for example, based on low, moderate, and high factor scores.

3.3.2. The Predictive Model

This step identifies the activity patterns of the neural networks predicting each of the three behavioral domains, quantified by the data reduction PCA step as factors: approach factor (aF), avoidance factor (vF), and control factor (cF). These behavioral domains are examined separately, but concurrently, using the same procedure. This step uses supervised ML tools. The ML algorithms (such as support vector machine model or random forest model) implement iterative computations to train the computer to recognize the neural patterns that optimally predict the behavioral factor scores (aF, vF, and cF). In other words, the goal of these analyses is to produce the most efficient (low-cost, low-noise) predictive model of a given behavior using neural activity patterns as predictors. The neural inputs (i.e., predictors) to the model consist of resting state connectivity (iFC) measures, in the form of weights between hubs (e.g., ventral striatum to ventromedial prefrontal cortex), and regional blood-oxygen-level dependent (BOLD) activations during task-related fMRI (Figure 4). These input data are scalar, since a single variable (beta for activation, or Fisher-transformed Pearson correlation for connectivity) is extracted, and not the timeseries of BOLD activity/connectivity data. One advantage of ML methods is that multiple neural variables can be examined as predictors of a given behavior in a single model, without violating the assumptions of the statistical model (e.g., *t*-tests are conducted with the assumption that the data is normally distributed). In Figure 4, we present three equations for each behavioral domain (F, G, H). Each equation is unique to its behavioral domain in terms of the parameters (computed by the ML algorithms) that weigh the neural predictors. A higher weight signifies a more determinant role in predicting the behavior. The dominant predictors are those that also appear most determinant in decision trees (see comment below describing decision trees in more details), which maximize the output separation (subjects scoring high on the behavioral domain versus those scoring low). Furthermore, many ML models, by default, test interactions. For example, classification trees are a type of machine-learning model where the sample is partitioned in a sequence of steps (e.g., two steps: tree sequentially split by gender and then by family history of substance use).

We provide for the reader a comment, which describes decision trees in more details. *"A decision tree is s supervised learning algorithm, which attempts to classify or regress a dataset in a hierarchical fashion. As the name suggests, a decision tree has a tree-like architecture, with points (nodes) at which the tree splits into branches (edges). The split in the tree depends on the dimension that best separates the data. The criterion governing this split is defined by a cost function. The cost function computes the difference between the predefined label/score assigned to the datapoint and the prediction based on the split. The dimension, along which the cost function is minimized, becomes the node criterion. This process is then repeated in a recursive fashion, with the ends of the new branches becoming new nodes. A popular algorithm used in decision trees is the Recursive Binary splitting algorithm, where each node splits into 2 branches in a recursive fashion. An important consideration while using decision trees is to know when to stop the tree from growing any further and which splits to remove. A number of thumb rules can be used For example, one can predefine the maximum possible depth (length of the longest path) of the tree; or pre-set the minimum number of datapoints required in a branch before a split can occur; or get rid of the branches that do not impact the cost function too much."*

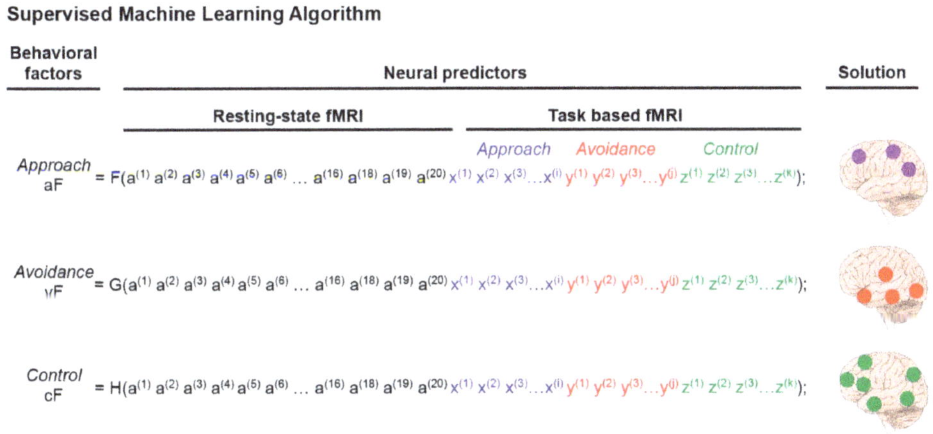

Supervised Machine Learning Algorithm

Behavioral factors	Neural predictors		Solution

Figure 4. Supervised machine-learning step. Supervised ML analysis to identify the networks predicting the three PCA factors of interest (aF, vF, cF). This algorithm computes the predictive value of the extracted neural measures. As such, it provides the components (nodes) of the neural networks that predict the behavioral factors previously identified by PCA (Figure 3). The predictive model can take the form of equations, F for aF, G for vF, and H for cF. The predictors are neuroimaging data. More specifically, a $^{(1)}$ is the first extracted value of the resting state functional magnetic resonance imaging (fMRI), up to a$^{(20)}$ which is the value of the last extracted measure that passes the significant threshold set for the resting state study (this number is arbitrary). The variable $x^{(1)}$ is the extracted value of the most significant regional activation of the approach-task-based fMRI, and (i) is the number of regions extracted from the reward-task fMRI scans; $y^{(1)}$ corresponds to the avoidance domain with (j) being the number of regional activations extracted from the avoidance-task based fMRI scans; and $z^{(1)}$ corresponds to the control domain with (k) being the number of regional activations extracted from the control-task fMRI scans. The brain illustrations on the right of the equations represent the solution of the ML analysis, which identifies the nodes (neural predictors) that best predict aF, vF, and cF, respectively (i.e., have the highest weight). The number of these regional activations (or nodes) is arbitrarily set to three for the approach factor, four for the avoidance factor, and six for the control factor. These nodes define the neural networks that best predict reactivity to the behavioral domains of the triadic model.

We present two simple fictitious examples of classification tree results in Figure 5. The first example (Figure 5A) uses demographic and clinical data to classify participants as high or low risk-takers. The model places gender at the top of the tree, i.e., first key variable that splits the sample in function of the propensity for risk-taking. It shows that males are more frequently high risk-takers than females. The second variable emerging as the next strongest predictor is family history of substance use. A positive family history of substance use strongly increases propensity for risk-taking in males, but less so in females. In other words, a positive family history confers risk that differs between males and females.

The second example (Figure 5B), also totally fictitious, is closer to the thematic of this paper, i.e., identify neural predictors of behavior. In this made-up example, the classification tree analysis reveals that approach behavior (e.g., aF) is most frequently (at the top of the tree) predicted by high ventral striatal (VS) response to reward, but only if the circuit's strength between VS and ventral medial PFC (vmPFC) is low, and the dorsolateral PFC (DLPFC) response is high. Machine learning would be able to identify this model, but linear models would not, unless the interaction term was specified (known a priori). With many potential interactions, it would be challenging for human researchers to consider all the possible interaction terms, but it is easy for a machine. Ultimately, a classification tree analysis would delineate the brain regions that matter in the modulation of approach behavior.

In the theoretical example of Figure 5B, the most powerful predictors are the VS, the vmPFC, and the dorsolateral PFC (DLPFC) (all fictitious examples).

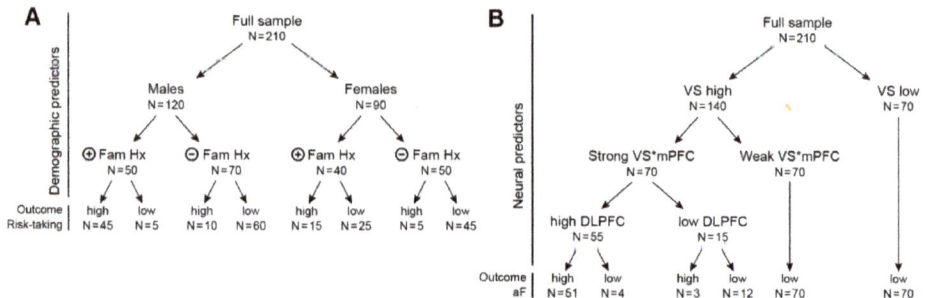

Figure 5. Two fictitious examples of solutions using classification tree algorithms. (**A**) Example 1 illustrates a ML classification of subjects into groups of high or low risk-takers (high versus low value of the outcome measure), in function of sex and family history of substance use (fmhx-su). The sample is composed of 120 males and 90 females. The modulation of risk-taking by fmhx-su is different in males and females. Males with a positive fmhx-su are more prone to be high risk-takers (45 of 50, 90%) compared to males without fmhx-su (10 of 70, 14%). However, this factor does not seem to be as determinant in females, 15 of 40 females (38%) compared to 5 of 45 (11%) without fmhx-su. (**B**) Example 2 illustrates a ML classification of individuals as a function of high versus low propensity for approach behavior (high aF versus low aF) using neural predictors. This tree shows that the ventral striatum (VS) is the strongest predictor of high aF. All the individuals with low VS have a low aF scores. In contrast, the association of high VS sensitivity with high aF is modulated by the connectivity of VS* the medial prefrontal cortex (mPFC), and by the activity of the dorsolateral prefrontal cortex (DLPFC). This tree clearly illustrates how such analysis can help clarify interactions among neural predictors of specific behaviors. VS = ventral striatum activation, VS*mPFC = intrinsic connectivity between VS and medial prefrontal cortex, DLPFC = dorsolateral prefrontal cortex.

3.3.3. Output of the Predictive Model of the Characterization of the Three Neural Systems

Taken together, the expected output of Question 1 is the delineation of the main nodes engaged (via activation or connectivity) in each of the three functional domains. In addition to providing the identity of these nodes, Question 1 also reveals patterns of interactions that predict the degree of behavioral propensity towards either approach, avoidance or control. Here, these patterns of interactions are not used in the subsequent analyses, although they are important to fully characterize the neural substrates of each behavioral domain. Analyses for Question 2 will focus on the main nodes identified in Question 1. For illustration, we will arbitrary assign nodes to each neural system: approach system, A1, A2, A3, avoidance system, V1, V2, V3, V4, and control system, C1, C2, C3, C4, C5, C6. In actuality, some nodes are likely to be common to two or all three systems, but, for simplicity, this situation is not considered.

3.4. Question 2: Dynamic Interactions among the Three Systems

Question 2 concerns how the neural predictors of all three behavioral domains (i.e., approach A1–A3, avoidance V1–V4, and control C1–C6) work together in each of the appetitive and aversive contexts. Indeed, the triadic model predicts that, in an appetitive context, the approach system will be active and more tightly intra-connected, whereas the avoidance system will tend to be silenced [7,72]. The opposite pattern would characterize the neural pattern in an aversive context (Figure 1). The control network would manifest different couplings with the approach versus avoidance system as a function of the appetitive versus aversive context. Clearly, the reality is more complex, particularly with expected interactions among nodes of the different neural systems, which we anticipate being able to characterize using ML strategies.

3.4.1. Question 2, Step 1

The neural predictors identified in Question 1 provide the basis for the input variables of this analysis (Figure 6). As a reminder, the fictitious results of Question 1 reveal three brain regions (A1–A3) that predict approach, four brain regions (V1–V4) for avoidance, and six brain regions (C1–C6) for control. The strategy to query Question 2 takes two steps: (1) the collection of all neural data from all three contexts (approach, avoidance, control), and (2) a supervised ML "categorization" analysis (Figure 6).

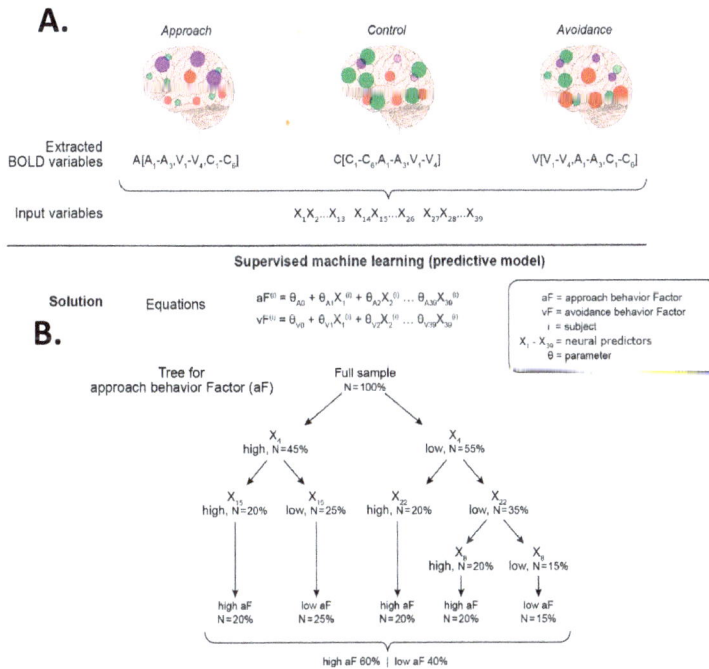

Figure 6. Strategy for addressing Question 2, Steps 1–2. Extraction of neural predictors and supervised ML to predict behavioral factors aF and vF. (**A**) Step 1: Neural data extraction. This step consists of gathering all potential neural predictors of the behavioral factors identified in Question 1 (Figure 4). These neural predictors (nodes) are now all extracted from every task-based fMRI scan (cognitive-task fMRI, avoidance-task fMRI, and approach-task fMRI). The brain illustrations show the activation maps of all the nodes of interest, the approach nodes (purple), the avoidance nodes (red), and the control nodes (green), in each task-based fMRI scan. The extraction of the blood-oxygen-level dependent (BOLD) signals for all regions of interest (ROIs) (13 per scan) are labelled X_1 through X_{39}. (**B**) Step 2: Supervised ML analysis. The extracted 39 ROIs variables (X_1–X_{39}) are the predictors used in two analyses, one for the approach domain and the other for the avoidance domain. Each analysis can be performed using two supervised algorithms. The first algorithm uses a linear model to estimate the strength of each neural predictor (theta weights). The second algorithm uses a decision tree to provide a hierarchical structure that informs more directly the interactions among neural predictors. The example shows the sample divided in two groups, one group with low aF scores, and the other group with high vF scores. The tree depicts four ROI with significant weights in predicting the groups. These ROI are ROI$_4$, ROI$_{15}$, ROI$_{22}$, and ROI$_8$, and their respective BOLD values are X_4, X_{15}, X_{22}, and X_8.

The first data collection step (Figure 6A) is a re-examination of the task-based fMRI scans, in order to extract the values of the neural predictors of all three contexts pooled together. In other words, the "approach" nodes (or regions of interest, ROI) A1–A4 are also extracted from the control- and avoidance-related scans, the "avoidance" ROIs V1–V3 from the control- and approach-related scans, and the "control" ROIs C1–C5 from the avoidance- and approach-related scans. Therefore, the number of potential neural predictors for Question 2 is tripled (3 approach + 4 avoidance + 6 control ROIs = 13 ROIs, whose activity is extracted from the reward-task fMRI + the negative-task fMRI + the cognitive-task fMRI, i.e., 13 × 3 = 39). Similar to Question 1, for simplicity, only scalar variables are used as input data, not timeseries.

3.4.2. Question 2, Step 2

In the second step (Figure 6B), the input data (*n* = 39) are categorized based on their predictive value of each behavioral domain. This analysis falls under the supervised ML approach, using learning algorithms of support vector machines or decision trees, as described in Question 1. To avoid confusion, the supervised ML algorithm, used in Question 1, identified the neural predictors from task-based and resting-state scans of approach, avoidance or control propensity. In Question 2, this ML algorithm is used to identify the neural predictors from the pooled neural predictors (*n* = 13 extracted from all three contexts, *n* = 13 × 3) of the propensity for approach, avoidance, and control separately. The result of this last analysis informs the patterns of interactions across the three neural systems that support the behavioral domains of the triadic model. These results would represent a major advance in knowledge of how brain systems work together to organize behavior.

Figure 6 illustrates two types of representations of the results. The equations provide measures of the strength of each neural predictor (theta weights). The trees provide a representation of the hierarchical power of the neural predictors to influence behavioral outcomes, informing more directly interactions among neural predictors.

3.5. Question 3: Maturation of the Triadic Neural System Dynamics

The strategy for Question 3 is a simple replication of the steps described above, but at each follow-up (e.g., 12 years old, 16 years old, and 20 years old). An example of a possible outcome is presented in Figure 7, which clearly shows how this process could inform the developmental trajectories not only of the triadic neural systems, but also of their interactions. We summarize the steps below:

(a) Step 1: Behavioral characterization. The predicted behavior outcome measures are computed as in Question 1 by conducting a factor analysis of all available behavioral data, at each follow-up.

(b) Step 2: Brain-behavior classification: This step gives rise to two types of results: trees that depict the hierarchical organization of predictors at each follow-up point and equations that quantify the contribution of each cluster to a given behavioral domain, respectively.

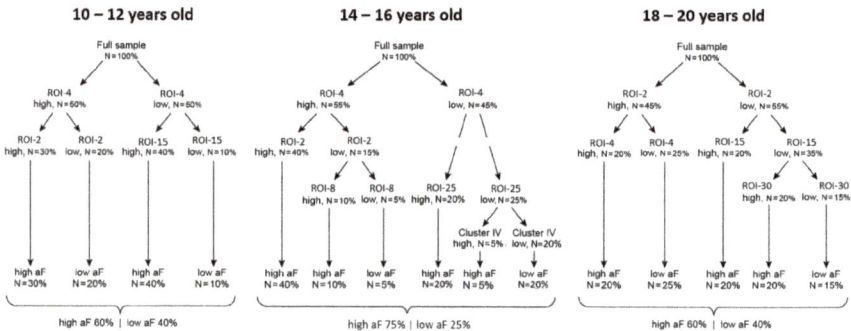

Figure 7. Decision trees across development. Fictitious examples of developmental analysis of neural predictors of behavior: examples of decision-trees at each follow-up. Changes in classification trees at different age groups inform the evolution of mechanisms underlying motivated behaviors of approach and avoidance.

4. Conclusions

In this paper we offer a preview of the potential contribution of the latest, so far most powerful, tools to help delineate how brain networks code motivated behaviors. This window into brain-behavior causal mechanisms can have invaluable implications for understanding developmental changes in health and diseases, and can provide critical guides for refining and extending research in this field. Specifically, the present work provides a guide that can serve to query the mechanisms underlying the contributions of prefrontal circuits to emotion regulation. Finally, findings that emerge from such an analytical approach can raise key questions that, in turn, can be examined in focused studies, or warrant a re-examination of previous data.

Author Contributions: All authors contributed significantly to the preparation of the manuscript

Funding: This research received no external funding.

Acknowledgments: This work was supported by the Intramural Research Program of the National Institute of Mental Health, project number ZIAMH002798 (clinical protocol 02-M-0321, NCT00047853) to C.G.

Conflicts of Interest: The authors declare no conflict of interest.

References

1. Casey, B.J.; Jones, R.M.; Hare, T.A. The adolescent brain. *Annu. N. Y. Acad. Sci.* **2008**, *1124*, 111–126. [CrossRef] [PubMed]
2. Ernst, M.; Pine, D.S.; Hardin, M. Triadic model of the neurobiology of motivated behavior in adolescence. *Psychol. Med.* **2006**, *36*, 299–312. [CrossRef] [PubMed]
3. Steinberg, L. A social neuroscience perspective on adolescent risk-taking. *Dev. Rev.* **2008**, *28*, 78–106. [CrossRef] [PubMed]
4. Steinberg, L. A dual systems model of adolescent risk-taking. *Dev. Psychobiol.* **2010**, *53*, 216–224. [CrossRef] [PubMed]
5. Vink, M.; Derks, J.M.; Hoogendam, J.M.; Hillegers, M.; Kahn, R.S. Functional differences in emotion processing during adolescence and early adulthood. *NeuroImage* **2014**, *91*, 70–76. [CrossRef] [PubMed]
6. Galvan, A. Adolescent development of the reward system. *Front. Hum. Neurosci.* **2010**, *4*, 6. [CrossRef]
7. Ernst, M. The triadic model perspective for the study of adolescent motivated behavior. *Brain Cogn.* **2014**, *89*, 104–111. [CrossRef]
8. Tversky, A.; Kahneman, D. Advances in prospect theory: Cumulative representation of uncertainty. *J. Risk Uncertain.* **1992**, *5*, 297–323. [CrossRef]
9. Elliot, A.J.; Covington, M.V. Approach and avoidance motivation. *Educ. Psychol. Rev.* **2001**, *13*, 73–92. [CrossRef]
10. Lammel, S.; Lim, B.K.; Malenka, R.C. Reward and aversion in a heterogeneous midbrain dopamine system. *Neuropharmacology* **2014**, *76*, 351–359. [CrossRef]
11. Mathews, A.; Mackintosh, B. A cognitive model of selective processing in anxiety. *Cogn. Ther. Res.* **1998**, *22*, 539–560. [CrossRef]
12. Brody, C.D.; Hanks, T.D. Neural underpinnings of the evidence accumulator. *Curr. Opin. Neurobiol.* **2016**, *37*, 149–157. [CrossRef]
13. Cisek, P.; Kalaska, J.F. Neural correlates of reaching decisions in dorsal premotor cortex: Specification of multiple direction choices and final selection of action. *Neuron* **2005**, *45*, 801–814 [CrossRef] [PubMed]
14. Rushworth, M.F.S.; Kolling, N.; Sallet, J.; Mars, R.B. Valuation and decision-making in frontal cortex: One or many serial or parallel systems? *Curr. Opin. Neurobiol.* **2012**, *22*, 946–955. [CrossRef] [PubMed]
15. Song, J.-H.; Nakayama, K. Hidden cognitive states revealed in choice reaching tasks. *Trends Cogn. Sci.* **2009**, *13*, 360–366. [CrossRef] [PubMed]
16. Burle, B.; Vidal, F.; Tandonnet, C.; Hasbroucq, T. Physiological evidence for response inhibition in choice reaction time tasks. *Brain Cogn.* **2004**, *56*, 153–164. [CrossRef] [PubMed]
17. Hunt, L.T.; Kolling, N.; Soltani, A.; Woolrich, M.W.; Rushworth, M.F.; Behrens, T.E. Mechanisms underlying cortical activity during value-guided choice. *Nat. Neurosci.* **2012**, *15*, 470–479. [CrossRef] [PubMed]

18. Strait, C.E.; Blanchard, T.C.; Hayden, B.Y. Reward value comparison via mutual inhibition in ventromedial prefrontal cortex. *Neuron* **2014**, *82*, 1357–1366. [CrossRef]
19. Usher, M.; McClelland, J.L. The time course of perceptual choice: The leaky, competing accumulator model. *Psychol. Rev.* **2001**, *108*, 550–592. [CrossRef]
20. Balleine, B.W.; O'Doherty, J.P. Human and rodent homologies in action control: Corticostriatal determinants of goal-directed and habitual action. *Neuropsychopharmacology* **2010**, *35*, 48–69. [CrossRef]
21. Berridge, K.C.; Kringelbach, M.L. Neuroscience of affect: Brain mechanisms of pleasure and displeasure. *Curr. Opin. Neurobiol.* **2013**, *23*, 294–303. [CrossRef] [PubMed]
22. Berridge, K.C.; Kringelbach, M.L. Pleasure systems in the brain. *Neuron* **2015**, *86*, 646–664. [CrossRef] [PubMed]
23. Berridge, K.C.; Robinson, T.E. Parsing reward. *Trends Neurosci.* **2003**, *26*, 507–513. [CrossRef]
24. Delgado, M.R.; Gillis, M.M.; Phelps, E.A. Regulating the expectation of reward via cognitive strategies. *Nat. Neurosci.* **2008**, *11*, 880–881. [CrossRef]
25. Delgado, M.R.; Jou, R.L.; Phelps, E.A. Neural systems underlying aversive conditioning in humans with primary and secondary reinforcers. *Front. Neurosci.* **2011**, *5*, 71. [CrossRef] [PubMed]
26. Saga, Y.; Tremblay, L. Ventral striatopallidal pathways involved in appetitive and aversive motivational processes. *Decis. Neurosci.* **2017**, 47–58. [CrossRef]
27. McCutcheon, J.E.; Ebner, S.R.; Loriaux, A.L.; Roitman, M.F. Encoding of aversion by dopamine and the nucleus accumbens. *Front. Neurosci.-Switz.* **2012**, *6*, 137. [CrossRef]
28. Anderson, A.K.; Phelps, E.A. Expression without recognition: Contributions of the human amygdala to emotional communication. *Psychol. Sci.* **2000**, *11*, 106–111. [CrossRef] [PubMed]
29. Mirenowicz, J.; Schultz, W. Preferential activation of midbrain dopamine neurons by appetitive rather than aversive stimuli. *Nature* **1996**, *379*, 449–451. [CrossRef] [PubMed]
30. Schultz, W. Behavioral dopamine signals. *Trends Neurosci.* **2007**, *30*, 203–210. [CrossRef]
31. Bromberg-Martin, E.S.; Matsumoto, M.; Hikosaka, O. Dopamine in motivational control: Rewarding, aversive, and alerting. *Neuron* **2010**, *68*, 815–834. [CrossRef] [PubMed]
32. Goode, T.D.; Maren, S. Role of the bed nucleus of the stria terminalis in aversive learning and memory. *Learn. Mem.* **2017**, *24*, 480–491. [CrossRef] [PubMed]
33. Maren, S. Parsing reward and aversion in the amygdala. *Neuron* **2016**, *90*, 209–211. [CrossRef] [PubMed]
34. Sanford, C.A.; Soden, M.E.; Baird, M.A.; Miller, S.M.; Schulkin, J.; Palmiter, R.D.; Clark, M.; Zweifel, L.S. A central amygdala CRF circuit facilitates learning about weak threats. *Neuron* **2017**, *93*, 164–178. [CrossRef] [PubMed]
35. Balleine, B.W.; Killcross, S. Parallel incentive processing: An integrated view of amygdala function. *Trends Neurosci.* **2006**, *29*, 272–279. [CrossRef] [PubMed]
36. Gottfried, J.A.; O'Doherty, J.; Dolan, R.J. Encoding predictive reward value in human amygdala and orbitofrontal cortex. *Science* **2003**, *301*, 1104–1107. [CrossRef]
37. Murray, E.A. The amygdala, reward and emotion. *Trends Cogn. Sci.* **2007**, *11*, 489–497. [CrossRef]
38. Tye, K.M.; Cone, J.J.; Schairer, W.W.; Janak, P.H. Amygdala neural encoding of the absence of reward during extinction. *J. Neurosci.* **2010**, *30*, 116–125. [CrossRef]
39. Wassum, K.M.; Izquierdo, A. The basolateral amygdala in reward learning and addiction. *Neurosci. Biobehav. Rev.* **2015**, *57*, 271–283. [CrossRef]
40. Kragel, P.A.; LaBar, K.S. Decoding the nature of emotion in the brain. *Trends Cogn. Sci.* **2016**, *20*, 444–455. [CrossRef]
41. Murphy, F.C.; Nimmo-Smith, I.; Lawrence, A.D. Functional neuroanatomy of emotions: A meta-analysis. *Cogn. Affect. Behav. Neurosci.* **2003**, *3*, 207–233. [CrossRef]
42. Banich, M.T. Executive function. *Curr. Dir. Psychol. Sci.* **2009**, *18*, 89–94. [CrossRef]
43. Petrides, M. Lateral prefrontal cortex: Architectonic and functional organization. *Philos. Trans. R. Soc. Lond. Ser. B Biol. Sci.* **2005**, *360*, 781–795. [CrossRef] [PubMed]
44. Christoff, K.; Gabrieli, J.D.E. The frontopolar cortex and human cognition: Evidence for a rostrocaudal hierarchical organization within the human prefrontal cortex. *Psychobiology* **2000**, *28*, 168–186. [CrossRef]
45. Stuss, D.T.; Alexander, M.P. Is there a dysexecutive syndrome? *Philos. Trans. R. Soc. Lond. Ser. B Biol. Sci.* **2007**, *362*, 901–915. [CrossRef]

46. Kouneiher, F.; Charron, S.; Koechlin, E. Motivation and cognitive control in the human prefrontal cortex. *Nat. Neurosci.* **2009**, *12*, 939–945. [CrossRef] [PubMed]

47. LeDoux, J.; Daw, N.D. Surviving threats: Neural circuit and computational implications of a new taxonomy of defensive behaviour. *Nat. Rev. Neurosci.* **2018**, *19*, 269–282. [CrossRef] [PubMed]

48. Ernst, M.; Nelson, E.E.; Jazbec, S.; McClure, E.B.; Monk, C.S.; Leibenluft, E.; Blair, J.; Pine, D.S. Amygdala and nucleus accumbens in responses to receipt and omission of gains in adults and adolescents. *NeuroImage* **2005**, *25*, 1279–1291. [CrossRef]

49. Smith, A.R.; Chein, J.; Steinberg, L. Impact of socio-emotional context, brain development, and pubertal maturation on adolescent risk-taking. *Horm. Behav.* **2013**, *64*, 323–332. [CrossRef]

50. Sturman, D.A.; Moghaddam, B. The neurobiology of adolescence: Changes in brain architecture, functional dynamics, and behavioral tendencies. *Neurosci. Biobehav. Rev.* **2011**, *35*, 1704–1712. [CrossRef]

51. Ernst, M.; Daniele, T.; Frantz, K. New perspectives on adolescent motivated behavior: Attention and conditioning. *Dev. Cogn. Neurosci.* **2011**, *1*, 377–389. [CrossRef] [PubMed]

52. Silvers, J.A.; McRae, K.; Gabrieli, J.D.; Gross, J.J.; Remy, K.A.; Ochsner, K.N. Age-related differences in emotional reactivity, regulation, and rejection sensitivity in adolescence. *Emotion* **2012**, *12*, 1235–1247. [CrossRef]

53. Hare, T.A.; Tottenham, N.; Galvan, A.; Voss, H.U.; Glover, G.H.; Casey, B.J. Biological substrates of emotional reactivity and regulation in adolescence during an emotional go-nogo task. *Biol. Psychiatry* **2008**, *63*, 927–934. [CrossRef] [PubMed]

54. Quevedo, K.M.; Benning, S.D.; Gunnar, M.R.; Dahl, R.E. The onset of puberty: Effects on the psychophysiology of defensive and appetitive motivation. *Dev. Psychopathol.* **2009**, *21*, 27–45. [CrossRef] [PubMed]

55. Dwyer, D.B.; Falkai, P.; Koutsouleris, N. Machine learning approaches for clinical psychology and psychiatry. *Annu. Rev. Clin. Psychol.* **2018**, *14*, 91–118. [CrossRef]

56. Foster, K.R.; Koprowski, R.; Skufca, J.D. Machine learning, medical diagnosis, and biomedical engineering research–commentary. *Biomed. Eng. Online* **2014**, *13*, 94–103. [CrossRef]

57. Bzdok, D.; Meyer-Lindenberg, A. Machine learning for precision psychiatry: Opportunities and challenges. *Biol. Psychiatry: Cogn. Neurosci. Neuroimaging* **2018**, *3*, 223–230. [CrossRef] [PubMed]

58. Iniesta, R.; Stahl, D.; McGuffin, P. Machine learning, statistical learning and the future of biological research in psychiatry. *Psychol. Med.* **2016**, *46*, 2455–2465. [CrossRef] [PubMed]

59. IMAGEN. Welcome to the IMAGEN Study. Available online: https://imagen-europe.com/ (accessed on 25 January 2019).

60. CONNECTOME. Connectome Coordination Facility. Available online: https://www.humanconnectome.org (accessed on 25 January 2019).

61. NCANDA. National Consortium on Alcohol and Neurodevelopment in Adolescence. Available online: http://ncanda.org (accessed on 25 January 2019).

62. ABCD. Adolescent Brain Cognitive Development Study. Available online: https://abcdstudy.org (accessed on 25 January 2019).

63. Marcus, D.S.; Harms, M.P.; Snyder, A.Z.; Jenkinson, M.; Wilson, J.A.; Glasser, M.F.; Barch, D.M.; Archie, K.A.; Burgess, G.C.; Ramaratnam, M.; et al. Human Connectome Project informatics: Quality control, database services, and data visualization. *NeuroImage* **2013**, *80*, 202–219. [CrossRef] [PubMed]

64. Jernigan, T.L.; Brown, S.A. Introduction. *Dev. Cogn. Neurosci.* **2018**, *32*, 1–3. [CrossRef]

65. Deng, L.; Yu, D. Deep Learning: Methods and Applications. *Found. Trends Signal* **2014**, *7*, 197–387. [CrossRef]

66. LeCun, Y.; Bengio, Y.; Hinton, G. Deep learning. *Nature* **2015**, *521*, 436–444. [CrossRef] [PubMed]

67. Marblestone, A.H.; Wayne, G.; Kording, K.P. Toward an integration of deep learning and neuroscience. *Front. Comput. Neurosci.* **2016**, *10*, 1–41. [CrossRef] [PubMed]

68. Tarca, A.L.; Carey, V.J.; Chen, X.W.; Romero, R.; Draghici, S. Machine learning and its applications to biology. *PLoS Comput. Biol.* **2007**, *3*, e116. [CrossRef] [PubMed]

69. Varoquaux, G.; Craddock, R.C. Learning and comparing functional connectomes across subjects. *NeuroImage* **2013**, *80*, 405–415. [CrossRef] [PubMed]

70. Varoquaux, G.; Raamana, P.R.; Engemann, D.A.; Hoyos-Idrobo, A.; Schwartz, Y.; Thirion, B. Assessing and tuning brain decoders: Cross-validation, caveats, and guidelines. *NeuroImage* **2017**, *145*, 166–179. [CrossRef] [PubMed]

71. Gleason, P.M.; Boushey, C.J.; Harris, J.E.; Zoellner, J. Publishing nutrition research: A review of multivariate techniques—Part 3: Data reduction methods. *J. Acad. Nutr. Diet.* **2015**, *115*, 1072–1082. [CrossRef]
72. Ernst, M.; Spear, L.P. Reward systems. In *Handbook of Developmental Social Neuroscience*; de Haan, M., Gunnar, M.R., Eds.; Guilford Press: New York, NY, USA, 2009; pp. 324–341.

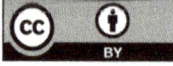

brain sciences

MDPI

Article

Decreased Neuron Density and Increased Glia Density in the Ventromedial Prefrontal Cortex (Brodmann Area 25) in Williams Syndrome

Linnea Wilder [1], Kari L. Hanson [1], Caroline H. Lew [1], Ursula Bellugi [2] and Katerina Semendeferi [1,*

[1]   Department of Anthropology, Social Sciences Building Rm. 210, University of California, San Diego, 9500 Gilman Drive, La Jolla, CA 92093-0532, USA; llwilder@ucsd.edu (L.W.), k1hanson@ucsd.edu (K.L.H.), cfhorton@ucsd.edu (C.H.L.)
[2]   Laboratory for Cognitive Neuroscience, Salk Institute for Biological Studies, 10010 N. Torrey Pines Rd., La Jolla, CA 92037, USA; bellugi@salk.edu
*   Correspondence: ksemende@ucsd.edu; Tel.: +1-858-822-0750

Received: 25 September 2018; Accepted: 27 November 2018; Published: 29 November 2018

Abstract: Williams Syndrome (WS) is a neurodevelopmental disorder caused by a deletion of 25–28 genes on chromosome 7 and characterized by a specific behavioral phenotype, which includes hypersociability and anxiety. Here, we examined the density of neurons and glia in fourteen human brains in Brodmann area 25 (BA 25), in the ventromedial prefrontal cortex (vmPFC), using a postmortem sample of five adult and two infant WS brains and seven age-, sex- and hemisphere-matched typically developing control (TD) brains. We found decreased neuron density, which reached statistical significance in the supragranular layers, and increased glia density and glia to neuron ratio, which reached statistical significance in both supra- and infragranular layers. Combined with our previous findings in the amygdala, caudate nucleus and frontal pole (BA 10), these results in the vmPFC suggest that abnormalities in frontostriatal and frontoamygdala circuitry may contribute to the anxiety and atypical social behavior observed in WS.

Keywords: Williams Syndrome; neuron density; glia density; ventromedial prefrontal cortex

1. Introduction

Williams Syndrome (WS) is a rare (<1 in 7500) neurodevelopmental disorder resulting from a deletion of approximately 25–28 genes on chromosome band 7q11.23 [1]. Individuals with WS have a specific and well defined cognitive and behavioral phenotype. The cognitive profile of WS is characterized by deficits in global IQ and spatial processing, and relatively preserved language and face processing. However, even in these relatively spared skills, WS individuals demonstrate delayed and abnormal development, along with atypical cognitive processing during some language and face tasks [2,3]. WS behavior is marked by high levels of sociability and anxiety. WS individuals have a high drive to engage in social interactions with others, and a tendency to approach even unfamiliar individuals to engage them in conversation [4,5]. In striking contrast to this, Autism Spectrum Disorders (ASD) are characterized often by social avoidance [6,7]. Unlike WS, ASD are genetically complex and heterogenous [6,7]. Interestingly, however, duplication of the WS gene deletion appears to cause ASD in a small subset of cases, demonstrating the range of behavioral effects that alterations at this locus can cause [8].

Abnormalities in the structure and function of the prefrontal cortex (PFC) have been demonstrated in imaging studies of WS. Overall cortical surface area, including surface area in two regions linked to emotion processing and social behavior, the orbital and medial prefrontal cortices, is decreased in WS. Cortical thickness, however, appears increased in these regions, and relative to brain size, total gray matter volume may also be increased in the orbital and medial prefrontal cortices in WS [9–11]. Functional imaging studies (fMRI) provide evidence of deficits in behavioral inhibition in WS. WS subjects had slower response times on an inhibition task than TD controls and displayed lower levels of activation in the striatum and frontal cortex [12]. These abnormalities in fronto-striatal circuitry, and deficits in behavioral inhibition may relate to WS hypersociability, which has been described as an inability to inhibit the desire to approach and engage with others [13,14]. In a functional imaging study examining response to threat, WS individuals displayed lower levels of activation in the amygdala and ventromedial prefrontal cortex vmPFC while viewing threatening faces, but higher levels of activation in these regions while viewing threatening scenes, compared to TD controls [15]. Atypical communication between frontal and limbic regions has been suggested as a possible factor in the high anxiety seen in WS [16]. At the cellular level, microstructural analyses of WS subjects demonstrated lower neuronal density in the infragranular layers of the rostral orbitofrontal cortex [17] An increase in the ratio of glia to neurons, and in the density of oligodendrocytes in WS, has been found in the in the medial caudate nucleus, a region that receives projections from the vmPFC [18,19]. In the amygdala of WS subjects, neuron number was higher in the lateral nucleus [20]. Taken together, these findings suggest that abnormalities in PFC cytoarchitecture, and altered prefrontal inhibitory control of the amygdala and striatum, may be linked to the atypical anxiety and social behavior characteristic of WS.

Here, we examined one area of the vmPFC, Brodmann area 25 (BA 25), that is critically involved in social behaviors and related functions of inhibition and decision making [21]. This area is heavily connected to several subcortical structures, including the amygdala and striatum, both of which are altered in WS, and in other disorders including autism [18,20,22–24]. Using postmortem tissue from ten adult and four infant subjects, seven WS and seven age, sex, and hemisphere matched typically developing (TD) controls, we measured the density of neurons and glia in the supragranular (II/III) and infragranular (V/VI) layers of BA 25 in the vmPFC to test whether the previously observed decreases in neuron density in WS are restricted to rostral orbitofrontal cortical areas, or if there are widespread alterations to the frontal cortex in WS.

2. Materials and Methods

2.1. Brain Tissue

We examined cortical tissue from BA 25 in the vmPFC in a total of fourteen postmortem human subjects, including five adult WS and five adult TD subjects, as well as two WS infant subjects and two TD infant subjects (Table 1). TD subjects were matched with WS subjects for age (110/114 and 234/245 days for infants, 18–43 years for adults), sex, and hemisphere (right), to control for possible cytoarchitectonic asymmetries and age and sex-related differences [25,26].

Table 1. Subject Information.

Subject	Age at Death	Sex	Hemisphere	PMI (h)	Cause of Death
WS 7	114 days	M	R	<30	Multiorgan failure
TD 5883	110 days	M	R	34	Sudden unexplained death in infancy
WS 2	245 days	F	R	N/A	Sudden infant death syndrome
TD 4392	234 days	F	R	13	Intussuseption of Meckel's diverticulum
WS 10	18 years	M	R	24	Cardiac complications
TD 4916	19 years	M	R	5	Drowning
WS 15	24 years	F	R	20	Pneumonia, Sepsis
TD 5350	25 years	F	R	26	Sepsis
WS 1	31 years	M	R	26	Cardiac complications
TD 5539	31 years	M	R	24	Acute drug intoxication
WS 14	42 years	F	R	18	Cardiac complications
TD 5445	42 years	F	R	10	Pulmonary thromboembolism
WS 9	43 years	F	R	12	Cardiac complications
TD 4636	43 years	F	R	19	Pulmonary thromboembolism

WS: Williams Syndrome; TD: typically developing control; PMI: post mortem interval in hours.

All subjects in the Bellugi Williams Syndrome Brain Collection are part of an ongoing donation-based program now run by the Laboratory for Human Comparative Neuroanatomy at UCSD (La Jolla, CA, USA).

2.2. Regions of Interest

The region of interest (ROI) was identified using anatomical landmarks and by the absence of any visible border between cortical layers II and III and between layers V and VI. BA 25 occupies a portion of the brain immediately caudal and ventral to genu of the corpus callosum. It is agranular, lacking a visible layer IV, and poorly laminated compared to surrounding cortical areas [27,28]. Cortical layers II/III and V/VI were analyzed as two distinct ROIs (Figure 1).

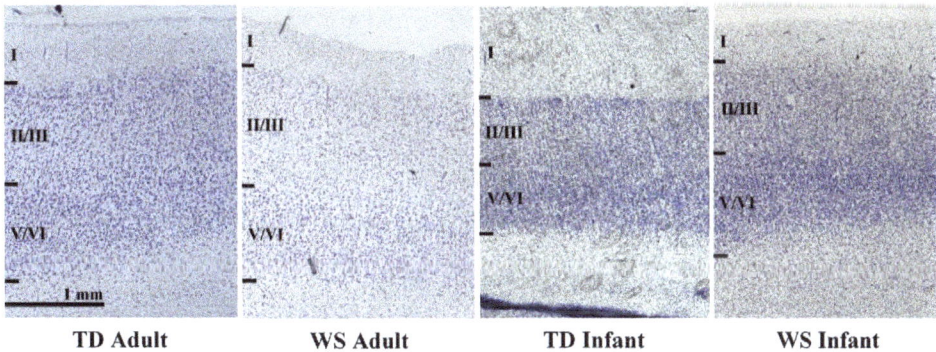

| TD Adult | WS Adult | TD Infant | WS Infant |

Figure 1. Microphotographs of Brodmann area 25 (BA 25) in adult and infant Williams Syndrome (WS) and typically developing control (TD). Images taken at 2×.

2.3. Processing of Tissue

Blocks of tissue containing BA 25 were extracted and cryoprotected using a series of 10%, 20%, and 30% sucrose solutions with 0.1 M phosphate buffer until saturated. Frozen tissue was cut on a Leica SM 2010R (Leica Biosystems, Wetzlar, Germany) sliding microtome into ten series of 40 micrometer (μm) thick sections in adult subjects. Due to the fragility of infant tissue, infant subjects were cut into five series of 80 μm thick sections. One series was rehydrated for 48 h in a neutral phosphate buffer, then mounted on gelatin-coated slides. Mounted sections were dried for 48 h at room temperature, then dehydrated in a 1:1 chloroform ethanol solution overnight. These sections were stained with a 0.25% thionine stain for Nissl substance to visualize cell bodies, rehydrated, submerged in xylenes or citrisolv for 15 min after staining, and then cover-slipped with permount. The remaining series were stored for use in later processing, including a variety of immunohistological staining experiments.

2.4. Unbiased, Design-Based Stereology

Data collection was performed using StereoInvestigator software (MBF Bioscience, Williston, VT, USA) on a Dell workstation receiving live video feed from an Optronics MicroFire color video camera (East Muskogee, OK, USA) attached to a Nikon Eclipse 80i microscope (Nikon Instruments, Melville, NY, USA) equipped with a Ludl MAC5000 stage (Ludl, Hawthorn, NY, USA) and a Heidenhain z-axis encoder (Heidenhain, Plymouth, MN, USA). To increase the accuracy and consistency of measurements across all subjects, we report neuron and glia density rather than number, a standard practice for data collection in the cortex [17,29–31].

All data were collected by a single rater (LW). Inter-rater reliability was ensured through repeated neuron density estimations on a sample previously reported in the literature to 95% concordance [17]. Sections were coded before data collection to blind the rater to diagnosis. Six sections per subject, spaced as equidistantly as allowed by individual section quality, were analyzed, representing the maximum extent of the area in the coronal plane. Neuron and glia densities in layers II/III and V/VI were estimated using the Optical Fractionator probe in StereoInvestigator. Two regions of interest per section, one bounding layers II/III and the other bounding layers V/VI, were drawn at a 1× magnification, consistent with previous work on WS cortex [17]. BA 25 in adults has no visible layer IV. Neurons and glia were counted using a 1.4 numerical aperture, 100× oil objective lens, with a grid size of 300 × 300 microns, a dissector height of 9 microns, and a counting frame of 85 × 85 microns. For infant subjects, a 50 × 50 micron counting frame was used. Within this frame, neurons and glia not touching the line of exclusion were counted using different markers. Cells were distinguished based on their morphology. Neurons were identified by the presence of a distinct nucleolus, and a lightly stained nucleus surrounded by cytoplasm. Glia were identified by their smaller size and lightly or darkly stained nucleus, with very little or no staining of the surrounding cytoplasm (Figure 2) [32]. For each ROI (layers II/III and layers V/VI, respectively), neuron and glia densities were calculated by dividing population estimate of each cell type by the planimetric volume estimate from the Optical Fractionator probe.

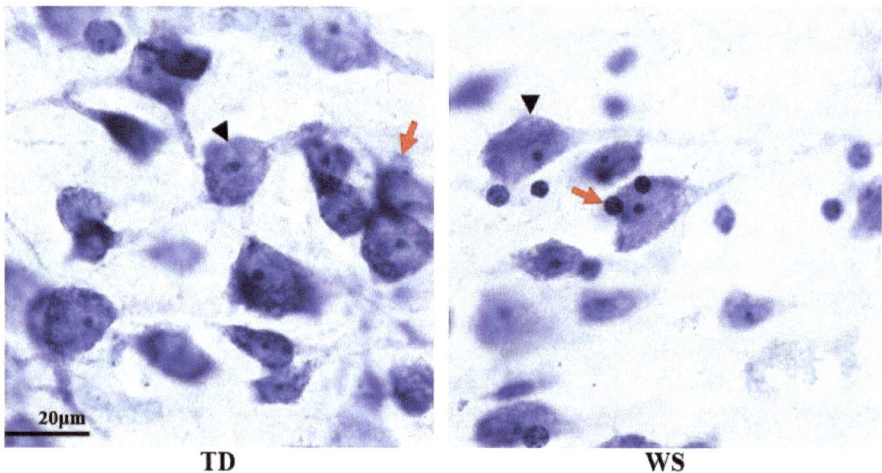

TD   **WS**

Figure 2. Microphotograph of BA 25 adult WS and TD. Neurons (black arrowheads) were distinguished from glia (red arrows) by their large size and distinctly stained nucleolus. Images taken at 100×.

2.5. Statistical Analysis

Standard two-tailed *t*-tests ($p < 0.05$) were used to compare neuron density, glia density, and glia to neuron ratio in WS and TD. Supragranular and infragranular layers were compared separately, as well as the average density of these layers combined. Percent difference in WS compared to TD was calculated as the difference in mean value of WS from TD, in relation to the mean TD value, for neuron density, glia density, and glia to neuron ratio, in each ROI.

3. Results

3.1. Adult Neuron Density

Results are summarized in Table 2 and Figure 3. In supragranular layers, neuron density was significantly decreased in WS compared to TD ($p = 0.046$, 17% decrease). Neuron density infragranular layers were decreased in WS, but this was not statistically significant ($p = 0.186$, 9% decrease).

Table 2. Mean Neuron Density (neurons/mm$^{3)}$ and Standard Deviation in BA 25.

Cortical Layers	II/III	V/VI
TD	30,882 ± 2537	36,506 ± 2567
WS	25,594 ± 4157	33,094 ± 4417
% Difference	−17%	−9%

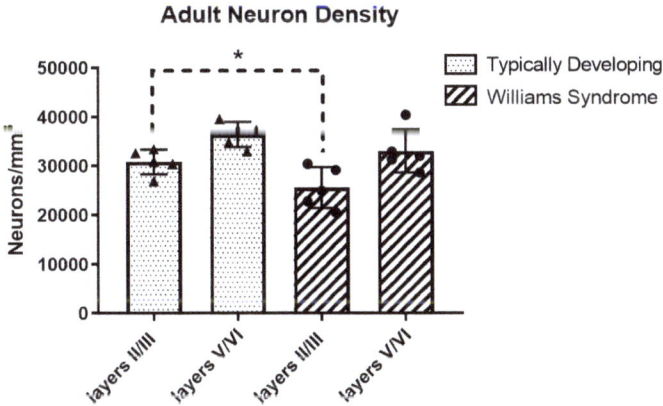

Figure 3. Mean neuron density in adults. * Statistically significant results.

3.2. Adult Glia Density and Glia to Neuron Ratio

Results are summarized in Tables 3 and 4, and Figure 4. Mean glia density was significantly increased in WS compared to TD, in both supragranular (83% increase, $p = 0.00007$) and infragranular (116% increase, $p = 0.000001$) layers. Glia to neuron ratio was also increased in WS compared to TD in supragranular (125% increase, $p = 0.003$) and infragranular (140%, $p = 0.0003$) layers.

Table 3. Mean Glia Density (glia/mm$^{3)}$ and Standard Deviation in BA 25.

Cortical Layers	II/III	V/VI
TD	18,756 ± 426	19,721 ± 465
WS	34,355 ± 2038	42,510 ± 1844
% Difference	+83%	+116%

Table 4. Glia to Neuron Ratio in BA 25.

Cortical Layers	II/III	V/VI
TD	0.61	0.54
WS	1.38	1.30
% Difference	+125%	+140%

Adult Glia Density

Adult Glia:Neuron Ratio

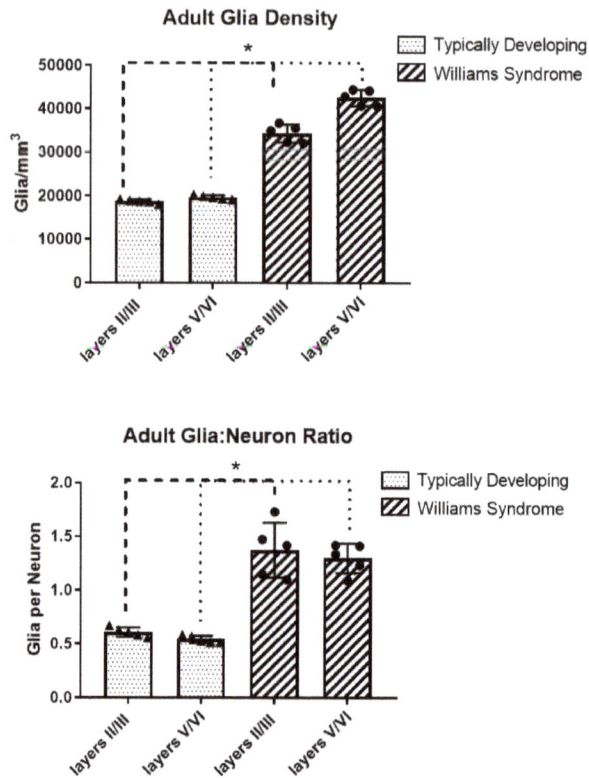

Figure 4. Mean glia density and glia to neuron ratio in adults. * Statistically significant results.

3.3. Infant Neuron Density, Glia Density, and Glia to Neuron Ratio

Results are summarized in Figure 5. In the 114 (WS) and 110 (TD) day-old subject pair, neuron density, glia density, and glia to neuron ratio were quite similar between the TD and WS subject in the supragranular layers (within 1%). In the infragranular layers, neuron density, glia density, and glia to neuron ratio were lower in the WS subject (33% lower, 55% lower, and 16% lower respectively). In the 234- and 245-day pair, across all layers, neuron density was lower (35% lower supragranular, 16% lower infragranular), and glia density (5% higher supragranular, 16% higher infragranular) and glia to neuron ratio (63% higher supragranular, 61% higher infragranular) were both higher in the WS subject.

Table 5 summarizes results for all ages.

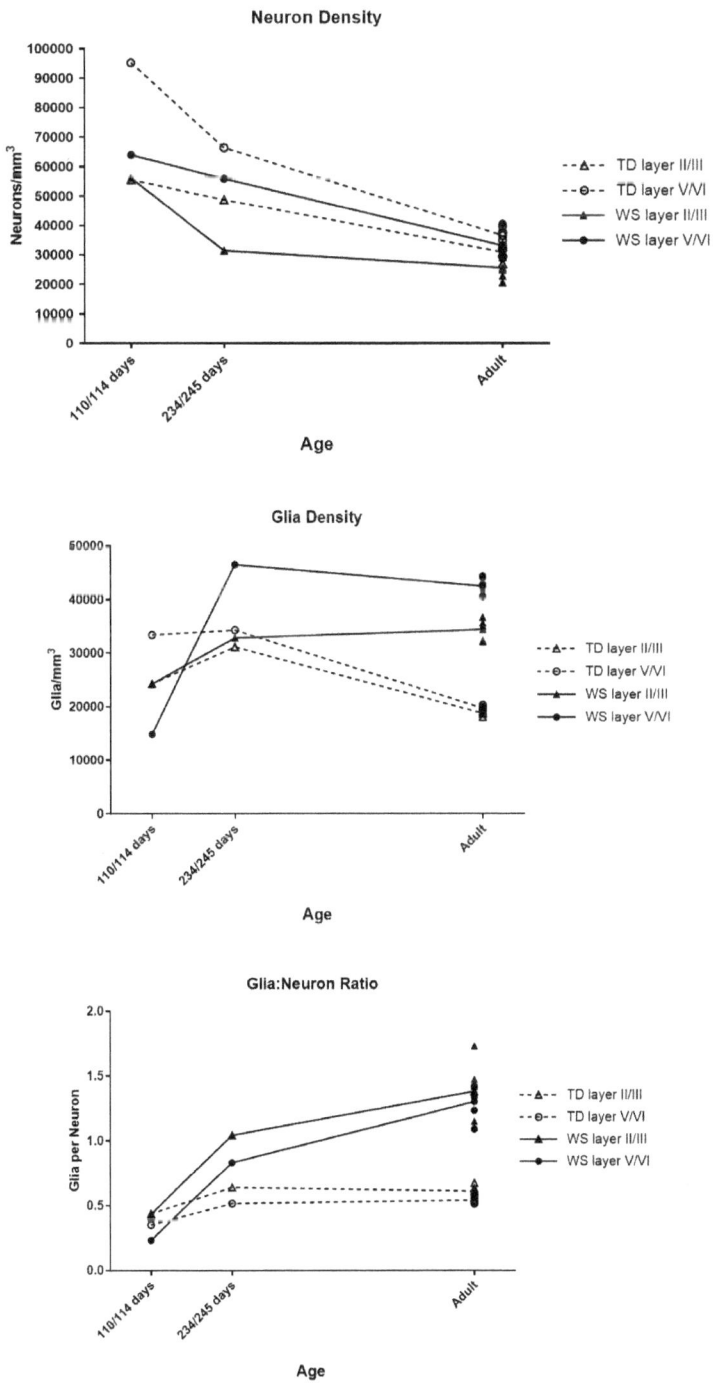

Figure 5. Neuron density, glia density, and glia to neuron ratio in infants.

Table 5. Summary table of results.

Age	Layer	Neuron Density	Glia Density
4 months	II/III	No difference	No difference
	V/VI	33% Lower	16% Lower
8 months	II/III	35% Lower	5% Higher
	V/VI	16% Lower	16% Higher
Adult	II/III	17% Lower *	83% Higher *
	V/VI	9% Lower	116% Higher *

* Statistically significant results.

4. Discussion

Very few histological studies of BA 25 in TD adults have been conducted [27,33,34], and none on infants. All data from these few adult studies are qualitative rather than quantitative. The present study provides the first quantitative data for neuron and glia density in TD adult and infant BA 25. Our findings demonstrate variation in cell density between cortical layers consistent with expected patterns based on adult TD brains from the limited reports available. Qualitative description of human BA 25, along with quantitative findings in macaques, show that caudal, agranular regions of the vmPFC, such as BA 25, are characterized by higher neuron density in infragranular layers compared to supragranular layers, and lower glia density than neuron density in all layers [27,28]. As expected, neuron density is much higher in infants than adults [35]. This study builds on previous research on the adult PFC in both TD and WS, a region implicated in the behavioral phenotype of the disorder, and is the first to examine the PFC in WS infants [9,17,35].

Adults: A previous postmortem histological study of WS, which included three of the same adult WS subjects utilized here, along with an additional three adult WS subjects and six adult TD controls, found decreased neuron density in BA 10 and 11 of the prefrontal cortex (PFC), with the greatest difference observed in the infragranular layers [17]. A study on the morphology of basal dendrites in adult WS subjects found that dendritic length and branching were compromised in the supragranular layers in BA 10 and 11, relative to more posterior areas of the cortex, BA 4, 3 and 18 [36]. Based on the above study, we expected to find decreased neuron density in BA 25 in WS adults compared to TD adults, which is consistent with our results. This difference was greater in supragranular layers than in infragranular layers. In the present study, we additionally found significant increases in glia density and glia to neuron ratio, in both supragranular and infragranular layers of BA 25 in WS adults. An increase in glia was also observed in the caudate nucleus in WS, which seems to be driven by an increase in oligodendrocytes [18].

Infants: As expected, in both the TD and WS infants, overall neuron density was lower in the eight-month-old subjects than in the four-month-old subjects. In the TD infants, this difference was greatest in infragranular layers, while in WS infants there was a greater decrease in supragranular layers. Additionally, glia density increased with age in both the TD and WS infants, although this increase was far greater in WS. In the older TD infant, both neuron density and glia density were elevated compared to adult TD subjects, but glia to neuron ratio was very close to the adult mean. In the older WS infant, neuron density was elevated compared to adult WS. However, overall glia density in this subject was similar to the WS adult mean, and glia to neuron ratio was much lower.

In the youngest infant pair examined here (about four months old), differences in both neuron and glia density between TD and WS appear almost exclusively in the infragranular layers. Additionally, this was the only pair examined in which the WS subject had lower glia density than the TD subject. In the older infant pair (about eight months old) examined here, differences in neuron and glia density occurred in a similar pattern as was seen in adults. There was a greater difference in neuron density in supragranular layers, and a greater difference in glia density in infragranular layers, suggesting that this pattern is not present at birth, but is established in infancy. At both time points in the infants, overall neuron density was lower in WS than TD, as it is in adults, but the difference in neuron density in the supragranular layers may develop postnatally, in infancy. In the four-month-old infant pair, glia density was lower in WS than in TD, in contrast to all other pairs examined. Although these results represent only two WS infants, one at each age point, this suggests there may be disruptions in prenatal gliogenesis or glial migration in WS, followed by a significant increase in glial cells which begins in infancy, and continues beyond the ages of the infants included in this study.

Here, we demonstrated decreased neuron density in WS compared to TD subjects starting in early infancy; and increased in glia density in WS older infants and adults compared to TDs, but not in the youngest infant pair examined. Although the exact mechanisms for the decrease in neuron density, and the differences in glia development observed here in BA 25 in WS are unknown, they may be due in part to the deletion of GTF2I, GTF2IRD1, and FZD9 genes crucially involved in neural development, cell division, and cell fate and neuroinflammatory processes increasing glia and decreasing neuronal survival [37–39]. Given that the decrease in neuron density in BA 25 is present even early in the first year of life, it likely results from a combination of deficient neurogenesis prenatally and increased apoptosis prenatally, possibly extending slightly into the postnatal period. WS neural progenitor cells (NPCs), differentiated from WS induced pluripotent stem cells (iPSCs), were found to have increased doubling time, resulting in a smaller population of NPCs, and increased levels of apoptosis compared to TD NPCs. FZD9 appears to be critically involved in these processes in WS. By restoring FZD9, both apoptosis and the doubling time of WS NPCs and apoptosis were reduced to a similar level as in TD controls, creating the same number of NPCs as TD controls [37].

The increase in glia density in BA 25 in WS could be due to excess production of glial cells, deficits in apoptosis, or disrupted migration. Glia have critical roles in neural development and neurological functions, affecting neuronal survival, and synapse formation, elimination, and functioning [40–42]. Changes in glia cells, or in the ratio of glia to neurons, can alter the typical course of neurodevelopment and the formation and functioning of neural circuits [43]. Abnormalities in glia cells have been linked to many neurological or neurodevelopmental disorders, including major depressive disorder, ASD, and schizophrenia [42–44]. Decreased glia density has been found in the orbitofrontal cortex of subjects with major depressive disorder, and increased microglia density has been found in the prefrontal cortex in both ASD and schizophrenia [45–47].

Deletion of FZD9 gene has been shown to affect neural progenitor cells through the canonical Wnt pathway, a pathway necessary to inhibit the differentiation of oligodendrocyte progenitor cells (OPCs) [37,38]. The proliferation of oligodendrocytes occurs in a series of successive waves, beginning prenatally, with later generated cells replacing earlier derived populations [38,48,49]. OPCs continue to proliferate while migrating to white matter until an appropriate density of OPCs has been reached [50]. OPCs remain proliferative in the subventricular zone throughout postnatal life, although cell turnover is low in typically developing adults [38,50].

In typical development, neural stem cells switch from neurogenic to gliogenic, producing astrocytes and then oligodendrocytes, in the prenatal period. The timing of this switch is critical. If the switch happens too early, it can result in overproduction of astrocytes and deficits in some neuronal populations. If it occurs too late, this can reduce the number of astrocytes produced, limiting the signals they provide for axonal guidance, neuronal survival, and synaptogenesis [43,51–53]. Chronic neuroinflammation, which is found in many neurological disorders, could cause increased density and activation of microglia, and potentially atrophy in astrocytes, leading to the excessive pruning of synapse and neuronal death. This may result in underconnectivity in the brain and contribute to the phenotypes of neurodevelopmental disorders [42,44,54]. Inflammation may also alter synaptic transmission through changes to astrocyte function, further affecting cognition and behavior [42].

In contrast to the findings in WS, increases in neuron number have been found in the PFC of young subjects with ASD, age range 2–16 years, with no significant difference in glia number [55]. Impaired connectivity between regions critical to social cognition and emotional regulation may be a common factor underlying some of the social and emotional abnormalities seen in both ASD and WS. In ASD, reduced fractional anisotropy was found in white matter adjacent to the vmPFC, and in the temporal lobe approaching the amygdala, suggesting disrupted connections between frontal and limbic brain regions [56]. Additionally, there is evidence of atypical activation of the vmPFC while evaluating emotional faces, as well as altered functional connectivity in fronto-striatal and fronto-amygdala circuits [57,58]. Although no differences were found in total glia number in the PFC, increased density, along with increased activation, of microglia has been demonstrated in the PFC in ASD [46]. The increased activation of microglia may reflect ongoing neuroinflammatory processes, which may contribute to loss of synaptic connections and under-connectivity in ASD [46].

Neuroinflammatory mechanisms could account for the increased glia density in WS. Although no studies have been conducted to examine microglia in WS specifically, chronic neuroinflammation is common in many neurodevelopmental disorders, including ASD and schizophrenia, and is often the cause of increased glia density [42,44,46,54]. The results from infant subjects suggest that the increased glia density in WS may develop over the first year of life, but it does not appear to be present before 4 months of age. It is not currently known if this increase is restricted to certain types of glia and to frontal and striatal regions, or if it represents a systemic perturbation of glia. Further investigation, utilizing immunohistochemical staining to determine what type of glia cells are affected, and examination of more brain regions in WS could help elucidate this matter.

The results presented here, combined with prior findings of decreased neuron density in BA 10 and 11 in WS, suggest that neuronal abnormalities in WS may be a common feature across the PFC [17]. Additionally, abnormalities have been reported in the striatum and the amygdala in WS, two subcortical structures heavily connected to BA 25 [18,20]. Together, these findings suggest that abnormalities in PFC cytoarchitecture, and altered prefrontal inhibitory control of the amygdala and striatum, may be linked to the atypical anxiety and social behaviors characteristic of WS.

Author Contributions: Conceptualization, L.W. and K.S.; Data curation, L.W.; Formal analysis, L.W.; Funding acquisition, K.S.; Investigation, L.W., K.L.H., and K.S.; Methodology, L.W., K.L.H. and C.H.L.; Resources, U.B. and K.S.; Writing—original draft, L.W.; Writing—review and editing, L.W. and K.S.

Funding: This research was funded by the National Institutes of Health, grant numbers P01 NICHD033113, 5R03MH103697, R56 MH109587.

Acknowledgments: We are extremely grateful to the tissue donors and their families, who made this research possible. WS human tissue was obtained under the Bellugi Williams Syndrome Brain Collection, now curated by K.S. and run by the Laboratory for Human Comparative Neuroanatomy at UCSD. TD human tissue was obtained from the NIH Neurobiobank at the University of Maryland, Baltimore, MD. We additionally thank past and present lab members, Chelsea Brown, Valerie Judd, Hailee Orfant, Kimberly Groeniger, Deion Cuevas, and Branka Hrvoj-Mihic for their help and support.

Conflicts of Interest: The authors declare no conflict of interest.

References

1. Strømme, P.; Bjømstad, P.G.; Ramstad, K. Prevalence Estimation of Williams Syndrome. *J. Child Neurol.* **2002**, *17*, 269–271. [CrossRef] [PubMed]
2. Bellugi, U.; Lichtenberger, L.; Jones, W.; Lai, Z.; St. George, M.I. The Neurocognitive Profile of Williams Syndrome: A Complex Pattern of Strengths and Weaknesses. *J Cognit. Neurosci.* **2000**, *12*, 7–29. [CrossRef]
3. Karmiloff-Smith, A.; Thomas, M.; Annaz, D.; Humphreys, K.; Ewing, S.; Brace, N.; Duuren, M.V.; Pike, G.; Grice, S.; Campbell, R. Exploring the Williams syndrome face-processing debate: The importance of building developmental trajectories. *J. Child Psychol. Psychiatry* **2004**, *45*, 1258–1274. [CrossRef] [PubMed]
4. Doyle, T.F.; Bellugi, U.; Korenberg, J.R.; Graham, J. "Everybody in the world is my friend" hypersociability in young children with Williams syndrome. *Am. J. Med. Genet. Part A* **2004**, *124A*, 263–273. [CrossRef] [PubMed]
5. Klein-Tasman, B.P.; Mervis, C.B. Distinctive Personality Characteristics of 8-, 9-, and 10-Year-Olds with Williams Syndrome. *Dev. Neuropsychol.* **2003**, *23*, 269–290. [CrossRef] [PubMed]

6. Geschwind, D.H. Genetics of autism spectrum disorders. *Trends Cognit. Sci.* **2011**, *15*, 409–416. [CrossRef] [PubMed]

7. Miles, J.H. Autism spectrum disorders—A genetics review. *Genet. Med.* **2011**, *13*, 278–294. [CrossRef] [PubMed]

8. Merla, G.; Brunetti-Pierri, N.; Micale, L.; Fusco, C. Copy number variants at Williams–Beuren syndrome 7q11.23 region. *Human Genet.* **2010**, *128*, 3–26. [CrossRef] [PubMed]

9. Fan, C.C.; Brown, T.T.; Bartsch, H.; Kuperman, J.M.; Hagler, D.J.; Schork, A.; Searcy, Y.; Bellugi, U.; Halgren, E.; Dale, A.M. Williams syndrome-specific neuroanatomical profile and its associations with behavioral features. *NeuroImage: Clin.* **2017**, *15*, 343–347. [CrossRef] [PubMed]

10. Meda, S.A.; Pryweller, J.R.; Thornton-Wells, T.A. Regional Brain Differences in Cortical Thickness, Surface Area and Subcortical Volume in Individuals with Williams Syndrome. *PLoS ONE* **2012**, *7*, e31913. [CrossRef]

11. Reiss, A.L.; Eckert, M.A.; Rose, F.E.; Karchemskiy, A.; Kesler, S.; Chang, M., Reynolds, M.F.; Kwon, H.; Galaburda, A. An Experiment of Nature: Brain Anatomy Parallels Cognition and Behavior in Williams Syndrome. *J. Neurosci.* **2004**, *24*, 5009–5015. [CrossRef] [PubMed]

12. Mobbs, D.; Eckert, M.A.; Mills, D.; Korenberg, J.; Bellugi, U.; Galaburda, A.M.; Reiss, A.L. Frontostriatal Dysfunction During Response Inhibition in Williams Syndrome. *Biol. Psychiatry* **2007**, *62*, 256–261. [CrossRef] [PubMed]

13. Jones, W.; Bellugi, U.; Lai, Z.; Chiles, M.; Reilly, J.; Lincoln, A.; Adolphs, R. II. Hypersociability in Williams Syndrome. *J. Cognit. Neurosci.* **2000**, *12*, 30–46. [CrossRef]

14. Porter, M.A.; Coltheart, M.; Langdon, R. The neuropsychological basis of hypersociability in Williams and Down syndrome. *Neuropsychologia* **2007**, *45*, 2839–2849. [CrossRef] [PubMed]

15. Meyer-Lindenberg, A.; Hariri, A.R.; Munoz, K.E.; Mervis, C.B.; Mattay, V.S.; Morris, C.A.; Berman, K.F. Neural correlates of genetically abnormal social cognition in Williams syndrome. *Nat. Neurosci.* **2005**, *8*, 991–993. [CrossRef] [PubMed]

16. Ng, R.; Brown, T.T.; Järvinen, A.M.; Erhart, M.; Korenberg, J.R.; Bellugi, U.; Halgren, E. Structural integrity of the limbic–prefrontal connection: Neuropathological correlates of anxiety in Williams syndrome. *Soc. Neurosci.* **2016**, *11*, 187–192. [CrossRef] [PubMed]

17. Lew, C.H.; Brown, C.; Bellugi, U.; Semendeferi, K. Neuron density is decreased in the prefrontal cortex in Williams syndrome. *Autism Res.* **2017**, *10*, 99–112. [CrossRef] [PubMed]

18. Hanson, K.L.; Lew, C.H.; Hrvoj-Mihic, B.; Groeniger, K.M.; Halgren, E.; Bellugi, U.; Semendeferi, K. Increased glia density in the caudate nucleus in williams syndrome: Implications for frontostriatal dysfunction in autism. *Dev. Neurobiol.* **2018**, *78*, 531–545. [CrossRef] [PubMed]

19. Ferry, A.T.; Öngür, D.; An, X.; Price, J.L. Prefrontal cortical projections to the striatum in macaque monkeys: Evidence for an organization related to prefrontal networks. *J. Comp. Neurol.* **2000**, *425*, 447–470. [CrossRef]

20. Lew, C.H.; Groeniger, K.M.; Bellugi, U.; Stefanacci, L.; Schumann, C.M.; Semendeferi, K. A postmortem stereological study of the amygdala in Williams syndrome. *Brain Struct. Funct.* **2018**, *223*, 1897–1907. [CrossRef] [PubMed]

21. Ruff, C.C.; Fehr, E. The neurobiology of rewards and values in social decision making. *Nat. Rev. Neurosci.* **2014**, *15*, 549–562. [CrossRef] [PubMed]

22. Barbas, H.; Zikopoulos, B. Sequential and parallel circuits for emotional processing in primate orbitofrontal cortex. *Orbitofront. Cortex* **2006**, *1*, 57–93.

23. Schumann, C.M.; Amaral, D.G. Stereological Analysis of Amygdala Neuron Number in Autism. *J. Neurosci.* **2006**, *26*, 7674–7679. [CrossRef] [PubMed]

24. Morgan, J.T.; Barger, N.; Amaral, D.G.; Schumann, C.M. Stereological Study of Amygdala Glial Populations in Adolescents and Adults with Autism Spectrum Disorder. *PLoS ONE* **2014**, *9*, e110356. [CrossRef] [PubMed]

25. Rentería, M.E. Cerebral Asymmetry: A Quantitative, Multifactorial, and Plastic Brain Phenotype. *Twin Res. Hum. Genet.* **2012**, *15*, 401–413. [CrossRef] [PubMed]

26. Zilles, K.; Schleicher, A.; Langemann, C.; Amunts, K.; Morosan, P.; Palomero-Gallagher, N.; Schormann, T.; Mohlberg, H.; Bürgel, U.; Steinmetz, H.; et al. Quantitative analysis of sulci in the human cerebral cortex: Development, regional heterogeneity, gender difference, asymmetry, intersubject variability and cortical architecture. *Hum. Brain Mapp.* **1997**, *5*, 218–221. [CrossRef]

27. Öngür, D.; Ferry, A.T.; Price, J.L. Architectonic subdivision of the human orbital and medial prefrontal cortex. *J. Comp. Neurol.* **2003**, *460*, 425–449. [CrossRef] [PubMed]

28. Dombrowski, S.M.; Hilgetag, C.C.; Barbas, H. Quantitative Architecture Distinguishes Prefrontal Cortical Systems in the Rhesus Monkey. *Cereb. Cortex* **2001**, *11*, 975–988. [CrossRef] [PubMed]

29. Benes, F.M.; Davidson, J.; Bird, E.D. Quantitative Cytoarchitectural Studies of the Cerebral Cortex of Schizophrenics. *Arch. Gen. Psychiatry* **1986**, *43*, 31–35. [CrossRef] [PubMed]

30. Oblak, A.L.; Rosene, D.L.; Kemper, T.L.; Bauman, M.L.; Blatt, G.J. Altered posterior cingulate cortical cyctoarchitecture, but normal density of neurons and interneurons in the posterior cingulate cortex and fusiform gyrus in autism. *Autism Res.* **2011**, *4*, 200–211. [CrossRef] [PubMed]

31. Smiley, J.F.; Konnova, K.; Bleiwas, C. Cortical thickness, neuron density and size in the inferior parietal lobe in schizophrenia. *Schizophr. Res.* **2012**, *136*, 43–50. [CrossRef] [PubMed]

32. García-Cabezas, M.Á.; John, Y.J.; Barbas, H.; Zikopoulos, B. Distinction of Neurons, Glia and Endothelial Cells in the Cerebral Cortex: An Algorithm Based on Cytological Features. *Front. Neuroanat.* **2016**, *10*. [CrossRef] [PubMed]

33. Mackey, S.; Petrides, M. Quantitative demonstration of comparable architectonic areas within the ventromedial and lateral orbital frontal cortex in the human and the macaque monkey brains. *Eur. J. Neurosci.* **2010**, *32*, 1940–1950. [CrossRef] [PubMed]

34. Mackey, S.; Petrides, M. Architecture and morphology of the human ventromedial prefrontal cortex. *Eur. J. Neurosci.* **2014**, *40*, 2777–2796. [CrossRef] [PubMed]

35. Huttenlocher, P.R. Morphometric study of human cerebral cortex development. *Neuropsychologia* **1990**, *28*, 517–527. [CrossRef]

36. Hrvoj-Mihic, B.; Hanson, K.L.; Lew, C.H.; Stefanacci, L.; Jacobs, B.; Bellugi, U.; Semendeferi, K. Basal Dendritic Morphology of Cortical Pyramidal Neurons in Williams Syndrome: Prefrontal Cortex and Beyond. *Front. Neurosci.* **2017**, *11*. [CrossRef] [PubMed]

37. Chailangkarn, T.; Trujillo, C.A.; Freitas, B.C.; Hrvoj-Mihic, B.; Herai, R.H.; Yu, D.X.; Brown, T.T.; Marchetto, M.C.; Bardy, C.; McHenry, L.; et al. A human neurodevelopmental model for Williams syndrome. *Nature* **2016**, *536*, 338–343. [CrossRef] [PubMed]

38. Mitew, S.; Hay, C.M.; Peckham, H.; Xiao, J.; Koenning, M.; Emery, B. Mechanisms regulating the development of oligodendrocytes and central nervous system myelin. *Neuroscience* **2014**, *276*, 29–47. [CrossRef] [PubMed]

39. Sakurai, T.; Dorr, N.P.; Takahashi, N.; McInnes, L.A.; Elder, G.A.; Buxbaum, J.D. Haploinsufficiency of Gtf2i, a gene deleted in Williams Syndrome, leads to increases in social interactions. *Autism Res.* **2011**, *4*, 28–39. [CrossRef] [PubMed]

40. Bayraktar, O.A.; Fuentealba, L.C.; Alvarez-Buylla, A.; Rowitch, D.H. Astrocyte Development and Heterogeneity. *Cold Spring Harb. Perspect. Biol.* **2015**, *7*, a020362. [CrossRef] [PubMed]

41. Molofsky, A.V.; Krenick, R.; Ullian, E.; Tsai, H.; Deneen, B.; Richardson, W.D.; Barres, B.A.; Rowitch, D.H. Astrocytes and disease: A neurodevelopmental perspective. *Genes. Dev.* **2012**, *26*, 891–907. [CrossRef] [PubMed]

42. Petrelli, F.; Pucci, L.; Bezzi, P. Astrocytes and Microglia and Their Potential Link with Autism Spectrum Disorders. *Front. Cell. Neurosci.* **2016**, *10*. [CrossRef] [PubMed]

43. Sloan, S.A.; Barres, B.A. Mechanisms of astrocyte development and their contributions to neurodevelopmental disorders. *Curr. Opin. Neurobiol.* **2014**, *27*, 75–81. [CrossRef] [PubMed]

44. Zhan, Y.; Paolicelli, R.C.; Sforazzini, F.; Weinhard, L.; Bolasco, G.; Pagani, F.; Vyssotski, A.L.; Bifone, A.; Gozzi, A.; Ragozzino, D.; et al. Deficient neuron-microglia signaling results in impaired functional brain connectivity and social behavior. *Nat. Neurosci.* **2014**, *17*, 400–406. [CrossRef] [PubMed]

45. Rajkowska, G.; Miguel-Hidalgo, J.J.; Wei, J.; Dilley, G.; Pittman, S.D.; Meltzer, H.Y.; Overholser, J.C.; Roth, B.L.; Stockmeier, C.A. Morphometric evidence for neuronal and glial prefrontal cell pathology in major depression. *Biol. Psychiatry* **1999**, *45*, 1085–1098. [CrossRef]

46. Morgan, J.T.; Chana, G.; Pardo, C.A.; Achim, C.; Semendeferi, K.; Buckwalter, J.; Courchesne, E.; Everall, I.P. Microglial Activation and Increased Microglial Density Observed in the Dorsolateral Prefrontal Cortex in Autism. *Biol. Psychiatry* **2010**, *68*, 368–376. [CrossRef] [PubMed]

47. Garey, L. When cortical development goes wrong: Schizophrenia as a neurodevelopmental disease of microcircuits. *J. Anat.* **2010**, *217*, 324–333. [CrossRef] [PubMed]

48. Kessaris, N.; Fogarty, M.; Iannarelli, P.; Grist, M.; Wegner, M.; Richardson, W.D. Competing waves of oligodendrocytes in the forebrain and postnatal elimination of an embryonic lineage. *Nat. Neurosci.* **2006**, *9*, 173–179. [CrossRef] [PubMed]

Brain Sci. **2018**, *8*, 209

49. Lee, J.C.; Mayer-Proschel, M.; Rao, M.S. Gliogenesis in the central nervous system. *Glia* **2000**, *30*, 105–121. [CrossRef]

50. Orentas, D.M.; Miller, R.H. Regulation of oligodendrocyte development. *Mol. Neurobiol.* **1998**, *18*, 247–259. [CrossRef] [PubMed]

51. Homem, C.C.F.; Repic, M.; Knoblich, J.A. Proliferation control in neural stem and progenitor cells. *Nat. Rev. Neurosci.* **2015**, *16*, 647–659. [CrossRef] [PubMed]

52. Kohwi, M.; Doe, C.Q. Temporal fate specification and neural progenitor competence during development. *Nat. Rev. Neurosci.* **2013**, *14*, 823–838. [CrossRef] [PubMed]

53. Ren, Q.; Yang, C.-P.; Liu, Z.; Sugino, K.; Mok, K.; He, Y.; Ito, M.; Nern, A.; Otsuna, H.; Lee, T. Stem Cell-Intrinsic, Seven-up-Triggered Temporal Factor Gradients Diversify Intermediate Neural Progenitors. *Curr. Biol.* **2017**, *27*, 1303–1313. [CrossRef] [PubMed]

54. Rodriguez, J.I.; Kern, J.K. Evidence of microglial activation in autism and its possible role in brain underconnectivity. *Neuron Glia Biol.* **2011**, *7*, 205–213. [CrossRef] [PubMed]

55. Courchesne, E.; Mouton, P.R.; Calhoun, M.E.; Semendeferi, K.; Ahrens-Barbeau, C.; Hallet, M.J.; Barnes, C.C.; Pierce, K. Neuron Number and Size in Prefrontal Cortex of Children with Autism. *JAMA* **2011**, *306*, 2001–2010. [CrossRef] [PubMed]

56. Barnea-Goraly, N.; Kwon, H.; Menon, V.; Eliez, S.; Lotspeich, L.; Reiss, A.L. White matter structure in autism: Preliminary evidence from diffusion tensor imaging. *Biol. Psychiatry* **2004**, *55*, 323–326. [CrossRef] [PubMed]

57. Di Martino, A.; Choi, E.Y.; Jones, R.M.; Castellanos, F.X.; Mukerji, A. *Imaging the Striatum in Autism Spectrum Disorder*; CRC Press: Boca Raton, FL, USA, 2016.

58. Monk, C.S.; Weng, S.-J.; Wiggins, J.L.; Kurapati, N.; Louro, H.M.C.; Carrasco, M.; Maslowsky, J.; Risi, S.; Lord, C. Neural circuitry of emotional face processing in autism spectrum disorders. *J. Psychiatry Neurosci.* **2010**, *35*, 105–114. [CrossRef] [PubMed]

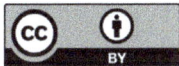

brain sciences

MDPI

Perspective

What Role Does the Prefrontal Cortex Play in the Processing of Negative and Positive Stimuli in Adolescent Depression?

Siyabend Kaya and Ciara McCabe *

School of Psychology and Clinical Language Sciences, University of Reading, Reading RG6 6AL, UK;
m.s.kaya@pgr.reading.ac.uk
* Correspondence: c.mccabe@reading.ac.uk; Tel.: +44-118-378-5450; Fax: +44-118-378-6715

Received: 27 March 2019; Accepted: 3 May 2019; Published: 7 May 2019

Abstract: This perspective describes the contribution of the prefrontal cortex to the symptoms of depression in adolescents and specifically the processing of positive and negative information. We also discuss how the prefrontal cortex (PFC) activity and connectivity during tasks and at rest might be a biomarker for risk for depression onset in adolescents. We include some of our recent work examining not only the anticipation and consummation of positive and negative stimuli, but also effort to gain positive and avoid negative stimuli in adolescents with depression. We find, using region of interest analyses, that the PFC is blunted in those with depression compared to controls across the different phases but in a larger sample the PFC is blunted in the anticipatory phase of the study only. Taken together, in adolescents with depression there is evidence for dysfunctional PFC activity across different studies and tasks. However, the data are limited with small sample sizes and inconsistent findings. Larger longitudinal studies with more detailed assessments of symptoms across the spectrum are needed to further evaluate the role of the PFC in adolescent depression.

Keywords: depression; adolescent; prefrontal cortex; neural; reward; positive and negative

1. Depression a Global Burden

Depression is currently reported as the most important cause of worldwide ill health. In the last 10 years, the depression rate has increased by more than 18% [1] and more than 300 million people worldwide now suffer from depression [1]. Unfortunately, a completely effective treatment has not been developed for individuals suffering from depression. Although current pharmacotherapy and psychotherapy helps many patients, they have limited efficacy and significant adverse effects [2].

Depression differs from the emotional fluctuations shown in daily life events, and long-term depression, in particular, can lead to serious health problems. It can prevent an individual from fulfilling his/her potential in school, in society, in family, and in work life. There are also high rates of depression in those that commit suicide and approximately 800,000 people die from suicide each year, with suicide being the second leading cause of death among 15–29-year-olds [1].

2. Adolescent Depression

Adolescent depression is defined by the diagnostic statistical manual (DSM) as having five or more symptoms present during a two week period; (1) depressed or irritable, cranky mood (outside being frustrated) or (2) loss of interest or pleasure and any three of the following: Significant weight loss or decrease in appetite (more than 5% of body weight in a month) or failure to meet expected weight gains, insomnia or hypersomnia, psychomotor agitation or retardation, fatigue or lack of energy, feelings of worthlessness or guilt, decreased concentration or indecisiveness, or recurrent thoughts of death or suicide [3].

Early onset depression, in particular during the adolescence period, has a destructive effect that predicts worse health outcomes in later life [2]. Therefore, understanding the underlying mechanisms of depression in adolescence is needed if we are to improve treatment and initiate prevention [4]. Adolescents experience dynamic changes in their social relations, thus leading to a very complex emotional life, while at the same time deal with hormonal and neural changes [5]. As adolescence is a time of fluctuating positive and negative emotional experiences, it is a vulnerable time for depression. However, as with adult depression described above, there is a heterogeneity in symptoms of adolescent depression and it is not entirely clear how they map to neurobiology [6]. One reason for this has been inconsistent use of questionnaires and assessments in research, which lack any specific detail about mood change in depression [7]. Understanding adolescent depression could benefit from more detailed measures of specific symptoms, e.g., anhedonia (the reduced experience of interest and pleasure), which is currently usually only assessed via its presence or absence and not in any detail from the adolescent experience [7]. In an attempt to do this, we recently collected information on the adolescent experience of depression and anhedonia through qualitative interviews and found that a number of adolescents described a blunting of all emotion (positive and negative) and not just positive emotion, which may have been expected [8]. However, this fits with the view of a recent meta-analysis also suggesting overall blunting in positive and negative emotions in depression [9]. Still yet, more needs to be done to illuminate the adolescent depression experience perhaps using experiential sampling methodology, which is the changes in symptoms during daily life, if we are to develop even more efficacious personalised treatments.

Recent methodological developments have led to significant improvements in understanding the neurobiological mechanisms of the emotional lives of adolescents [10,11]. Owing to these improvements, it is reported that in the course of adolescence, neural networks are reconstructed with both increases and decreases in white and grey matter, respectively [12,13]. These changes have been suggested as underlying age differences in behaviour for e.g., it is thought that adolescents are more sensitive to peer relationships than adults because they have more activation in areas involved in socialisation, such as the medial prefrontal cortex (mPFC), compared to adults [12].

3. Neurobiology of Depression

At the biological level, depression can have wide spread effects on the brain [14]. Studies old [15–17] and new [18–20] find that depression affects many brain regions. Prominent brain regions with both functional and structural differences in depression are the frontolimbic brain regions such as the amygdala, hypothalamus, and prefrontal cortex (PFC) [21,22] (for review, see References [23,24]). Dysfunctional connectivity between these regions via an amygdala–striatal–pallidial–thalamic–cingulate cortex circuit is also found dysfunctional in depression [14,25]. Interestingly, a recent review of voxel-level resting state functional connectivity (RSFC) suggests that the lateral orbitofrontal cortex, which projects to the ACC, has increased sensitivity to non-rewards in depression whereas the more medial orbitofrontal cortex reward system is underactive in depression [26]. Moreover, Rolls et al. in 2018 found that unmedicated patients with depression primarily had increased RSFC between the subcallosal anterior cingulate with the lateral orbitofrontal cortex, between the pregenual/supracallosal anterior cingulate and the medial orbitofrontal cortex, and between parts of the anterior cingulate with the inferior frontal gyrus, superior parietal lobule, and with early cortical visual areas. Further, this study reported that the RSFC was reduced in depressed patients that were medicated [26]. Interestingly, a recent study has also found that increased pretreatment pregenual anterior cingulate cortex activity to sad vs. happy faces was observed in responders relative to nonresponders, and that anterior cingulate cortex activity was able to predict response status at the level of the individual participant [27]. Given the importance of such networks of activity in the pathophysiology of depression and its treatment, how they might also act as predictors for adolescent depression could aid the identification of new targets for intervention approaches. In this respect, studies have emphasized that the PFC is one of the most important cortical brain regions in a network of regions in depression and is therefore a possible target for treatment and prevention in adolescents [28].

4. The Importance of the PFC

The role of the PFC in behaviours involving cognitive control and emotion processing has been well documented in adults (for review, see Reference [29]) and adolescents [30]. In summary, the dlPFC is mostly associated with cognitive processes such as target-oriented behaviours and attention control [31,32] while the vlPFC has a significant role in complex processes such as the self-regulation of emotion [19,33].The vmPFC, on the other hand, has been shown to play a role in the production of negative emotions [34–37].

Interestingly, during adolescence, the structural maturation of the PFC is suggested to underlie the maturation of emotion regulation strategies. Studies consistently find normative thinning of the grey matter during adolescence which has been identified as an adaptive process in longitudinal studies on cognition [38]. For example, Shaw et al. [39] found that adolescents that exhibited greater peak thickness around puberty, followed by greater cortical thinning into adulthood had superior intellectual abilities. Furthermore, greater cortical thinning of the left dlPFC and left vlPFC during adolescence has been found to predict greater use of cognitive reappraisal, the ability to negotiate emotionally stressful situations by being more optimistic, reinterpreting the stressful stimuli, and actively mending their negative mood, in healthy females [38]. These findings suggest that cortical maturation may play a role in the development of adaptive emotion regulation strategies during adolescence. Interestingly, dysfunction, by way of decreased perfusion in the PFC, has been reported in patients who attempted suicide. It is thought this PFC dysfunction might reduce problem-solving ability, increase negative emotions, and, finally, aid suicidal behaviour especially given the role of the orbitofrontal cortex in response inhibition [22,40].

5. The Role of the PFC in Depression and the Processing of Negative Stimuli

The mechanisms underpinning the processing of negative emotions have received attention, as low mood and negative thinking are thought to be maintaining characteristics of depression [41]. Negative emotional stimuli activate a broad network of brain regions, including the medial prefrontal (mPFC) and anterior cingulate (ACC) cortices and, although early reviews suggested a dorsal-caudal cognitive and ventral-rostral affective subdivision [42], more recent work suggests both subdivisions make key contributions to emotional processing. Specifically, dorsal-caudal regions of the ACC and mPFC are thought to be involved in appraisal and expression of negative emotion, whereas ventral-rostral portions of the ACC and mPFC seem to have a regulatory role with respect to limbic regions involved in generating emotional responses [43]. Examining these systems in relation to low mood, a study by Aoki and colleagues [44] using the neuroimaging tool optical topography, found that adults experiencing higher levels of negative moods showed lower levels of PFC activity during a verbal working memory task. This also replicated the results of their previous study based on an independent sample [45]. In another study using near infrared spectroscopy (NIRS), participants were asked to remember parts of their lives related to positive (happiness) and negative (anger) feelings, and at the same time, heart rate changes were measured. The authors found that changes in oxyhemoglobin in the bilateral PFC during silent recall of negative episodes were significantly larger than those during silent recall of positive episodes. The authors concluded that their results were important in showing that the PFC plays a key role in the cognitive control of particularly negative emotions [18].

As mentioned above, the dlPFC is thought to be involved in executive function and cognitive control over behaviour and action [46]. It has been found, using EEG, to have functional and structural asymmetry that correlates with depressive symptoms in healthy young adults, individuals with subclinical depression, and patients with depression [47]. Previous studies report that the left dlPFC is hypoactive for positive and the right dlPFC hyperactive for negative stimuli in depression [48] and a study by Siegle et al. [49] detected that depressed participants showed reduced dlPFC activity to negative words. Furthermore, the lateral orbitofrontal cortex (lOFC), which connects to the dlPFC, has been found to have a critical role in reversal learning and adapting behaviour based on the most positive outcome [50]. Recently, it has been posited that dysfunction of the lOFC "non-reward" circuit may lead to the generation of negative self-thoughts and reduced self-esteem apparent in depression [50,51].

6. PFC Markers of Risk for Depression and Early Life Stress (ELS)

To date, it is difficult to ascertain neural markers of risk for depression, e.g., it is not known which of the functional neuroanatomical differences seen in depressed patients predate and predict depression onset [52,53]. By examining adolescents, neurobiological studies can begin to address this issue, and studies have found heightened activity in the amygdala during facial-emotion recognition tasks [54] and greater connectivity between the amygdala and part of the PFC the subgenual anterior cingulate cortex [55]. Further, recent studies examining PFC connectivity and risk of depression by virtue of early life stress (ELS) find that adolescent females exhibited a positive association between ELS and ventrolateral prefrontal cortex (vlPFC) during implicit emotion regulation and both males and females exhibited an association between ELS and increased negative connectivity between right vlPFC and bilateral amygdala [56]. The authors suggest these results might reflect greater vlPFC activation in an emotion regulation context in response to stress i.e., under the stress accelerated hypothesis. This is where accelerated development of neural circuitry involved in emotion functioning is caused by stress and is adaptive in the short term [57]. Further, there is evidence in animal models of ELS-induced changes in mPFC function and developmental trajectory, which may be responsible for the emergence of both early-onset (during childhood and adolescence) and adulthood-onset anxiety and mood disorders [58,59]. In summary, studies find ELS, a risk factor for depression, affects PFC function in early puberty, thus indicating the importance of this region as a potential target for early intervention in those at risk.

7. PFC and Resting State Functional Connectivity (RSFC) in Adolescents with Depression

Studies have begun to examine RSFC in adolescents with depression and a recent study found that depressed adolescents showed significantly greater RSFC to left amygdala, bilateral supragenual ACC, but not with PFC. The results partially support the putative dual-system hypothesis believed to underlie disorders such as major depression i.e., an imbalance between "hot" limbic activity and "cold" PFC activity. The authors suggested that adolescents have aberrant, bottom-up processing in hot limbic regions without the concomitant differences in cognitive control in cold prefrontal regions, unlike in adults with depression. In addition, changes in functional connectivity were significantly associated with changes in symptom severity after cognitive behavioural therapy. This indicates that symptom recovery may be at least partially associated with normalization of RSFC in hot emotional brain systems, and their restoration is critical for successful therapeutic interventions [60]. We have also examined resting state functional connectivity (RSFC) in adolescents and the relationship between PFC connectivity and depression symptoms. We found decreased RSFC between the amygdala and the pgACC and hippocampus and precuneus in young people with depression symptoms. We also found decreased RSFC in the young people with depression symptoms between the pgACC and the putamen and between the dmPFC and the precuneus [61]. Further, the pgACC RSFC with the insula/orbitofrontal cortex correlated inversely with the anticipation of pleasure in all subjects. Increased RSFC was observed between the pgACC and the prefrontal cortex and the amygdala and the temporal pole in the young people with depression symptoms compared to those with no symptoms. As increased connectivity between the pgACC and the insula correlated with decreased ability to anticipate pleasure, we suggest this might be a mechanism underlying the risk of experiencing anhedonia, a suggested biomarker for depression [61]. In our more recent work, we also found that in a large sample of young people with a range of depression scores, both anhedonia and depression severity related to decreased dmPFC RSFC with the precuneus, a part of the default mode network.

However, we also found that increased dmPFC connectivity with the ACC/paracingulate gyrus related to anhedonia whereas increased RSFC with the frontal pole related to depression severity. This study is important as it shows us how we can dissociate symptoms in adolescents based on PFC RSFC [62]. In adolescents with depression, medial prefrontal cortical connectivity with brain regions involved in executive functioning, emotion regulation, and attention have been reported altered [28].

8. The Role of the PFC in Depression and the Processing of Positive Stimuli

In regard to positive processing specifically, studies have shown blunted neural responses that relate to positive affect [63] and depression symptoms in adolescents [64,65] and even young children [66]. Further, in relation to positive stimuli, studies of adolescents with depression report mostly decreased responses to monetary reward in regions like the ventral striatum, caudate, the dorsolateral and medial prefrontal cortex (PFC), orbitofrontal cortex (OFC), anterior cingulate cortex (ACC), and amygdala [67,68]. However, most neurobiological tasks of positive emotion processing (reward) do not examine the different phases of processing such as the anticipatory, motivational, and consummatory aspects of reward. This has led to inconsistencies across studies on reward in depression [69].

We have been interested in examining how young people at risk of depression respond to positive and negative stimuli both behaviourally and at the neural level. Furthermore, as recent behavioural data find that depressed adults have reduced effort expenditure for reward compared to healthy controls [70], we are also interested in how this is represented at the neural level. Therefore, to address this, we have developed an experimental model that examines the anticipation of a food reward and a consummatory phase where rewarding food is eaten. We have shown previously that those at risk of depression have decreased responses to anticipation and consummation (sight and taste of chocolate reward) in both ventral striatum and anterior cingulate cortex (ACC) [71]. We also showed that young people (16–21 years) with a family history of depression but no personal experience of depression had diminished neural responses in the orbitofrontal cortex (OFC) and the dorsal anterior cingulate cortex (dACC) to rewarding stimuli, sight, and taste combined in the at-risk group [72]. More recently, we have also shown that when examining neural activity between young people with depression symptoms and controls, using a region of interest analysis, regions like the pregenual ACC and ventral medial PFC were blunted across all positive and negative phases in adolescents with depression symptoms. We also found that whole brain analysis revealed further blunted activity in the precuneus and inferior frontal gyrus (during aversive anticipation) and hippocampus (during effort for reward) and ACC/frontal pole (during aversive consummation) in young people with depression symptoms. Further, we found a negative correlation between pgACC activity during reward consummation and anhedonia in adolescents with depression symptoms [73]. Although this was a comparatively small study, the results are in keeping with the meta-analysis and first quantitative review of emotional reactivity in depression that found consistent reductions in both positive AND negative reactivity [9] which supported our previous study [71]). This also fits with the recent hypothesis that as connectivity of the ACC, a hub for integrating cognitive, affective, and social information to guide self-regulation across domains, supports adaptive development of self-regulation during adolescence, disrupted maturation of ACC connectivity could contribute to the development of depression [74].

In our follow-up, much larger study currently under review, we found participants with depression symptoms invested less physical effort to gain the positive rewarding stimulus than controls and had blunted neural anticipation of positive and negative stimuli in the precuneus, insula, and PFC (left dlPFC and lOFC) and blunted neural effort for positive in the putamen [75]. As the dlPFC is involved in cognitive control and in executive functions [47], we suggest dysfunction in this region might indicate a mechanism by which reduced planning to gain positive and avoid negative stimuli might arise in those with depression symptoms. As the lOFC connects to the dlPFC, insula, and premotor areas [76] and has been found to have a critical role in reversal learning and adapting behaviour based on the most rewarding outcome [76], reduced lOFC activity might disrupt ability to switch behaviour, which, in those depressed, might affect preparation to gain reward or avoid aversion.

9. Conclusions

Taken together, the literature on the neural activity related to positive and negative emotion processing is limited in adolescent psychopathology [7,64]. Depression, notwithstanding decades of studies, is a serious disorder with early onset in adolescence indicating worse long-term outcomes, yet the neural basis of adolescent depression is not yet fully understood [7]. Although the PFC is a key region implicated in the processing of positive and negative emotion, some inconsistencies in direction of effects are present in the literature [23,77]. Therefore, in order to understand the role of PFC in adolescent depression, further studies are needed that examine the processing of positive and negative stimuli in a dimensional fashion across the spectrum, in line with an RDoC type approach. Further, it would also be of interest to examine how adolescents regulate their emotion processing in relation to PFC activity over time and depression onset [30]. Adolescence is an important time, in which both physical and mental changes are experienced. Although studies have shown that the PFC region is implicated in depression in adults, less is known about how the PFC impacts upon negative and positive moods in the adolescent period. Knowing how the PFC is involved in major symptoms like anhedonia could allow us to develop more targeted interventions for youth depression.

Author Contributions: S.K. and C.M. wrote the manuscript.

Funding: No specific funding was used for this work.

Conflicts of Interest: S.K. and C.M. report no conflicts of interest.

References

1. WHO. Depression. Available online: https://www.who.int/news-room/fact-sheets/detail/depression (accessed on 22 April 2019).
2. Harrington, R.; Fudge, H.; Rutter, M.; Pickles, A.; Hill, J. Adult outcomes of childhood and adolescent depression: I. Psychiatric status. *Arch. Gen. Psychiatry* **1990**, *47*, 465–473. [CrossRef] [PubMed]
3. American Psychiatric Association. *Diagnostic and Statistical Manual of Mental Disorders*, 5th ed.; American Psychiatric Association Publishing: Washington, DC, USA, 2013.
4. Davey, C.G.; Yücel, M.; Allen, N.B. The emergence of depression in adolescence: Development of the prefrontal cortex and the representation of reward. *Neurosci. Biobehav. Rev.* **2008**, *32*, 1–19. [CrossRef] [PubMed]
5. Guyer, A.E.; Silk, J.S.; Nelson, E.E. The neurobiology of the emotional adolescent: From the inside out. *Neurosci. Biobehav. Rev.* **2016**, *70*, 74–85. [CrossRef] [PubMed]
6. Blom, E.H.; Ho, T.C.; Connolly, C.G.; LeWinn, K.Z.; Sacchet, M.D.; Tymofiyeva, O.; Weng, H.Y.; Yang, T.T. The neuroscience and context of adolescent depression. *Acta Paediatr.* **2016**, *105*, 358–365.
7. McCabe, C. Linking anhedonia symptoms with behavioural and neural reward responses in adolescent depression. *Behav. Sci.* **2018**, *22*, 143–151. [CrossRef]
8. Watson, R.; Harvey, K.; McCabe, C. Understanding anhedonia: A qualitative study exploring loss of interest and pleasure in adolescent depression. *Eur. Child Adolesc. Psychiatry* **2019**. under review.
9. Bylsma, L.M.; Morris, B.H.; Rottenberg, J. A meta-analysis of emotional reactivity in major depressive disorder. *Clin. Psychol.* **2008**, *28*, 676–691. [CrossRef]
10. Gabbay, V.; Johnson, A.R.; Alonso, C.M.; Evans, L.K.; Babb, J.S.; Klein, R.G. Anhedonia, but not Irritability, Is Associated with Illness Severity Outcomes in Adolescent Major Depression. *J. Child Adolesc. Psychopharmacol.* **2015**, *25*, 194–200. [CrossRef] [PubMed]
11. Casey, B.J. Beyond Simple Models of Self-Control to Circuit-Based Accounts of Adolescent Behavior. *Annu. Psychol.* **2015**, *66*, 295–319. [CrossRef]
12. Dumontheil, I. Adolescent brain development. *Behav. Sci.* **2016**, *10*, 39–44. [CrossRef]
13. Giorgio, A.; Watkins, K.; Chadwick, M.; James, S.; Winmill, L.; Douaud, G.; De Stefano, N.; Matthews, P.M.; Smith, S.; Johansen-Berg, H.; et al. Longitudinal changes in grey and white matter during adolescence. *NeuroImage* **2010**, *49*, 94–103. [CrossRef]
14. Pandya, M.; Altinay, M.; Malone, D.A.; Anand, A. Where in the brain is depression? *Curr. Psychiatry Rep.* **2012**, *14*, 634–642. [CrossRef]

15. Bremner, J.D.; Narayan, M.; Anderson, E.R.; Staib, L.H.; Miller, H.L.; Charney, D.S. Hippocampal volume reduction in major depression. *Am. J. Psychiatry* **2000**, *157*, 115–118. [CrossRef]

16. McEwen, B.S. Effects of adverse experiences for brain structure and function. *Biol. Psychiatry* **2000**, *48*, 721–731. [CrossRef]

17. Öngür, D.; Drevets, W.C.; Price, J.L. Glial reduction in the subgenual prefrontal cortex in mood disorders. *Proc. Natl. Acad. Sci. USA* **1998**, *95*, 13290–13295. [CrossRef] [PubMed]

18. Compare, A.; Brugnera, A.; Adorni, R.; Sakatani, K. Effects of Positive and Negative Mood Induction on the Prefrontal Cortex Activity Measured by Near Infrared Spectroscopy. *Adv. Exp. Med. Biol.* **2016**, *923*, 151–157.

19. Kim, J.U.; Weisenbach, S.L.; Zald, D.H. Ventral prefrontal cortex and emotion regulation in aging: A case for utilizing transcranial magnetic stimulation. *Int. J. Geriatr. Psychiatry* **2018**, *34*, 215–222. [CrossRef]

20. Ozawa, S.; Matsuda, G.; Hiraki, K. Negative emotion modulates prefrontal cortex activity during a working memory task: a NIRS study. *Front. Hum. Neurosci.* **2014**, *8*. [CrossRef] [PubMed]

21. Gao, L.; Cai, Y.; Wang, H.; Wang, G.; Zhang, Q.; Yan, X. Probing prefrontal cortex hemodynamic alterations during facial emotion recognition for major depression disorder through functional near-infrared spectroscopy. *J. Neural Eng.* **2019**, *16*, 026026. [CrossRef]

22. Noda, Y.; Zomorrodi, R.; Vila-Rodríguez, F.; Downar, J.; Farzan, F.; Cash, R.F.; Rajji, T.K.; Daskalakis, Z.J.; Blumberger, D.M. Impaired neuroplasticity in the prefrontal cortex in depression indexed through paired associative stimulation. *Depress. Anxiety* **2018**, *35*, 448–456. [CrossRef] [PubMed]

23. Hulvershorn, L.A.; Cullen, K.; Anand, A. Toward Dysfunctional Connectivity: A Review of Neuroimaging Findings in Pediatric Major Depressive Disorder. *Brain Imaging Behav.* **2011**, *5*, 307–328. [CrossRef] [PubMed]

24. Drevets, W.C.; Price, J.L.; Furey, M.L. Brain structural and functional abnormalities in mood disorders: implications for neurocircuitry models of depression. *Anat. Embryol.* **2008**, *213*, 93–118. [CrossRef]

25. Price, J.L.; Drevets, W.C. Neural circuits underlying the pathophysiology of mood disorders. *Trends Cogn. Sci.* **2012**, *16*, 61–71. [CrossRef]

26. Rolls, E.T.; Cheng, W.; Gong, W.; Qiu, J.; Zhou, C.; Zhang, J.; Lv, W.; Ruan, H.; Wei, D.; Cheng, K.; et al. Functional Connectivity of the Anterior Cingulate Cortex in Depression and in Health. *Cereb Cortex* **2018**, *1*, 14. [CrossRef]

27. Godlewska, B.R.; Browning, M.; Norbury, R.; Igoumenou, A.; Cowen, P.J.; Harmer, C.J. Predicting Treatment Response in Depression: The Role of Anterior Cingulate Cortex. *Int. J. Neuropsychopharmacol.* **2018**, *21*, 988–996. [CrossRef]

28. Kerestes, R.; Davey, C.G.; Stephanou, K.; Whittle, S.; Harrison, B.J. Functional brain imaging studies of youth depression: A systematic review. *NeuroImage Clin.* **2014**, *4*, 209–231. [CrossRef]

29. Thiruchselvam, R.; Todd, R.; Christoff, K.; Dixon, M.L. Emotion and the prefrontal cortex: An integrative review. *Psychol. Bull.* **2017**, *143*, 1033–1081.

30. Caballero, A.; Granberg, R.; Tseng, K.Y. Mechanisms contributing to prefrontal cortex maturation during adolescence. *Neurosci. Biobehav. Rev.* **2016**, *70*, 4–12. [CrossRef]

31. Albert, K.M.; Potter, G.G.; Boyd, B.D.; Kang, H.; Taylor, W.D. Brain network functional connectivity and cognitive performance in major depressive disorder. *J. Psychiatr.* **2019**, *110*, 51–56. [CrossRef]

32. Miller, E.K.; Cohen, J.D. An integrate theory of prefrontal cortex function. *Annu. Rev. Neurosci.* **2001**, *24*, 167–202. [CrossRef]

33. Ochsner, K.N.; Gross, J.J. The cognitive control of emotion. *Trends Cogn. Sci.* **2005**, *9*, 242–249. [CrossRef] [PubMed]

34. Diekhof, E.K.; Geier, K.; Falkai, P.; Gruber, O. Fear is only as deep as the mind allows: A coordinate-based meta-analysis of neuroimaging studies on the regulation of negative affect. *Neuroimage* **2011**, *58*, 275–285. [CrossRef]

35. Hiser, J.; Koenigs, M. The Multifaceted Role of the Ventromedial Prefrontal Cortex in Emotion, Decision Making, Social Cognition, and Psychopathology. *Biol. Psychiatry* **2018**, *83*, 638–647. [CrossRef]

36. Koenigs, M.; Grafman, J.H. The functional neuroanatomy of depression: Distinct roles for ventromedial and dorsolateral prefrontal cortex. *Behav. Brain* **2009**, *201*, 239–243. [CrossRef]

37. Vaidya, A.R.; Fellows, L.K. Ventromedial frontal lobe damage affects interpretation, not exploration, of emotional facial expressions. *Cortex* **2019**, *113*, 312–328. [CrossRef] [PubMed]

38. Vijayakumar, N.; Whittle, S.; Yücel, M.; Dennison, M.; Simmons, J.; Allen, N.B. Thinning of the lateral prefrontal cortex during adolescence predicts emotion regulation in females. *Soc. Cogn. Affect. Neurosci.* **2014**, *9*, 1845–1854. [CrossRef] [PubMed]

39. Shaw, P.; Greenstein, D.; Lerch, J.; Clasen, L.; Lenroot, R.; Gogtay, N.; Evans, A.; Rapoport, J.; Giedd, J. Intellectual ability and cortical development in children and adolescents. *Nat. Cell Boil.* **2006**, *440*, 676–679. [CrossRef]

40. Desmyter, S.; Van Heeringen, C.; Audenaert, K. Structural and functional neuroimaging studies of the suicidal brain. *Prog. Neuro-Psychopharmacol. Boil. Psychiatry* **2011**, *35*, 796–808. [CrossRef]

41. Beck, A.T. The Evolution of the Cognitive Model of Depression and Its Neurobiological Correlates. *Am. J. Psychiatry* **2008**, *165*, 969–977. [CrossRef]

42. Bush, G.; Luu, P.; Posner, M.I. Cognitive and emotional influences in anterior cingulate cortex. *Trends Cogn. Sci.* **2000**, *4*, 215–222. [CrossRef]

43. Etkin, A.; Egner, T.; Kalisch, R. Emotional processing in anterior cingulate and medial prefrontal cortex. *Trends Cogn. Sci.* **2011**, *15*, 85–93. [CrossRef]

44. Aoki, R.; Sato, H.; Katura, T.; Matsuda, R.; Koizumi, H. Correlation between prefrontal cortex activity during working memory tasks and natural mood independent of personality effects: An optical topography study. *Psychiatry Res. Neuroimaging* **2013**, *212*, 79–87. [CrossRef]

45. Aoki, R.; Sato, H.; Katura, T.; Utsugi, K.; Koizumi, H.; Matsuda, R.; Maki, A. Relationship of negative mood with prefrontal cortex activity during working memory tasks: An optical topography study. *Neurosci. Res.* **2011**, *70*, 189–196. [CrossRef]

46. Hoshi, E. Functional specialization within the dorsolateral prefrontal cortex: A review of anatomical and physiological studies of non-human primates. *Neurosci. Res.* **2006**, *54*, 73–84. [CrossRef]

47. Liu, W.; Mao, Y.; Wei, D.; Yang, J.; Du, X.; Xie, P.; Qiu, J. Structural Asymmetry of Dorsolateral Prefrontal Cortex Correlates with Depressive Symptoms: Evidence from Healthy Individuals and Patients with Major Depressive Disorder. *Neurosci. Bull.* **2016**, *32*, 217–226. [CrossRef]

48. Murphy, F.C.; Nimmo-Smith, I.; Lawrence, A.D. Functional neuroanatomy of emotions: A meta-analysis. *Cogn. Affect. Behav. Neurosci.* **2003**, *3*, 207–233. [CrossRef]

49. Siegle, G.J.; Steinhauer, S.R.; E Thase, M.; Stenger, V.; Carter, C.S. Can't shake that feeling: event-related fMRI assessment of sustained amygdala activity in response to emotional information in depressed individuals. *Biol. Psychiatry* **2002**, *51*, 693–707. [CrossRef]

50. Fettes, P.; Schulze, L.; Downar, J. Cortico-Striatal-Thalamic Loop Circuits of the Orbitofrontal Cortex: Promising Therapeutic Targets in Psychiatric Illness. *Front. Syst. Neurosci.* **2017**, *11*, 1898. [CrossRef]

51. Rolls, E.T. A non-reward attractor theory of depression. *Neurosci. Biobehav. Rev.* **2016**, *68*, 47–58. [CrossRef]

52. Barnes, J. *Essential Biological Psychology*; SAGE Publications Ltd: London, UK, 2013.

53. Zaremba, D.; Dohm, K.; Redlich, R.; Grotegerd, D.; Strojny, R.; Meinert, S.; Burger, C.; Enneking, V.; Förster, K.; Repple, J.; et al. Association of Brain Cortical Changes With Relapse in Patients With Major Depressive Disorder. *JAMA Psychiatry* **2018**, *75*, 484. [CrossRef]

54. Yang, T.T.; Simmons, A.N.; Matthews, S.C.; Tapert, S.F.; Frank, G.K.; Max, J.E.; Bischoff-Grethe, A.; Lansing, A.E.; Brown, G.; Strigo, I.A.; et al. Adolescents With Major Depression Demonstrate Increased Amygdala Activation. *J. Am. Acad. Child Adolesc. Psychiatry* **2010**, *49*, 42–51.

55. Ho, T.C.; Yang, G.; Wu, J.; Cassey, P.; Brown, S.D.; Hoang, N.; Chan, M.; Connolly, C.G.; Henje-Blom, E.; Duncan, L.G.; et al. Functional connectivity of negative emotional processing in adolescent depression. *J. Affect. Disord.* **2014**, *155*, 65–74. [CrossRef]

56. Colich, N.L.; Williams, E.S.; Ho, T.C.; King, L.S.; Humphreys, K.L.; Price, A.N.; Ordaz, S.J.; Gotlib, I.H. The association between early life stress and prefrontal cortex activation during implicit emotion regulation is moderated by sex in early adolescence. *Dev. Psychopathol.* **2017**, *29*, 1851–1864. [CrossRef]

57. Callaghan, B.L.; Tottenham, N. The Stress Acceleration Hypothesis: effects of early-life adversity on emotion circuits and behavior. *Behav. Sci.* **2016**, *7*, 76–81. [CrossRef]

58. Chocyk, A.; Majcher-Maślanka, I.; Dudys, D.; Przyborowska, A.; Wędzony, K. Impact of early-life stress on the medial prefrontal cortex functions—A search for the pathomechanisms of anxiety and mood disorders. *Pharmacol. Rep.* **2013**, *65*, 1462–1470. [CrossRef]

59. Arnsten, A.; Datta, D. Loss of Prefrontal Cortical Top-Down Regulation with Uncontrollable Stress: Molecular Mechanisms, Changes with Age, and Relevance to Treatment. *Brain Sci.* **2019**, submitted.

60. Zhang, F. Resting-State Functional Connectivity Abnormalities in Adolescent Depression. *EBioMedicine* **2017**, *17*, 20–21. [CrossRef]

61. Rzepa, E.; McCabe, C. Decreased anticipated pleasure correlates with increased salience network resting state functional connectivity in adolescents with depressive symptomatology. *J. Psychiatr. Res.* **2016**, *82*, 40–47. [CrossRef]

62. Rzepa, E.; McCabe, C. Anhedonia and depression severity dissociated by dmPFC resting-state functional connectivity in adolescents. *J. Psychopharmacol.* **2018**, *32*, 1067–1074. [CrossRef]

63. Forbes, E.E.; Hariri, A.R.; Martin, S.L.; Silk, J.S.; Moyles, D.L.; Fisher, P.M.; Brown, S.M.; Ryan, N.D.; Birmaher, B.; Axelson, D.A.; et al. Altered striatal activation predicting real-world positive affect in adolescent major depressive disorder. *Am. J. Psychiatry* **2009**, *166*, 64–73. [CrossRef]

64. Auerbach, R.P.; Admon, R.; Pizzagalli, D.A. Adolescent Depression: Stress and Reward Dysfunction. *Harv. Rev. Psychiatry* **2014**, *22*, 139–148. [CrossRef]

65. Hanson, J.L.; Hariri, A.R.; Williamson, D.E. Blunted ventral striatum development in adolescence reflects emotional neglect and predicts depressive symptoms. *Boil. Psychiatry* **2015**, *78*, 598–605. [CrossRef]

66. Belden, A.C.; Irvin, K.; Hajcak, G.; Kappenman, E.S.; Kelly, D.; Karlow, S.; Luby, J.L.; Barch, D.M. Neural Correlates of Reward Processing in Depressed and Healthy Preschool-Age Children. *J. Am. Acad. Child Adolesc. Psychiatry* **2016**, *55*, 1081–1089. [CrossRef]

67. Forbes, E.E.; May, J.C.; Siegle, G.J.; Ladouceur, C.D.; Ryan, N.D.; Carter, C.S.; Birmaher, B.; Axelson, D.A.; Dahl, R.E. Reward-Related Decision-Making in Pediatric Major Depressive Disorder: An fMRI Study. *J. Child Psychol. Psychiatry* **2006**, *47*, 1031–1040. [CrossRef]

68. Forbes, E.E.; Dahl, R.E. Research review: Altered reward function in adolescent depression: What, when and how? *J. Child Psychol. Psychiatry* **2012**, *53*, 3–15. [CrossRef]

69. Argyropoulos, S.V.; Nutt, D.J. Anhedonia revisited: Is there a role for dopamine-targeting drugs for depression? *J. Psychopharmacol.* **2013**, *27*, 869–877. [CrossRef]

70. Yang, X.-H.; Huang, J.; Zhu, C.-Y.; Wang, Y.-F.; Cheung, E.F.; Chan, R.C.; Xie, G.-R. Motivational deficits in effort-based decision making in individuals with subsyndromal depression, first-episode and remitted depression patients. *Psychiatry Res.* **2014**, *220*, 874–882. [CrossRef]

71. McCabe, C.; Cowen, P.J.; Harmer, C.J. Neural representation of reward in recovered depressed patients. *Psychopharmacology* **2009**, *205*, 667–677. [CrossRef] [PubMed]

72. McCabe, C.; Woffindale, C.; Harmer, C.J.; Cowen, P.J. Neural Processing of Reward and Punishment in Young People at Increased Familial Risk of Depression. *Biol. Psychiatry* **2012**, *72*, 588–594. [CrossRef]

73. Rzepa, E.; Fisk, J.; McCabe, C. Blunted neural response to anticipation, effort and consummation of reward and aversion in adolescents with depression symptomatology. *J. Psychopharmacol.* **2017**, *31*, 303–311. [CrossRef]

74. Lichenstein, S.D.; Verstynen, T.; Forbes, E.E. Adolescent brain development and depression: A case for the importance of connectivity of the anterior cingulate cortex. *Neurosci. Biobehav. Rev.* **2016**, *70*, 271–287. [CrossRef] [PubMed]

75. Rzepa, E.; McCabe, C. Dimensional Anhedonia and the Adolescent brain: Reward and Aversion Anticipation, Effort and Consummation. Available online: https://www.biorxiv.org/content/10.1101/473835v1.full (accessed on 19 November 2018).

76. Kringelbach, M.L. The functional neuroanatomy of the human orbitofrontal cortex: evidence from neuroimaging and neuropsychology. *Prog. Neurobiol.* **2004**, *72*, 341–372. [CrossRef] [PubMed]

77. Bendall, R.C.A.; Thompson, C. Emotion does not influence prefrontal cortex activity during a visual attention task. A functional near-infrared specroscopy study. In Proceedings of the 5th Annual International Conference Proceedings on Cognitive and Behavioural Psychology, Singapore, 22–23 February 2016.

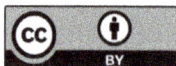

brain
sciences

MDPI

Review

Positive and Negative Emotion Regulation in Adolescence: Links to Anxiety and Depression

Katherine S. Young [1,*], Christina F. Sandman [2] and Michelle G. Craske [2,3]

[1] Social, Genetic and Development Psychiatry (SGDP) Centre, Institute of Psychology, Psychiatry and Neuroscience, King's College, London SE5 8AF, UK
[2] Department of Psychology, University of California, Los Angeles (UCLA), Los Angeles, CA 90095, USA; christysandman@ucla.edu (C.F.S.); MCraske@mednet.ucla.edu (M.G.C.)
[3] Department of Psychiatry and Biobehavioral Sciences, University of California, Los Angeles (UCLA), Los Angeles, CA 90095, USA
* Correspondence: katherine.s.young@kcl.ac.uk; Tel.: +44-0207-848-0865

Received: 11 February 2019; Accepted: 26 March 2019; Published: 29 March 2019

Abstract: Emotion regulation skills develop substantially across adolescence, a period characterized by emotional challenges and developing regulatory neural circuitry. Adolescence is also a risk period for the new onset of anxiety and depressive disorders, psychopathologies which have long been associated with disruptions in regulation of positive and negative emotions. This paper reviews the current understanding of the role of disrupted emotion regulation in adolescent anxiety and depression, describing findings from self-report, behavioral, peripheral psychophysiological, and neural measures. Self-report studies robustly identified associations between emotion dysregulation and adolescent anxiety and depression. Findings from behavioral and psychophysiological studies are mixed, with some suggestion of specific impairments in reappraisal in anxiety. Results from neuroimaging studies broadly implicate altered functioning of amygdala-prefrontal cortical circuitries, although again, findings are mixed regarding specific patterns of altered neural functioning. Future work may benefit from focusing on designs that contrast effects of specific regulatory strategies, and isolate changes in emotional regulation from emotional reactivity. Approaches to improve treatments based on empirical evidence of disrupted emotion regulation in adolescents are also discussed. Future intervention studies might consider training and measurement of specific strategies in adolescents to better understand the role of emotion regulation as a treatment mechanism.

Keywords: anxiety; depression; adolescence; emotion regulation; fMRI; psychophysiology; psychological treatment

---

1. Introduction

Emotion regulation is defined broadly as the capacity to manage one's own emotional responses. This includes strategies to increase, maintain, or decrease the intensity, duration, and trajectory of positive and negative emotions [1–3]. Learning to regulate emotions is a key socio-emotional skill that allows flexibility in emotionally-evocative situations. There are clear developmental shifts in how we manage emotional responses. In early childhood, emotions are frequently expressed and external support is sought (e.g., from a caregiver [4]). In adolescence, there is typically a decreased reliance on parental support and limited efficacy of adaptive internal emotion regulation [5]. As individuals mature into adulthood, emotional experiences are increasingly effectively managed through internal regulatory strategies [6]. Disruptions to emotion regulation capacities in adulthood are central to theories of how anxiety and depressive disorders manifest and are maintained [7,8]. These theories suggest that reduced capacities to downregulate heightened negative affect are common to both anxiety and depression, whereas reduced ability to regulate positive affect may be more specific to depressive disorders [9]. Many psychological interventions for anxiety and depression include cognitive or behavioral strategies that aim to improve abilities to regulate emotion [10,11].

Emotion regulation capacities develop substantially across adolescence. Studies of typically developing individuals suggest limited efficacy of internal regulatory strategies in early adolescence, shifting towards increased use of adaptive strategies and decreased use of maladaptive strategies with age [5,12]. This development coincides with changes in social environment and brain structure. Adolescence is a period of life with various emotional challenges, such as new academic or work-place pressures, increasing importance of peer and romantic relationships, and reduced dependence on family support [13]. Heightened emotional reactivity, increased risk-taking, and impulsive behaviors are also characteristic of adolescence [14]. This is coupled with ongoing neurobiological development among circuitries implicated in the management of emotional processes (for a review, see [15]). Investigation of normative development is ongoing, but current theories focus around maturation in activity and connectivity among the prefrontal cortex, striatum and amygdala across adolescence [16,17]. These models propose that increasing prefrontal control over emotionally reactive subcortical regions enhances capacities to regulate negative emotions (particularly fear) and manage impulsive tendencies (reward and approach [15,16,18]).

Adolescence is a period of heightened risk for the onset of anxiety disorders and depression [19,20]. It is well-established that stressful life events and childhood adversity are substantial risk factors for future psychopathology [21]. There is also evidence suggesting that the capacity to regulate emotional reactions to these events may play a mediating role [22,23]. Given increased independence and novel demands during adolescence relative to childhood, adolescents may have a particular need to regulate their emotions in response to stressors. Failure to do so may confer risk for mental health problems. Thus, emotion regulation may be one important piece of a complex puzzle in terms of risk for anxiety and depression. The current paper addresses the evidence linking disrupted emotion regulation to the development of anxiety and depression in adolescence. This question has been investigated across different levels of analysis including self-report, behavioral, peripheral psychophysiological and neural measures. Repeated observations across multiple levels of analysis increase the reliability and validity of observed associations and may improve precision in understanding dysfunction and disease course [24,25]. Here we review the consistency of evidence across multiple modalities and highlight discrepancies and gaps in the literature.

A major challenge in the study of emotion regulation is definition and operationalization of the construct. In this review, we focus on evidence from the most widely-used measures of emotion regulation, rather than providing an exhaustive list of all possible measures. We begin with an overview of methodological approaches to studying emotion regulation most frequently used in adolescents. We then review evidence across levels of analysis supporting claims of a link between negative and positive emotion regulation capacities with anxiety and depression (summarized in Table 1; note that as a narrative rather than a systematic review, we provide a selection of findings of interest, rather than an exhaustive list of all findings in this area). Next, we discuss how these findings have informed current and emerging interventions targeting emotion regulation and their potential for adolescent populations. Finally, we provide an overview of discrepancies and gaps in current research and directions for future work that may enhance our understanding of the development of emotion (dys)regulation among adolescents at risk for anxiety and depression.

Table 1. Reviewed evidence investigating links between emotion regulation and anxiety and depression in adolescence. Findings are organized according to negative and positive emotion regulation, and by methodology. (dlPFC: dorsolateral prefrontal cortex; dmPFC: dorsomedial prefrontal cortex; IFG: inferior frontal gyrus; IFL: inferior frontal lobule; MFG: middle frontal gyrus; PFC: prefrontal cortex; RSA: respiratory sinus arrhythmia; SFG: superior frontal gyrus; vlPFC: ventrolateral PFC).

Self-Report	Behavioral	Psychophysiological	Neural (fMRI)
Normative Age–Related Changes			
Increased use of 'adaptive' strategies, less use of 'maladaptive' strategies with age [5,12].	Reappraisal, but not distraction, improves linearly with age (ability does not always correlate with self-reported everyday use [26–28]).	Some evidence of age-related changes in RSA across adolescence [29].	Reduced amygdala reactivity with age [30–32], greater inverse PFC–amygdala connectivity, indicating better 'top-down' regulation [34,35].
Negative Emotion Regulation			
Associations with symptoms of anxiety			
More use of 'maladaptive' and less use of 'adaptive' strategies in anxiety disorders [36,37]. Social anxiety linked to reduced 'emotional clarity', reduced acceptance [38], and increased rumination [39].	Impaired reappraisal generation in anxiety disorders [40,41]. No differences in 'amplifying' or 'suppressing' expressive behaviors [42].	Greater number of visual fixations during negative images [43] and greater pupil dilation when 'upregulating' response to negative images [44] in adolescents with anxiety disorders.	Positive amygdala–vlPFC connectivity during affect labeling predicted future anxiety symptoms [45].
Associations with symptoms of depression			
More use of 'maladaptive', less use of 'adaptive' strategies in depression [36]. Specifically, less use of reappraisal [46], reduced acceptance [47] and higher suppression [48].	Mixed findings for reappraisal efficacy [49–51] in adolescents with depression.	Changes in RSA with age, linked to better 'acceptance', 'impulse control' and 'ability to use emotion regulation strategies' [52] in individuals with depression and conduct problems. RSA predicts more maladaptive emotion regulation in previously depressed adolescents [53]. Limited evidence of direct relationship between RSA and depression [54,55].	Evidence of disrupted activation and connectivity across emotion regulation neural circuitry (e.g., amygdala, PFC) in depression, but specific patterns of effects vary across studies ([49–51,56], see Figure).
Impacts link between stress and psychopathology			
Self-blame, catastrophizing, and rumination mediates the association between stress and depression [57]; rumination and impulsive responding links stress and internalizing symptoms [58].	Cognitive reappraisal mediates link between depressive symptoms and 'emotional recovery' from an experimental stressor [59].	RSA mediates the association between stress and anxiety [55].	Amygdala–vlPFC connectivity during incidental emotion regulation mediates the relationship between rumination and depressive symptoms [60].
Positive Emotion Regulation			
Associations with symptoms of anxiety			
Not investigated	Not investigated	Greater number of visual fixations during positive images in adolescents with anxiety disorders [43].	Not investigated
Associations with symptoms of depression			
Lower levels and shorter duration of positive affect [61,62], parental and self 'dampening' of positive emotions [63], lack of parental 'enhancing' [64] associated with depressive symptoms.	Reduced persistence of positive affect in conflict situation [65], low maternal positivity [66], and increased maternal dampening [67] associated with depressive symptoms.	Not investigated	Reduced activation of ventral striatum and PFC in response to reward (Forbes, 2011 #123 [68]), regulation not investigated
Impacts link between stress and psychopathology			
Not investigated	Not investigated	Not investigated	Not investigated

2. Overview of Measures of Emotion Regulation

Theoretical models of emotion regulation provide organizational frameworks within which to assess different strategies for regulation. The most widely used framework is the 'process model of emotion regulation' [2,11] which differentiates strategies along the timeline of a developing (negative) emotional response. A basic distinction in this model is between: (1) antecedent-focused strategies that manage the generation of an emotional reaction before it occurs, and (2) response-focused strategies that are invoked during an ongoing emotional reaction. A common antecedent-focused strategy is cognitive reappraisal, the process by which individuals consider a situation in a different way with the goal of managing their response when faced with that situation (e.g., when waiting for a friend to return a message, thinking 'they are busy' rather than thinking 'they don't like me'). Reappraisal is considered an adaptive regulatory strategy. A common response-focused strategy is expressive suppression, whereby individuals try to reduce or 'suppress' facial, vocal, or other expressions of the emotions they are currently experiencing. Expressive suppression is considered to be a maladaptive regulatory strategy. There are also numerous other strategies that impact the duration and intensity of negative emotions, such as problem solving, acceptance (considered to be adaptive) and rumination (maladaptive). Cognitive strategies for the regulation of positive emotions are not as widely discussed, but some focus on 'enhancing' and 'dampening', often in the context of interpersonal regulation between parents and children. Enhancing describes parental reactions of enthusiasm, encouragement or validation, whereas dampening refers to a focus on potential negative aspects of a situation, raising concerns and minimizing positive aspects [69].

3. Self-Report Measures of Emotion Regulation

A widely used self-report measure is the Emotion Regulation Questionnaire (ERQ) that follows the organizational principles of the process model of emotion regulation and has subscales for reappraisal and expressive suppression [70]. Other questionnaires assess different combinations of emotion regulation strategies, such as the Difficulties in Emotion Regulation Scale (DERS; [71]), the Cognitive Emotion Regulation Questionnaire (CERQ; [72]) and the *Fragebogen zur Erhebung der Emotionsregulation bei Kindern und Jugenlichen* (FEEL-KJ [73]). The varying content of these widely used self-report measures highlights inconsistencies with which the term 'emotion regulation' is used and limits the extent to which data across studies can be combined (see Table 2 for subscale comparison across measures). There are fewer standardized self-report measures available for positive emotion regulation. One such measure is the 'responses to positive affect' scale, which consists of three sub-scales: dampening, self-focused positive rumination and emotion-focused positive rumination [74].

Table 2. Overview of subscales across self-report measures of negative emotion regulation. Strategies are informally categorized as 'adaptive', 'maladaptive' or 'uncategorized' (describing more general emotion regulation behavior, rather than specific strategies). ERQ: Emotion Regulation Questionnaire; DERS: Difficulties in Emotion Regulation Scale; CERQ: Cognitive Emotion Regulations Questionnaire; FEEL-KJ: *Fragebogen zur Ehrebung her Emotionsregulation bei Kindern und Jugenlichen*.

ERQ	DERS	CERQ	FEEL-KJ
Adaptive Strategies			
Reappraisal		Positive reappraisal	Revaluation
	Non-acceptance	Acceptance	Acceptance
		Putting in perspective	
		Positive refocusing	
		Refocus on planning	
			Problem solving
			Cognitive problem solving
			Distraction
			Forgetting
			Humor enhancement

Table 2. *Cont.*

ERQ	DERS	CERQ	FEEL-KJ
Maladaptive Strategies			
Expressive suppression			Emotional control
		Self-blame	Self-devaluation
		Other-blame	
		Rumination	Rumination
		Catastrophizing	
			Giving-up
Uncategorized			
	Goal-directed behavior		
	Impulse control		Aggressive actions
	Emotional awareness		
	Accessing regulation strategies		
	Emotional clarity		
			Withdrawal
			Social support
			Expression

Retrospective self-report questionnaires are criticized for the likelihood of over-generalized responding, the assumption that people are conscious of how they regulate their emotions and bias in memory effects (remembering most recent and/or salient experiences [75]; Table 3 lists methodological limitations of techniques discussed). Overcoming limitations based on memory, experience sampling methodologies aim to capture responses to experiences during, or close in time to, real life events through high density self-reporting (multiple times per day). This approach offers richer data on emotional experiences and often encompasses both positive and negative affect. Existing studies using this approach assess emotion regulation through self-report of strategy use and duration of emotional experiences (i.e., 'emotional recovery'). However, 'emotional recovery' may be influenced by factors other than regulation, including emotional intensity or situational changes. This type of approach therefore prevents discrete measurement of emotional *reactivity* from emotional *regulation* (for a theoretical discussion of this issue, see [76]).

Table 3. Comparison of the methodological limitations of different study designs used to assess emotion regulation across levels of analysis. SR: self-report; Beh: behavioral; PP: peripheral psychophysiological; Neu: neural.

	SR: Questionnaire	SR: Experience Sampling	Beh: Stressful Situation	Beh: Observed Interactions	Beh/PP/Neu: Spontaneous Regulation	Beh/PP/Neu: Deliberate Regulation	Neu: Implicit Regulation
Methodological Limitation							
Varying content across measures	x			x			
Limited assessment of positive vs. negative affect	x		x		x	x	x
Retrospective bias	x						
Socially desirable responding	x	x	x	x		x	
Conflates emotional reactivity and regulation		x	x	x	x		
Assumes accurate insight into regulatory strategy	x	x					
Lacks ecological validity					x	x	x

4. Behavioral Assessment of Emotion Regulation

Observational approaches can be used to examine responses, for example: during in vivo stress inductions (e.g., Trier Social Stress Task [77] or mock job interviews [46,59]); between pairs of individuals in spontaneous interactions; or during prescribed stress-inducing or rewarding situations [65,66,78]. Participants' behavioral and verbal responses are coded and classified according to regulatory strategy and subjective affect ratings can be collected to measure emotional recovery. As with self-report measures, these approaches too may be influenced by socially desirable responding and lack the capacity to separate reactivity from regulation.

Computer-based methods of assessing emotion regulation behaviors involve presenting participants with affectively evocative images (such as from the International Affective Picture System [79]) and asking them to rate the strength of their emotional reaction. In some variants, participants passively view images to assess 'automatic' or 'spontaneous' regulation, other variants aim to enhance ecological validity by swapping affective images for descriptions of ambiguous situations (e.g., mother is late to come home [40]). While providing a degree of experimental control unavailable in observational studies, these 'spontaneous regulation' paradigms still cannot dissociate emotional reactivity from regulation, conflating assessment of the strength of an emotional response with the ability to regulate this response. Stronger 'deliberate regulation' designs compare ratings from passive 'reactivity' trials with active 'regulatory' trials in which participants are instructed to down- or up-regulate their emotional response. This approach offers a within-subjects inspection of the impact of deliberate emotion regulation using predetermined strategies. A potential drawback of this approach, however, is response bias in affect ratings where individuals may report reduced negative affect as a consequence of following task instructions rather than successful regulation per se. In some studies participants are trained to use specific strategies (such as reappraisal, distancing or suppression), although there is variability in the extensiveness of pre-task training and participant proficiency in strategy usage across studies.

5. Peripheral Psychophysiological Indicators of Emotion Regulation

Peripheral psychophysiological studies of emotion regulation use similar designs to those described above for behavioral assessments, so the limitations of those designs also apply to methods described here. Investigation of peripheral psychophysiological correlates of emotion regulation encompass a range of measures. Cardiac and respiratory measures include heart-rate variability and respiratory sinus arrhythmia (RSA; variation in heart rate within a breath cycle). Greater variation in heart rate and RSA are considered indicative of greater physiological adaptation to emotional stimuli (i.e., more effective regulation [80]). Ocular measures include pupil dilation, a measure of arousal or 'cognitive effort' [81], and visual fixation patterns, which demonstrate areas of attentional focus (and have also been suggested to indicate prefrontal cortex activation [82]). Facial electromyography (EMG) of the startle blink reflex and corrugator muscle activation are used as measures of negative emotional arousal [83]. Skin conductance levels and responses are used as a measure of emotional arousal at a chronic, or stimulus-evoked level, respectively [84]. These measures offer the potential for objective, low-cost biological markers of emotion regulation. However, they largely suffer from a lack of specificity in relation to psychological constructs, making the functional significance of differences observed difficult to interpret [85].

6. Neural Measures of Emotion Regulation

Neuroimaging studies using functional Magnetic Resonance Imaging (fMRI) to investigate neural correlates of emotion regulation have primarily used deliberate regulation paradigms. Across studies to date, instructions for regulation vary from broad approaches (e.g., 'decrease') to specific strategies (e.g., 'distance' or 'reappraise'). One concern with fMRI designs is that due to timing constraints, participants are often given a short period of time (approximately eight seconds) to implement a strategy per image, raising potential concerns of ecological validity. A different approach used in fMRI studies are measures of 'incidental regulation', such as affect labeling [86,87]. Unlike study designs assuming 'automatic' regulation, studies of 'incidental' regulation investigate processes wherein a specific task may lead to emotion regulation, without the deliberate intention of doing so. For example, in the affect labeling task, participants view images of emotional facial expressions and are asked to label the emotion they see. Affect labeling has been shown to decrease experienced negative emotions and is also common across forms of psychotherapy [86]. As many individuals may be unaware of their emotion regulation strategies, the incidental nature of affect labeling may be helpful in addressing/circumventing limitations of self-report methodologies. One criticism of this approach, however, is that individuals do not intend to regulate when labeling (i.e., the goal is implicit), so it may not be considered a true form of emotion regulation. Despite this concern, studies using this task have demonstrated that affect labeling recruits neural circuitries implicated in emotion regulation in healthy adults, such as reduced amygdala activation, and increased inverse ventrolateral prefrontal cortex (vlPFC)–amygdala connectivity [86,87]. Because affect labeling robustly activates this circuitry in healthy samples, it offers an objective comparison of potential biological differences in psychopathology during incidental emotion regulation.

7. Relationships between Emotion Regulation Abilities and Symptoms of Anxiety and Depression in Adolescents

7.1. Findings from Self-Report Studies

Analyses of self-reported data consistently identify associations between emotion regulation abilities and symptoms of anxiety and depression in adolescents. For example, less use of cognitive reappraisal and greater use of expressive suppression was associated with higher symptoms of depression [46,48], and higher levels of rumination were associated with greater symptoms of social anxiety [39]. This was recently confirmed in a meta-analysis of 35 studies in adolescents (aged 13–18 years), demonstrating that compared to healthy individuals, those with anxiety and depressive disorders engaged in less reappraisal, problem solving, and acceptance (adaptive regulatory strategies) and more avoidance, suppression and rumination (maladaptive strategies [36]). Of these associations, the strongest effects were observed for reduced acceptance and increased avoidance and rumination across both anxiety and depression, with little evidence of specific disruptions linked to either disorder. Other work has sought to investigate patterns of disrupted emotion regulation specific to individual anxiety disorders. One study suggested greater deficits in emotional clarity and non-acceptance of emotions in social anxiety disorder compared to generalized anxiety disorder (using the DERS [38]). However, another found no differences between groups of adolescents with different anxiety disorder diagnoses (using the FEEL-KJ [37]). While use of different questionnaires across studies may explain differences in effects observed, there is no strong evidence of specific deficits in emotion regulation resulting in specific symptom profiles within anxiety disorders.

Relatively few studies have examined the role of positive emotion regulation in relation to symptoms of anxiety and depression. One study in which parents reported on adolescent affect found that parents of depressed adolescents rated shorter durations of 'happy' affect in their children, compared to parents of non-depressed adolescents [61]. However, this study did not investigate strategies for maintaining or dampening positive affect, limiting the ability to differentiate disruptions in regulation from reactivity. Other studies have focused on interpersonal aspects of emotion regulation, showing that self-reported parental dampening, or a lack of parental enhancing of positive affect, was related to prospective increases in adolescent depression, potentially via their own dampening of positive affect [63,64]. The extent to which these findings are specific to symptoms of depression, rather than more general psychopathology remains unexplored.

Studies using experience sampling methodologies are beginning to examine relationships between daily experiences of emotion, regulation strategies and symptoms of anxiety and depression. One such study in adolescents aged 13–16 years over a 21-day period showed that symptoms of depression were related to reduced *variance* in reported emotional state (including happiness, depression, anger and anxiety), an effect that was associated with the 'acceptance' subscale of the DERS [47]. A study that collected data over two weekends using nine daily self-reports of emotional events and self-rated emotion regulation in a sample of 12–17 year-olds found no association between momentary use of emotion regulation strategies and depression in girls, but an inverse relationship between acceptance and depression in boys [88]. These types of approach hold much promise for examining daily life experiences of emotion regulation, but further work is required to standardize analytic approaches and investigate other factors that may influence these relationships potentially explaining the mixed findings observed to date.

Beyond simple correlations of co-occurring emotion regulation deficits and symptoms of anxiety and depression, it has been suggested that disrupted emotion regulation is a risk factor for the development of psychopathology [89,90]. Confirming this effect, meta-analytic data suggests that disrupted self-reported emotion regulation abilities predict subsequent diagnosis of anxiety or depression [36]. Critically, the same analyses did not find that psychopathology predicted subsequent disruptions to emotion regulation. This unidirectional relationship was also observed in a large (N = 1065) study of adolescents aged 11–14 years [75]. Although this study showed that while a latent construct of 'emotion dysregulation' (combining multiple subscales) predicted symptoms of anxiety, aggression and disordered eating behaviors, depression was predicted only by rumination, expression of anger and expression of sadness. While highlighting the differing effects that can be observed with varying definitions of emotion regulation, this work does provide support for the notion that disrupted emotion regulation is a risk factor for future psychopathology.

Emotion regulation has also been proposed as a mediating variable between a risk factor (e.g., early life adversity) and the development of psychopathology. Mediator variables hold the potential to identify factors that might be altered through intervention to reduce the risk of psychopathology. Studies investigating the mediating role of emotion regulation in adolescents suggest that increased use of maladaptive emotion regulation strategies may mediate the association between adversity and psychopathology. These studies found: (1) an effect of self-blame, catastrophizing, and rumination on the relationship between stressful life events and symptoms of depression [57]; and (2) a role for rumination and impulsive responding on the relationship between childhood maltreatment and symptoms of internalizing psychopathology [58]. What these studies do not indicate is whether higher levels of adaptive strategies reduce the risk of psychopathology following early life adversity.

7.2. Findings from Behavioral Studies

Across studies using deliberate emotion regulation paradigms, there is some evidence suggesting that anxiety is associated with reduced use of reappraisal, while findings for depression are mixed. Considering first anxiety, anxious adolescents were shown to have heightened emotional reactivity to negative images and impairments in generating reappraisals when cued [40,41]. However, in trials where they did successfully generate reappraisals, anxious adolescents were able to effectively reduce their negative affect to a similar degree as their non-anxious counterparts. Deficits in reappraisal generation corresponded both with less frequent self-reported everyday use of reappraisal and lower reappraisal self-efficacy (i.e., the belief that reappraisal would improve their feelings), suggesting a combination of real and perceived deficits in adaptive emotion regulation. Classification of anxious adolescents' verbal responses to ambiguous situations according to regulatory strategy showed reduced spontaneous use of reappraisal and problem solving and increased use avoidance and help-seeking strategies with no differences in attentional deployment (distraction) or behavioral response modulation (suppression) [40]. Together, these findings suggest that reappraisal may be an effective yet underutilized strategy in adolescents with anxiety. Another study assessing abilities to suppress or amplify expressive behaviors in response to positive and negative images found no effects of anxiety or depression [42], suggesting impairments observed may be specific to reappraisal skills.

Studies investigating reappraisal ability have demonstrated mixed effects for adolescent depression. All studies to date with behavioral affect rating data have used deliberate emotion regulation paradigms while participants also underwent fMRI (neural results are discussed below). Two studies found no difference in reappraisal success (difference in average affect ratings for 'look' minus 'decrease' trials in samples aged 13–17 [49] and aged 15 [50]), but a third study in a sample of 15–25 year-olds showed poorer reappraisal success in adolescents with depression compared to healthy controls [51]. One difference between studies that may contribute to the discrepancy in findings is depression severity, with deficits in reappraisal observed in a sample with more severe depressive symptoms (and an older age range). It is possible that depression severity impedes the effectiveness of reappraisal, although it remains unclear whether this is due to deficits in reappraisal generation or implementation. Future work directly comparing these processes in adolescents with anxiety, depression and mixed diagnoses would be helpful to delineate the nature of any differences associated with specific disorders.

Behavioral studies of interpersonal positive emotion regulation highlight an association between depressive symptoms and shorter duration of positive affect. In one study, adolescents and their parents completed a trivia game which was rigged to provide positive feedback, followed by a 'conflict task' in which families discussed previously identified 'family issues' [65]. While there was no association between depressive symptoms and observed positive affect during the reward task, there was an association with the 'persistence' of positive affect, defined as the maintenance of positive affect in a negative situation. Other findings suggest links between parental and adolescent emotion regulation, with reduced maternal positivity and increased dampening related to reduced maintenance of positive affect [66] and higher adolescent depressive symptomatology [67]. However, these studies did not assess self-focused regulatory strategies that may contribute to positive affect persistence, again impacting the ability to dissociate disruptions to emotion regulation from disrupted emotional reactivity.

As suggested in the self-report literature, there is emerging behavioral evidence that emotion regulation may impact the association between stressful experiences and psychopathology. In one study examining this effect, adolescents completed a social stress task (a mock job interview), provided distress ratings before and after the task, and completed self-report measures of cognitive reappraisal (using the ERQ) and depressive symptoms. Among those reporting higher levels of depressive symptoms, greater self-reported tendency to use cognitive reappraisal was associated with faster 'emotional recovery' (difference in distress ratings from before to 30 min after the task [59]). These findings indirectly suggest that the ability to use cognitive reappraisal in the face of social stressors may buffer the impact of depressive symptoms on emotional reactivity and recovery. However, it is important to note that in-vivo emotion regulation was not directly assessed during the stress task. Findings from self-report studies suggest that emotion regulation following stressful life events may impact the likelihood of developing psychopathology, while this study suggests a relationship in the opposite direction, that self-reported general emotion regulation tendencies may affect the impact of depression upon emotional reactivity/recovery. A variant on this paradigm in which participants are instructed to use reappraisal or other specific strategies in different conditions would allow a more direct investigation of the efficacy of each strategy. This would also help clarify the direction of these relationships, which would be useful in improving understanding of the developmental etiology of depression in adolescents (e.g., clarifying emotional reactivity or recovery as a vulnerability factor or a symptom of depression).

7.3. Findings from Studies of Peripheral Psychophysiology

Studies of peripheral psychophysiological indicators of emotion regulation in adolescents have sought to identify specific patterns of disruption linked to anxiety and depression. One small study in anxious youth ($N = 27$, aged 8–17 years) demonstrated that the number of fixations during negatively and positively valenced pictures (relative to neutral pictures) was greater among individuals with anxiety disorders, compared to healthy individuals [43]. The authors suggest that as visual fixations have been shown to correlate with activation of the prefrontal cortex [82], these findings may indicate that anxious adolescents were trying to regulate their responses even in the absence of instructions to do so. However, given that there were no differences in visual fixations when participants were instructed to regulate, this interpretation seems unlikely. The same study also found greater pupil dilation during negative compared to neutral pictures when instructed to 'upregulate' emotional responses in anxious, but not healthy adolescents [43]. As pupil dilation is considered an index of arousal this might suggest anxious adolescents experience more intense emotions when deliberately upregulating. However, the general nature of instructions prevents conclusions regarding the type of strategy employed, or whether, for example, adolescents with anxiety engage maladaptive regulatory strategies more readily than healthy adolescents. In addition, it is important to note that using psychophysiological measures to make inferences about emotional states is a form of 'reverse inference', and the lack of specificity between emotional experiences and peripheral psychophysiological markers caution against this type of conclusion.

Whereas research in children suggests a predictive relationship between RSA and future anxiety and depression (e.g., [54,91]), findings from studies in adolescents are mixed. A large study of 11-year-olds (N = 1653) found no correlation between RSA and concurrent or future depressive symptoms assessed at age 13 [55]. The same study did, however, identify an interaction with life stress such that among individuals who experienced higher levels of stressful life events, higher RSA was associated with reduced self-reported anxiety [55]. Other work has suggested that atypical RSA patterns (either higher or lower) are associated with maladaptive regulatory strategies, which in turn are predictive of future depressive episodes in older adolescents with a history of depression (although RSA did not directly predict depression recurrence [53]). In another study, change over time in RSA predicted emotion regulation abilities in a sample of 8-12 year-olds with varying levels of depression and conduct problems [52]. Improving physiological responses to emotional challenges over time, i.e., increased RSA during a sad mood induction, was associated with fewer self-reported difficulties in emotion regulation, particularly in relation to 'accepting', 'impulse control' and 'ability to use emotion regulation strategies'. RSA is often considered a specific measure of emotion regulation, yet it has also been shown to vary according to individual differences in emotional reactivity [80] which limits interpretations that can be made with this measure.

Investigating the effects of sustaining positive affect, a study of young adults (18–21 year-olds) involved a reward task, followed by a mood induction film clip that was positive, negative or neutral [92]. Reporting higher positive emotion during the reward task was associated with a faster return to physiological baseline (based on heart rate measures) when subsequently viewing a neutral film clip, but slower return to baseline when subsequently viewing a positive film clip. This study suggests that individual differences in reactivity to reward are related to physiological differences in adaptation to subsequent mood induction stimuli to maintain (positive clip) or reduce (neutral clip) positive affective states. However, this study did not examine the impact of intentional regulation of positive affect, which would be of much interest to investigate whether individuals can generate a 'sustained' positive valence state, and how this relates to symptoms of psychopathology.

Overall, evidence from psychophysiological studies linking emotion dysregulation to anxiety and depression is preliminary and highly varied in experimental methodology and sample characteristics, making comparisons across studies difficult. Addressing some of these challenges, a recent study concurrently used a range of measures to assess emotion reactivity and regulation during presentation of valenced images [44]. In a sample of young adolescents, measures of corrugator and startle EMG and skin conductance were assessed while participants were instructed to 'maintain' or 'discontinue' their emotional responses. Corrugator EMG activity was sensitive to valence (positive vs. negative stimuli), while startle EMG and skin conductance was sensitive to regulation instruction. This approach offers promise for identifying reliable indicators of emotion regulation across development and how they may be disrupted in adolescent anxiety and depression.

7.4. Findings from fMRI Studies

In normative adolescent neural development, the maturation of prefrontal regions supporting emotion regulation lags behind limbic regions involved in emotion generation (for a review, see [15]). Most studies observe linear decreases in amygdala reactivity to affective stimuli with age [30–32], alongside linear increases in dorsomedial prefrontal cortex (dmPFC) recruitment [33]. Age-related improvements in cognitive regulation of emotion are also associated with reduced amygdala activation [34,93] as well as increases in inverse coupling (i.e., negative correlation in functional connectivity) between the PFC and amygdala [34]. A shift from positive to inverse amygdala–PFC connectivity occurs from childhood to adolescence [30]. By mid-adolescence, most youth display inverse amygdala–PFC connectivity, with stronger inverse connectivity corresponding to lower symptoms of anxiety in a non-clinical sample [30,94]. Evidence across fMRI studies suggests that disruptions in the same cortico-limbic circuitry during emotion regulation are implicated in anxiety and depression in adolescents.

Studies reviewed above described mixed findings as to whether adolescents with depression demonstrated disrupted abilities to reduce ratings of negative affect during instructed reappraisal [49–51]. In contrast, functional MRI data from the same studies have consistently found evidence of aberrant prefrontal activation and connectivity during deliberate emotion regulation. However, the specific regions implicated and disruptions in connectivity observed vary across studies (see Figure 1). Three out of four extant studies found evidence of heightened amygdala reactivity or greater amygdala–PFC connectivity during regulation in adolescents with depression [50,51,56]. However, the study which did not observe these findings was the largest (with the greatest power to detect effects) and did not find robust evidence of altered amygdala reactivity or connectivity, instead demonstrating changes in connectivity between dorsal regions of prefrontal cortex and inferior frontal regions [49]. Studies of depression in adults generally support a model of heightened activation in cognitive control regions and impaired subcortical down-regulation [95–98], which has been interpreted as an effortful yet ineffective attempt to regulate. In adolescents, connectivity between subregions of PFC may also play a role. Further investigation of inconsistencies across studies, perhaps by utilizing measures of emotion regulation from other levels of analysis, would be useful in determining the role of regulatory circuitry in adolescent depression. Importantly, no studies have investigated neural differences in up-regulation of positive emotions in adolescents with depression, which is an important avenue for future research given the relevance of the positive affect system in major depressive disorder.

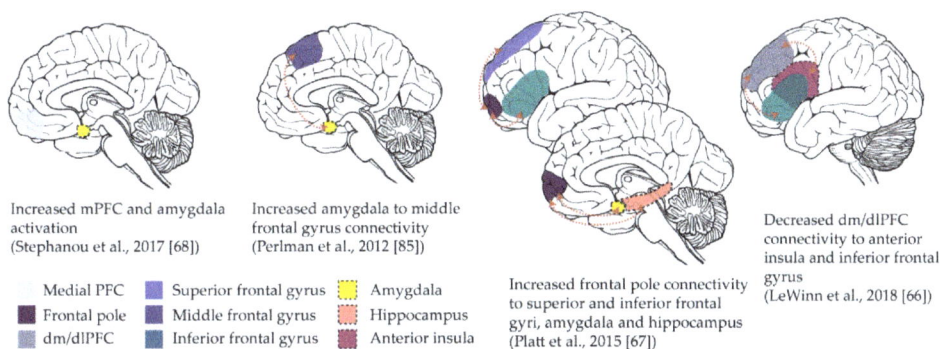

Increased mPFC and amygdala activation (Stephanou et al., 2017 [68])

Increased amygdala to middle frontal gyrus connectivity (Perlman et al., 2012 [85])

Increased frontal pole connectivity to superior and inferior frontal gyri, amygdala and hippocampus (Platt et al., 2015 [67])

Decreased dm/dlPFC connectivity to anterior insula and inferior frontal gyrus (LeWinn et al., 2018 [66])

Medial PFC	Superior frontal gyrus	Amygdala
Frontal pole	Middle frontal gyrus	Hippocampus
dm/dlPFC	Inferior frontal gyrus	Anterior insula

Figure 1. Patterns of altered neural activation and connectivity during emotion regulation in adolescents with depression. Overall, studies to date have demonstrated altered activation and connectivity in the amygdala and across regions of prefrontal cortex. The directionality of effects (greater or lesser in depressed compared to non-depressed participants), and the specific set of regions involved however varies across studies. (PFC: prefrontal cortex, dm/dlPFC: dorsomedial/dorsolateral PFC).

fMRI investigations of emotion regulation in adolescents with anxiety have been more limited than in depression, with no studies of deliberate reappraisal to date. However, activation across similar circuitry during incidental emotion regulation may prospectively predict the development of anxiety symptoms. For example, in a sample of ninth grade females (mean age 15), positive amygdala–vlPFC connectivity during an incidental emotion regulation task (affect labeling [87]) predicted future symptoms of anxiety in the following 9 months [45]. Interestingly, childhood negative emotionality (assessed by parent, teacher, and self-report from grades 2–7) related to positive amygdala–right vlPFC connectivity in ninth grade, but only in girls with low levels of cognitive control (assessed by Brief Rating Inventory of Executive Functioning reports from grades 5–7). The authors suggested that individual differences in negative emotionality and cognitive control may be respective risk or resilience factors for 'less mature' positive connectivity between the amygdala and PFC, and in turn anxiety.

Similar to behavioral and self-reported findings, there is some evidence that neural measures of emotion regulation ability (cortico-limbic functional connectivity) may influence the association between stress and depression. After completing an incidental emotion regulation task [87], a sample of adolescent females (mean age 15) underwent a social stress manipulation by completing the Cyberball task [99] in which they were unknowingly excluded from a virtual game of catch. Positive amygdala vlPFC connectivity during incidental emotion regulation was associated with greater self-reported 'stress-reactive rumination' (following the Cyberball task) and mediated the relationship between self-reported rumination and depressive symptoms [60]. The retrospective self-report of depression and lack of temporal precedence limits these findings from a developmental psychopathology perspective, but highlights a potential mediating mechanism that could be investigated longitudinally in future research.

Taken together, these studies suggest that adolescents with anxiety and depression exhibit differences in neural functioning compared to non-depressed peers during deliberate emotion regulation. Evidence to date suggests that some of these differences may be similar to disruptions in emotion regulation neural circuitries observed in adults, although no studies have yet directly compared samples of adolescents and adults with anxiety or depression. Existing models of emotion regulation make inferences based on directional connectivity between prefrontal and subcortical brain regions. However, as functional connectivity analyses are correlational, it is ultimately impossible to interpret directionality (i.e., whether inverse connectivity indicates prefrontal down-regulation of affective regions). A less common yet promising analytical approach is 'effective connectivity' (e.g., dynamic causal modeling or Granger causality), which can be used to determine effective connectivity, or the directional influence of one region upon another. For example, one study using this technique demonstrated that adults with social anxiety disorder display impaired bidirectional amygdala–vmPFC effective connectivity while perceiving affective stimuli [100]. Use of this approach, and other advanced analytic techniques, may allow more direct investigation of proposed models of neural circuitry dysfunction during emotion regulation in adolescents with psychopathology.

8. Clinical Implications for Interventions in Adolescents

Understanding emotion regulation in adolescents with anxiety and depression is critical for improving the efficacy of existing treatments and informing the development of novel interventions. Promoting adaptive emotion regulation is a central component of most evidence-based psychotherapies for adolescent anxiety and depression, although different skills are emphasized across modalities. Cognitive Behavioral Therapy (CBT), emphasizes cognitive restructuring and promotes the use of reappraisal, while 'third wave' psychotherapies (e.g., mindfulness-based cognitive therapy, dialectical behavioral therapy [101]) focus on acceptance and decentering to regulate emotions. Most studies of psychotherapy effectiveness include both children and adolescents in combined samples, with age relating to better treatment outcomes [102]. Older adolescents may be better able to benefit from CBT possibly due to more developed cognitive and social skills, consistent with age-related improvements in emotion regulation ability in healthy adolescents [26,27]. It remains unknown whether emotion regulation skills taught in mindfulness-based versus cognitive behavioral approaches are better suited for certain individuals across development, highlighting the importance of age effects and treatment matching in future research.

As intervention packages typically contain several elements, it can be difficult to tease apart the 'active ingredients' of treatments. In line with the National Institute of Mental Health's (NIMH) shift in clinical trials to an experimental therapeutic paradigm [103], a priority for intervention research is to test specific mechanisms of action that account for meaningful clinical change. Emotion regulation is a prime candidate for such mechanistic studies. This has been the goal in more recent treatments that specifically focus on enhancing emotion (e.g., Contextual Emotion Regulation Therapy [104], Emotion Regulation Therapy [105]). Changes in decentering and reappraisal through Emotion Regulation Therapy temporally preceded reductions in anxiety and depression in young adults, suggesting a potential mechanism [106]. Future work should extend and tailor these treatments to adolescent populations.

Other mechanistic work aiming to distil the effects of individual treatment components has focused on briefer computerized trainings designed to change attentional or interpretational biases believed to contribute to anxiety and depression [107]. In line with the process model of emotion regulation [2], Cognitive Bias Modification aims to tap into antecedent-focused regulatory processes such as attentional deployment (Attention Bias Modification) and interpretation/reappraisal (Interpretation Bias Modification). Although these approaches have been shown to effectively retrain biases, estimates of the effects on clinical outcomes in adults are modest [108]. Recent adaptations that train attention toward positive stimuli show promise in reducing symptoms of anxiety and depression in children [109,110]. As reviewed above, adolescents with anxiety and depression may have specific deficits in the generation of reappraisals. More open-ended modifications of interpretation bias training may therefore be helpful in improving this ability.

Few interventions target positive emotion regulation in adolescence and adults alike, mirroring the relative dearth of research in this domain. Designed specifically to treat anhedonia in adults, Positive Affect Treatment (PAT [111]) promotes positive emotion through a variety of behavioral, cognitive, and experiential exercises. For example, rather than challenging negative thoughts as in traditional CBT, PAT promotes identifying positive aspects of situations (i.e., finding the silver lining). Through its treatment components, PAT likely both induces and augments positive affect, involving both bottom-up and top-down processes (i.e., emotional reactivity and regulation). Future research might adapt similar interventions for adolescents. Given the link between adolescent depressive symptoms and reduced positive emotion persistence [65,66] novel interventions may focus on techniques that sustain positive affect in the presence of stress and train recovery after stressful events.

Intervention studies also offer a powerful approach to investigating mechanisms of treatment action. Increasingly, neuroimaging measures have been included in trials of psychological interventions, with mounting evidence suggesting changes in functioning and connectivity in amygdala-prefrontal circuitry following CBT [112,113]. To date, there have been no studies of interventions with adolescents assessing neural mechanisms of interventions using emotion regulation tasks. Neuroscientific research of treatment mechanisms has started to lead to the development of novel treatment approaches, such as repeated transcranial magnetic stimulation (rTMS [114]) and neurofeedback [115,116], which hold promise for altering activation of emotion regulation neural circuitries.

9. Summary and Directions for Future Research

From the literature reviewed above (summarized in Table 1), there is a consistent body of evidence from self-report studies that disruptions to emotion regulation capacities are associated with greater likelihood of experiencing anxiety and depression in adolescence. There is also evidence suggesting that these disruptions to emotion regulation are predictive, rather than sequelae, of future psychopathology. To date, there is no strong evidence relating specific regulatory strategies with specific diagnoses or symptom profiles, suggesting that altered capacities in this domain confer a more general risk for psychopathology.

In contrast, findings from behavioral studies suggest that anxiety in adolescence may be specifically related to a reduced spontaneous use of reappraisal regulatory strategies. However, given that there are far fewer behavioral than self-report studies in this domain and that behavioral studies have less comprehensively assessed all forms of emotion regulation across different diagnoses, the specificity of this effect may not be as clear as it appears. There is no consensus from behavioral research as to whether depression is linked to disruptions in regulation of negative affect, with some studies showing reduced reappraisal efficacy and others not showing this effect. One finding that does appear more consistent is the reduced duration of positive affect among adolescents with depression, although the extent to which this is tied to deficits in cognitive regulatory strategies has not been investigated.

Findings from peripheral psychophysiological measures are limited, and effects observed are also mixed. There is some preliminary evidence from individual studies, but the variance in methods used prevents commentary on consensus of findings in this area. There has been a relative proliferation of functional MRI studies assessing disrupted emotion regulation neural circuitry. On the whole, these studies have identified differences in activation and functional connectivity between amygdala and prefrontal cortical brain regions in adolescents with depression. Studies of anxiety suggest that disruptions in neural functioning may precede onset of symptomatology. Although overall findings from neuroimaging studies point to disruptions in similar circuitries, individual studies show different spatial patterns of effects. A challenge to future work in this area is to establish greater specificity in models of emotion regulation neural circuitry, including tests of effective connectivity that can begin to investigate probable direction of information flow.

Across studies of self-report, behavioral, and neural measures of emotion regulation reviewed, there were findings indicating relationships between reactivity to stressful events, emotion dysregulation and psychopathology. Findings from self-report studies suggest that emotion regulation skills may mediate the effects between early life adversity and subsequent psychopathology, while evidence from other levels of analysis present less clear directionality. It may be that disruptions to emotion reactivity and regulation are vulnerability factors for the development of future psychopathology, or that these problems arise as symptoms of specific disorders.

Future Directions

As demonstrated in Table 1, there are clear gaps in current research on associations between emotion regulation and psychopathology in adolescents. One particular discrepancy is the greater focus on regulation of negative emotions, compared to positive emotions. Both the theory and (self-report) measurement tools available are more established for negative compared to positive regulation. Approaches used to investigate regulatory skills in behavioral, psychophysiological and neural levels of analysis however, may be just as appropriate for the study of positive emotion regulation. Some of the studies reviewed used multiple techniques to investigate emotion regulation across different levels of analysis. This should be encouraged in future work, particularly in the integration of newer techniques, such as ecological momentary assessment, to allow investigation of how findings observed in retrospective self-report or lab-based studies relate to daily life experiences.

As noted throughout, many of the studies reviewed also rely on indirect measures of emotion regulation, wherein responses to emotional stimuli are measured and the magnitude or duration of response is considered evidence of regulation. More stringent study designs use direct comparisons of instructed strategies which can help to disentangle effects of emotional *reactivity* from *regulation*. The instructions provided and regulatory strategies used in these studies is somewhat varied, but overall has focused on reappraisal, with less research investigating other regulatory skills (e.g., acceptance). Studies also vary in the use of emotional stimuli, but there has been a lack of discussion of whether there may be some strategies that are more appropriate than others for certain stimuli. For example, reappraisal may be an appropriate strategy for social stimuli, but less appropriate when responding to a moral violation (e.g., [27]).

There are also some individual difference variables that may be of much value to understanding the development of emotion regulation capacities. These include gender, pubertal status and cognitive abilities. Each of these have been suggested to impact the relationship between emotion regulation and psychopathology (e.g., [117–119]) and may be of interest in future work. Finally, further work investigating mechanisms of psychological interventions targeting emotion regulation abilities may be a particularly promising approach. This would allow a well-controlled investigation of whether training to enhance cognitive strategies for emotion regulation in adolescents mediates the impact of psychological therapies on symptoms of anxiety and depression.

Author Contributions: K.S.Y. and C.F.S. reviewed literature, all authors contributed to writing of the manuscript.

Funding: This research received no external funding.

Conflicts of Interest: The authors declare no conflict of interest.

References

1. Parrott, W.G. Beyond hedonism: Motives for inhibiting good moods. In *Handbook of Mental Control*; Wegner, D.M., Pennebaker, J.W., Eds.; Englewood Cliffs: Prentice Hall, NJ, USA, 1993; pp. 278–308.
2. Gross, J.J. Emotion regulation: Affective, cognitive, and social consequences. *Psychophysiology* **2002**, *39*, 281–291. [CrossRef] [PubMed]
3. Koole, S.L. The psychology of emotion regulation: An integrative review. *Cognit. Emot.* **2009**, *23*, 4–41. [CrossRef]
4. Kopp, C.B. Regulation of distress and negative emotions: A developmental view. *Dev. Psychol.* **1989**, *25*, 343. [CrossRef]
5. Zimmermann, P.; Iwanski, A. Emotion regulation from early adolescence to emerging adulthood and middle adulthood: Age differences, gender differences, and emotion-specific developmental variations. *Int. J. Behav. Dev.* **2014**, *38*, 182–194. [CrossRef]
6. Gross, J.J. Emotion regulation in adulthood: Timing is everything. *Curr. Direct. Psychol. Sci.* **2001**, *10*, 214–219. [CrossRef]
7. Clark, L.A.; Watson, D. Tripartite model of anxiety and depression: Psychometric evidence and taxonomic implications. *J. Abnorm. Psychol.* **1991**, *100*, 316. [CrossRef]
8. Hofmann, S.G.; Sawyer, A.T.; Fang, A.; Asnaani, A. Emotion dysregulation model of mood and anxiety disorders. *Depression Anxiety* **2012**, *29*, 409–416. [CrossRef]
9. Werner-Seidler, A.; Banks, R.; Dunn, B.D.; Moulds, M.L. An investigation of the relationship between positive affect regulation and depression. *Behav. Res. Therapy* **2013**, *51*, 46–56. [CrossRef]
10. Berking, M.; Wupperman, P.; Reichardt, A.; Pejic, A.; Dippel, A.; Znoj, H. Emotion-regulation skills as a treatment target in psychotherapy. *Behav. Res. Therapy* **2008**, *46*, 1230–1237. [CrossRef]
11. Gross, J.J. The emerging field of emotion regulation: An integrative review. *Rev. Gen. Psychol.* **1998**, *2*, 271. [CrossRef]
12. Gullone, E.; Hughes, E.K.; King, N.J.; Tonge, B. The normative development of emotion regulation strategy use in children and adolescents: A 2-year follow-up study. *J. Child Psychol. Psychiatry* **2010**, *51*, 567–574. [CrossRef]
13. Casey, B.; Duhoux, S.; Cohen, M.M. Adolescence: What do transmission, transition, and translation have to do with it? *Neuron* **2010**, *67*, 749–760. [CrossRef]
14. Steinberg, L. A social neuroscience perspective on adolescent risk-taking. *Dev. Rev.* **2008**, *28*, 78–106. [CrossRef]
15. Ahmed, S.P.; Bittencourt-Hewitt, A.; Sebastian, C.L. Neurocognitive bases of emotion regulation development in adolescence. *Dev. Cognit. Neurosci.* **2015**, *15*, 11–25. [CrossRef] [PubMed]
16. Ernst, M. The triadic model perspective for the study of adolescent motivated behavior. *Brain Cognit.* **2014**, *89*, 104–111. [CrossRef] [PubMed]
17. Somerville, L.H.; Casey, B. Developmental neurobiology of cognitive control and motivational systems. *Curr. Opin. Neurobiol.* **2010**, *20*, 236–241. [CrossRef]
18. Casey, B.; Heller, A.S.; Gee, D.G.; Cohen, A.O. Development of the emotional brain. *Neurosci. Lett.* **2017**, *693*, 29–34. [CrossRef]
19. Beesdo, K.; Pine, D.S.; Lieb, R.; Wittchen, H.-U. Incidence and risk patterns of anxiety and depressive disorders and categorization of generalized anxiety disorder. *Arch. Gen. Psychiatry* **2010**, *67*, 47–57. [CrossRef] [PubMed]

20. Lee, F.S.; Heimer, H.; Giedd, J.N.; Lein, E.S.; Sestan, N.; Weinberger, D.R.; Casey, B.J. Adolescent mental health—opportunity and obligation. *Science* **2014**, *346*, 547–549. [CrossRef]
21. Kessler, R.C.; McLaughlin, K.A.; Green, J.G.; Gruber, M.J.; Sampson, N.A.; Zaslavsky, A.M.; Aguilar-Gaxiola, S.; Alhamzawi, A.O.; Alonso, J.; Angermeyer, M. Childhood adversities and adult psychopathology in the WHO World Mental Health Surveys. *Br. J. Psychiatry* **2010**, *197*, 378–385. [CrossRef] [PubMed]
22. Coates, A.A.; Messman-Moore, T.L. A structural model of mechanisms predicting depressive symptoms in women following childhood psychological maltreatment. *Child Abuse Negl.* **2014**, *38*, 103–113. [CrossRef] [PubMed]
23. Stevens, N.R.; Gerhart, J.; Goldsmith, R.E.; Heath, N.M.; Chesney, S.A.; Hobfoll, S.E. Emotion regulation difficulties, low social support, and interpersonal violence mediate the link between childhood abuse and posttraumatic stress symptoms. *Behav. Therapy* **2013**, *44*, 152–161. [CrossRef] [PubMed]
24. Cuthbert, B.N.; Insel, T.R. Toward the future of psychiatric diagnosis: The seven pillars of RDoC. *BMC Med.* **2013**, *11*, 126. [CrossRef]
25. Sun, M.; Vinograd, M.; Miller, G.A.; Craske, M.G. Research Domain Criteria (RDoC) and Emotion Regulation. In *Emotion Regulation and Psychopathology in Children and Adolescents*; Essau, C.A., LeBlanc, S.S., Ollendick, T.H., Eds.; Oxford University Press: Oxford, UK, 2017; p. 79.
26. Silvers, J.A.; McRae, K.; Gabrieli, J.D.; Gross, J.J.; Remy, K.A.; Ochsner, K.N. Age-related differences in emotional reactivity, regulation, and rejection sensitivity in adolescence. *Emotion* **2012**, *12*, 1235–1247. [CrossRef] [PubMed]
27. Theurel, A.; Gentaz, E. The regulation of emotions in adolescents: Age differences and emotion-specific patterns. *PLoS ONE* **2018**, *13*, e0195501. [CrossRef] [PubMed]
28. Tottenham, N.; Hare, T.A.; Casey, B.J. Behavioral assessment of emotion discrimination, emotion regulation, and cognitive control in childhood, adolescence, and adulthood. *Front. Psychol.* **2011**, *2*, 39. [CrossRef] [PubMed]
29. Hollenstein, T.; McNeely, A.; Eastabrook, J.; Mackey, A.; Flynn, J. Sympathetic and parasympathetic responses to social stress across adolescence. *Dev. Psychobiol.* **2012**, *54*, 207–214. [CrossRef] [PubMed]
30. Gee, D.G.; Humphreys, K.L.; Flannery, J.; Goff, B.; Telzer, E.H.; Shapiro, M.; Hare, T.A.; Bookheimer, S.Y.; Tottenham, N. A developmental shift from positive to negative connectivity in human amygdala–prefrontal circuitry. *J. Neurosci.* **2013**, *33*, 4584–4593. [CrossRef]
31. Swartz, J.R.; Carrasco, M.; Wiggins, J.L.; Thomason, M.E.; Monk, C.S. Age-related changes in the structure and function of prefrontal cortex–amygdala circuitry in children and adolescents: A multi-modal imaging approach. *Neuroimage* **2014**, *86*, 212–220. [CrossRef] [PubMed]
32. Decety, J.; Michalska, K.J.; Kinzler, K.D. The contribution of emotion and cognition to moral sensitivity: A neurodevelopmental study. *Cereb. Cortex* **2011**, *22*, 209–220. [CrossRef] [PubMed]
33. Silvers, J.A.; Insel, C.; Powers, A.; Franz, P.; Hellon, C.; Martin, R.E.; Weber, J.; Mischel, W.; Casey, B.J.; Ochsner, K.N. The transition from childhood to adolescence is marked by a general decrease in amygdala reactivity and an affect-specific ventral-to-dorsal shift in medial prefrontal recruitment. *Dev. Cognit. Neurosci.* **2017**, *25*, 128–137. [CrossRef] [PubMed]
34. Silvers, J.A.; Insel, C.; Powers, A.; Franz, P.; Hellon, C.; Martin, R.E.; Weber, J.; Mischel, W.; Casey, B.J.; Ochsner, K.N. vlPFC–vmPFC–amygdala interactions underlie age-related differences in cognitive regulation of emotion. *Cereb. Cortex* **2016**, *27*, 3502–3514. [CrossRef] [PubMed]
35. Gee, D.G.; Gabard-Durnam, L.; Telzer, E.H.; Humphreys, K.L.; Goff, B.; Shapiro, M.; Flannery, J.; Lumian, D.S.; Fareri, D.S.; Caldera, C. Maternal buffering of human amygdala-prefrontal circuitry during childhood but not during adolescence. *Psychol. Sci.* **2014**, *25*, 2067–2078. [CrossRef]
36. Schäfer, J.Ö.; Naumann, E.; Homes, E.A.; Tuschen-Caffier, B.; Samson, A.C. Emotion regulation strategies in depressive and anxiety symptoms in youth: A meta-analytic review. *J. Youth Adolesc.* **2017**, *46*, 261–276. [CrossRef] [PubMed]
37. Keil, V.; Asbrand, J.; Tuschen-Caffier, B.; Schmitz, J. Children with social anxiety and other anxiety disorders show similar deficits in habitual emotional regulation: Evidence for a transdiagnostic phenomenon. *Eur. Child Adolesc. Psychiatry* **2017**, *26*, 749–757. [CrossRef]
38. Mathews, B.L.; Kerns, K.A.; Ciesla, J.A. Specificity of emotion regulation difficulties related to anxiety in early adolescence. *J. Adolesc.* **2014**, *37*, 1089–1097. [CrossRef] [PubMed]

39. Jose, P.E.; Wilkins, H.; Spendelow, J.S. Does social anxiety predict rumination and co-rumination among adolescents? *J. Clin. Child Adolesc. Psychol.* **2012**, *41*, 86–91. [CrossRef]
40. Carthy, T.; Horesh, N.; Apter, A.; Gross, J.J. Patterns of emotional reactivity and regulation in children with anxiety disorders. *J. Psychopathol. Behav. Assess.* **2010**, *32*, 23–36. [CrossRef]
41. Carthy, T.; Horesh, N.; Apter, A.; Edge, M.D.; Gross, J.J. Emotional reactivity and cognitive regulation in anxious children. *Behav. Res. Therapy* **2010**, *48*, 384–393. [CrossRef]
42. Henry, J.D.; Castellini, J.; Moses, E.; Scott, J.G. Emotion regulation in adolescents with mental health problems. *J. Clin. Exp. Neuropsychol.* **2016**, *38*, 197–207. [CrossRef]
43. De Witte, N.A.; Sütterlin, S.; Braet, C.; Mueller, S.C. Psychophysiological correlates of emotion regulation training in adolescent anxiety: Evidence from the novel PIER task. *J. Affect. Disord.* **2017**, *214*, 89–96. [CrossRef] [PubMed]
44. Latham, M.D.; Cook, N.; Simmons, J.G.; Byrne, M.L.; Kette, J.W.L.; Schwartz, O.; Vijayakumar, N.; Whittle, S.; Allen, N.B. Physiological correlates of emotional reactivity and regulation in early adolescents. *Biol. Psychol.* **2017**, *127*, 229–238. [CrossRef]
45. Davis, M.M.; Miernicki, M.E.; Telzer, E.H.; Rudolph, K.D. The contribution of childhood negative emotionality and cognitive control to anxiety-linked neural dysregulation of emotion in adolescence. *J. Abnorm. Child Psychol.* **2018**. [CrossRef]
46. Shapero, B.G.; Abramson, L.Y.; Alloy, L.B. Emotional reactivity and internalizing symptoms: Moderating role of emotion regulation. *Cognit. Therapy Res.* **2016**, *40*, 328–340. [CrossRef]
47. Lydon-Staley, D.M.; Xia, M.; Mak, H.W.; Fosco, G.M. Adolescent emotion network dynamics in daily life and implications for depression. *J. Abnorm. Child Psychol.* **2018**. [CrossRef]
48. Larsen, J.K.; Vermulst, A.A.; Elsinga, R.; English, T.; Gross, J.J.; Hofman, E.; Scholte, R.H.J.; Engels, R.C.M.E. Social coping by masking? Parental support and peer victimization as mediators of the relationship between depressive symptoms and expressive suppression in adolescents. *J. Youth Adolesc.* **2012**, *41*, 1628–1642. [CrossRef] [PubMed]
49. LeWinn, K.Z.; Strigo, I.A.; Connolly, C.G.; Ho, T.C.; Tymofiyeva, O.; Sacchet, M.D.; Weng, H.Y.; Blom, E.H.; Simmons, A.N.; Yang, T.T. An exploratory examination of reappraisal success in depressed adolescents: Preliminary evidence of functional differences in cognitive control brain regions. *J. Affect. Disord.* **2018**, *240*, 155–164. [CrossRef] [PubMed]
50. Platt, B.; Campbell, C.A.; James, A.C.; Murphy, S.E.; Cooper, M.J.; Lau, J.Y.F. Cognitive reappraisal of peer rejection in depressed versus non-depressed adolescents: Functional connectivity differences. *J. Psychiatr. Res.* **2015**, *61*, 73–80. [CrossRef]
51. Stephanou, K.; Davey, C.G.; Kerestes, R.; Whittle, S.; Harrison, B.J. Hard to look on the bright side: Neural correlates of impaired emotion regulation in depressed youth. *Soc. Cognit. Affect. Neurosci.* **2017**, *12*, 1138–1148. [CrossRef] [PubMed]
52. Vasilev, C.A.; Crowell, S.E.; Beauchaine, T.P.; Mead, H.K.; Katzke-Kopp, L.M. Correspondence between physiological and self-report measures of emotion dysregulation: A longitudinal investigation of youth with and without psychopathology. *J. Child Psychol. Psychiatry* **2009**, *50*, 1357–1364. [CrossRef]
53. Kovács, M.; Yaroslavsky, I.; Rottenberg, J.; George, C.J.; Kiss, E.; Halas, K.; Dochnal, R.; Benák, I.; Baji, I.; Vetro, A. Maladaptive mood repair, atypical respiratory sinus arrhythmia, and risk of a recurrent major depressive episode among adolescents with prior major depression. *Psychol. Med.* **2016**, *46*, 2109–2119. [CrossRef] [PubMed]
54. Gentzler, A.L.; Santucci, A.K.; Kovacs, M.; Fox, N.A. Respiratory sinus arrhythmia reactivity predicts emotion regulation and depressive symptoms in at-risk and control children. *Biol. Psychol.* **2009**, *82*, 156–163. [CrossRef] [PubMed]
55. Bosch, N.M.; Riese, H.; Ormel, J.; Verhulst, F.; Oldehinkel, A.J. Stressful life events and depressive symptoms in young adolescents: Modulation by respiratory sinus arrhythmia? The TRAILS study. *Biol. Psychol.* **2009**, *81*, 40–47. [CrossRef] [PubMed]
56. Perlman, G.; Simmons, A.N.; Wu, J.; Hahn, K.S.; Tapert, S.F.; Max, J.E.; Paulus, M.P.; Brown, G.G.; Frank, G.K.; Campbell-Sills, L. Amygdala response and functional connectivity during emotion regulation: A study of 14 depressed adolescents. *J. Affect. Disord.* **2012**, *139*, 75–84. [CrossRef] [PubMed]

57. Stikkelbroek, Y.; Bodden, D.H.M.; Kleinjan, M.; Reijnders, M.; van Baar, A.L. Adolescent depression and negative life events, the mediating role of cognitive emotion regulation. *PLoS ONE* **2016**, *11*, e0161062. [CrossRef]

58. Heleniak, C.; Jenness, J.L.; Vander Stoep, A.; McCauley, E.; McLaughlin, K.A. Childhood maltreatment exposure and disruptions in emotion regulation: A transdiagnostic pathway to adolescent internalizing and externalizing psychopathology. *Cognit. Therapy Res.* **2016**, *40*, 394–415. [CrossRef]

59. Shapero, B.G.; Stange, J.P.; McArthur, B.A.; Abramson, L.Y.; Alloy, L.B. Cognitive reappraisal attenuates the association between depressive symptoms and emotional response to stress during adolescence. *Cognit. Emot.* **2018**. [CrossRef]

60. Fowler, C.H.; Miernicki, M.E.; Rudolph, K.D.; Telzer, E.H. Disrupted amygdala-prefrontal connectivity during emotion regulation links stress-reactive rumination and adolescent depressive symptoms. *Dev. Cognit. Neurosci.* **2017**, *27*, 99–106. [CrossRef]

61. Sheeber, L.B.; Allen, N.B.; Leve, C.; Davis, B.; Shortt, J.W.; Katz, L.F. Dynamics of affective experience and behavior in depressed adolescents. *J. Child Psychol. Psychiatry* **2009**, *50*, 1419–1427. [CrossRef]

62. Silk, J.S.; Forbes, E.E.; Whalen, D.J.; Jakubcak, J.L.; Thompson, W.K.; Ryan, N.D.; Axelson, D.A.; Birmaher, B.; Dahl, R.E. Daily emotional dynamics in depressed youth: A cell phone ecological momentary assessment study. *J. Exp. Child Psychol.* **2011**, *110*, 241–257. [CrossRef]

63. Raval, V.V.; Luebbe, A.M.; Sathiyaseelan, A. Parental socialization of positive affect, adolescent positive affect regulation, and adolescent girls' depression in India. *Soc. Dev.* **2018**. [CrossRef]

64. Nelis, S.; Bastin, M.; Raes, F.; Bijttebier, P. How do my parents react when I feel happy? Longitudinal associations with adolescent depressive symptoms, anhedonia, and positive affect regulation. *Soc. Dev.* **2018**. [CrossRef]

65. Fussner, L.M.; Luebbe, A.M.; Bell, D.J. Dynamics of positive emotion regulation: Associations with youth depressive symptoms. *J. Abnorm. Child Psychol.* **2015**, *43*, 475–488. [CrossRef]

66. Yap, M.B.; Schwartz, O.S.; Byrne, M.L.; Simmons, J.G.; Allen, N.B. Maternal positive and negative interaction behaviors and early adolescents' depressive symptoms: Adolescent emotion regulation as a mediator. *J. Res. Adolesc.* **2010**, *20*, 1014–1043. [CrossRef]

67. Yap, M.B.; Allen, N.B.; Ladouceur, C.D. Maternal socialization of positive affect: The impact of invalidation on adolescent emotion regulation and depressive symptomatology. *Child Dev.* **2008**, *79*, 1415–1431. [CrossRef] [PubMed]

68. Forbes, E.E. fMRI studies of reward processing in adolescent depression. *Neuropsychopharmacology* **2011**, *36*, 372. [CrossRef]

69. Gilbert, K.E. The neglected role of positive emotion in adolescent psychopathology. *Clin. Psychol. Rev.* **2012**, *32*, 467–481. [CrossRef]

70. Gross, J.J.; John, O.P. Individual differences in two emotion regulation processes: Implications for affect, relationships, and well-being. *J. Personal. Soc. Psychol.* **2003**, *85*, 348. [CrossRef]

71. Gratz, K.L.; Roemer, L. Multidimensional assessment of emotion regulation and dysregulation: Development, factor structure, and initial validation of the difficulties in emotion regulation scale. *J. Psychopathol. Behav. Assess.* **2004**, *26*, 41–54. [CrossRef]

72. Garnefski, N.; Kraaij, V.; Spinhoven, P. Negative life events, cognitive emotion regulation and emotional problems. *Personal. Individ. Differ.* **2001**, *30*, 1311–1327. [CrossRef]

73. Cracco, E.; van Durme, K.; Braet, C. Validation of the FEEL-KJ: An instrument to measure emotion regulation strategies in children and adolescents. *PLoS ONE* **2015**, *10*, e0137080. [CrossRef] [PubMed]

74. Feldman, G.C.; Joormann, J.; Johnson, S.L. Responses to positive affect: A self-report measure of rumination and dampening. *Cognit. Therapy Res.* **2008**, *32*, 507. [CrossRef] [PubMed]

75. McLaughlin, K.A.; Hatzenbuehler, M.L.; Mennin, D.S.; Nolen-Hoeksema, S. Emotion dysregulation and adolescent psychopathology: A prospective study. *Behav. Res. Therapy* **2011**, *49*, 544–554. [CrossRef]

76. Gross, J.J.; Barrett, F.L. Emotion generation and emotion regulation: One or two depends on your point of view. *Emot. Rev.* **2011**, *3*, 8–16. [CrossRef]

77. Kirschbaum, C.; Pirke, K.-M.; Hellhammer, D.H. The 'Trier Social Stress Test'–a tool for investigating psychobiological stress responses in a laboratory setting. *Neuropsychobiology* **1993**, *28*, 76–81. [CrossRef]

78. Hops, H.; Biglan, A.; Tolman, A.; Arthur, J.; Longoria, N. *Living in Family Environments (LIFE) Coding System: Manual for Coders (Revised)*; Oregon Research Institute: Eugene, OR, USA, 1995.

79. Bradley, M.M.; Codispoti, M.; Cuthbert, B.N.; Lang, P.J. Emotion and motivation I: Defensive and appetitive reactions in picture processing. *Emotion* **2001**, *1*, 276. [CrossRef] [PubMed]
80. Butler, E.A.; Wilhelm, F.H.; Gross, J.J. Respiratory sinus arrhythmia, emotion, and emotion regulation during social interaction. *Psychophysiology* **2006**, *43*, 612–622. [CrossRef]
81. Cohen, N.; Moyal, N.; Henik, A. Executive control suppresses pupillary responses to aversive stimuli. *Biol. Psychol.* **2015**, *112*, 1–11. [CrossRef] [PubMed]
82. van Reekum, C.M.; Johnstone, T.; Urry, H.L.; Thurow, M.E.; Schaefer, H.S.; Alexander, A.L.; Davidson, R.J. Gaze fixations predict brain activation during the voluntary regulation of picture-induced negative affect. *Neuroimage* **2007**, *36*, 1041–1055. [CrossRef]
83. Ray, R.D.; McRae, K.; Ochsner, K.N.; Gross, J.J. Cognitive reappraisal of negative affect: Converging evidence from EMG and self report. *Emotion* **2010**, *10*, 587. [CrossRef] [PubMed]
84. Society for Psychophysiological Research Ad Hoc Committee on Electrodermal Measures; Boucsein, W.; Fowles, D.C.; Grimnes, S.; Ben-Shakhar, G.; Roth, W.T.; Dawson, M.E.; Filion, D.L. Publication recommendations for electrodermal measurements. *Psychophysiology* **2012**, *49*, 1017–1034. [CrossRef]
85. Tomarken, A.J. A psychometric perspective on psychophysiological measures. *Psychol. Assess.* **1995**, *7*, 387. [CrossRef]
86. Torre, J.B.; Lieberman, M.D. Putting feelings into words: Affect labeling as implicit emotion regulation. *Emot. Rev.* **2018**, *10*, 116–124. [CrossRef]
87. Lieberman, M.D.; Eisenberger, N.I.; Crocket, M.J.; Tom, S.M.; Pfeifer, J.H.; Way, B.M. Putting feelings into words. *Psychol. Sci.* **2007**, *18*, 421–428. [CrossRef] [PubMed]
88. Lennarz, H.K.; Hollenstein, T.; Lichtwarck-Aschoff, A.; Kuntsche, E.; Granic, I. Emotion regulation in action: Use, selection, and success of emotion regulation in adolescents' daily lives. *Int. J. Behav. Dev.* **2018**. [CrossRef] [PubMed]
89. Gotlib, I.H.; Joormann, J. Cognition and depression: Current status and future directions. *Annu. Rev. Clin. Psychol.* **2010**, *6*, 285–312. [CrossRef] [PubMed]
90. Dvir, Y.; Ford, J.D.; Hill, M.; Frazier, J.A. Childhood maltreatment, emotional dysregulation, and psychiatric comorbidities. *Harv. Rev. Psychiatry* **2014**, *22*, 149. [CrossRef] [PubMed]
91. Hinnant, J.B.; El-Sheikh, M. Children's externalizing and internalizing symptoms over time: The role of individual differences in patterns of RSA responding. *J. Abnorm. Child Psychol.* **2009**, *37*, 1049. [CrossRef]
92. Gilbert, K.E.; Nolen-Hoeksema, S.; Gruber, J. I don't want to come back down: Undoing versus maintaining of reward recovery in older adolescents. *Emotion* **2016**, *16*, 214. [CrossRef]
93. Stephanou, K.; Davey, C.G.; Kerestes, R.; Whittle, S.; Pujol, J.; Yücel, M.; Fornito, A.; López-Solà, M.; Harrison, B.J. Brain functional correlates of emotion regulation across adolescence and young adulthood. *Hum. Brain Mapp.* **2016**, *37*, 7–19. [CrossRef]
94. Wu, M.; Kujawa, A.; Lu, L.H.; Fitzgerald, D.A.; Klumpp, H.; Fitzgerald, K.D.; Monk, C.S.; Phan, K.L. Age-related changes in amygdala–frontal connectivity during emotional face processing from childhood into young adulthood. *Hum. Brain Mapp.* **2016**, *37*, 1684–1695. [CrossRef]
95. Johnstone, T.; van Reekum, C.M.; Urry, H.L.; Kalin, N.H.; Davidson, R.J. Failure to regulate: Counterproductive recruitment of top-down prefrontal-subcortical circuitry in major depression. *J. Neurosci.* **2007**, *27*, 8877–8884. [CrossRef] [PubMed]
96. Beauregard, M.; Paquette, V.; Le, J. Dysfunction in the neural circuitry of emotional self-regulation in major depressive disorder. *Neuroreport* **2006**, *17*, 843–846. [CrossRef]
97. Greening, S.G.; Osuch, E.A.; Williamson, P.C.; Mitchell, D.G.V. The neural correlates of regulating positive and negative emotions in medication-free major depression. *Soc. Cognit. Affect. Neurosci.* **2013**, *9*, 628–637. [CrossRef] [PubMed]
98. Erk, S.; Mikscl, A.; Stier, S.; Ciaramidaro, A.; Gapp, V.; Weber, B.; Walter, H. Acute and sustained effects of cognitive emotion regulation in major depression. *J. Neurosci.* **2010**, *30*, 15726–15734. [CrossRef]
99. Williams, K.D.; Cheung, C.K.; Choi, W. Cyberostracism: Effects of being ignored over the Internet. *J. Personal. Soc. Psychol.* **2000**, *79*, 748. [CrossRef]
100. Sladky, R.; Höflich, A.; Külböck, M.; Kraus, C.; Baldinger, P.; Moser, E.; Lanzenberger, R.; Windishberger, C. Disrupted effective connectivity between the amygdala and orbitofrontal cortex in social anxiety disorder during emotion discrimination revealed by dynamic causal modeling for fMRI. *Cereb. Cortex* **2013**, *25*, 895–903. [CrossRef] [PubMed]

101. Hayes, S.C.; Hofmann, S.G. The third wave of cognitive behavioral therapy and the rise of process-based care. *World Psychiatry* **2017**, *16*, 245. [CrossRef] [PubMed]

102. Reynolds, S.; Wilson, C.; Austin, J.; Hooper, L. Effects of psychotherapy for anxiety in children and adolescents: A meta-analytic review. *Clin. Psychol. Rev.* **2012**, *32*, 251–262. [CrossRef]

103. Insel, T.R.; Gogtay, N. National Institute of Mental Health clinical trials: New opportunities, new expectations. *JAMA Psychiatry* **2014**, *71*, 745–746. [CrossRef]

104. Kovacs, M.; Sherrill, J.; George, C.J.; Pollock, M.; Tumuluru, R.V.; Ho, V. Contextual emotion-regulation therapy for childhood depression: Description and pilot testing of a new intervention. *J. Am. Acad. Child Adolesc. Psychiatry* **2006**, *45*, 892–903. [CrossRef] [PubMed]

105. Mennin, D.S.; Fresco, D.M. Emotion regulation therapy. In *Handbook of Emotion Regulation*; Gross, J.J., Ed.; Guilford Publications: New York, NY, USA, 2014; pp. 469–490.

106. O'Toole, M.S.; Renna, M.E.; Mennin, D.S.; Fresco, D.M. Changes in decentering and reappraisal temporally precede symptom reduction during Emotion Regulation Therapy for generalized anxiety disorder with and without co-occurring depression. *Behav. Therapy* **2019**, in press. [CrossRef]

107. Hertel, P.T.; Mathews, A. Cognitive Bias Modification: Past Perspectives, Current Findings, and Future Applications. *Perspect. Psychol. Sci.* **2011**, *6*, 521–536. [CrossRef]

108. Cristea, I.A.; Kok, R.N.; Cuijpers, P. Efficacy of cognitive bias modification interventions in anxiety and depression: Meta-analysis. *Br. J. Psychiatry* **2015**, *206*, 7–16. [CrossRef]

109. Waters, A.M.; Zimmer-Gembeck, M.J.; Craske, M.G.; Pine, D.S.; Bradley, B.P.; Mogg, K. A Preliminary Evaluation of a Home-based, Computer-delivered Attention Training Treatment for Anxious Children Living in Regional Communities. *J. Exp. Psychopathol.* **2016**, *7*, 511–527. [CrossRef]

110. Waters, A.M.; Zimmer-Gembeck, M.J.; Craske, M.G.; Pine, D.S.; Bradley, B.P.; Mogg, K. Look for good and never give up: A novel attention training treatment for childhood anxiety disorders. *Behav. Res. Therapy* **2015**, *73*, 111–123. [CrossRef] [PubMed]

111. Craske, M.G.; Meuret, A.E.; Ritz, T.; Treanor, M.; Dour, H.J. Treatment for anhedonia: A neuroscience driven approach. *Depression Anxiety* **2016**, *33*, 927–938. [CrossRef] [PubMed]

112. Young, K.S.; Craske, M.G. The Cognitive Neuroscience of Psychological Treatment Action in Depression and Anxiety. *Curr. Behav. Neurosci. Rep.* **2018**, *5*, 13–25. [CrossRef]

113. Young, K.S.; Burklund, L.J.; Torre, J.B.; Saxbe, D.; Lieberman, M.D.; Craske, M.G. Treatment for social anxiety disorder alters functional connectivity in emotion regulation neural circuitry. *Psychiatry Res. Neuroimaging.* **2017**, *261*, 44–51. [CrossRef] [PubMed]

114. De Wit, S.; Van der Werf, Y.D.; Mataix-Cols, D.; Trujillo, J.P.; Van Oppen, P.; Veltman, D.J.; van den Heuvel, O.A. Emotion regulation before and after transcranial magnetic stimulation in obsessive compulsive disorder. *Psychol. Med.* **2015**, *45*, 3059–3073. [CrossRef]

115. Nicholson, A.A.; Rabellino, D.; Densmore, M.; Frewen, P.A.; Paret, C.; Kluetsch, R.; Schmahl, C.; Théberge, J.; Neufeld, R.W.J.; McKinnon, M.C. The neurobiology of emotion regulation in posttraumatic stress disorder: Amygdala downregulation via real-time fMRI neurofeedback. *Hum. Brain Mapp.* **2017**, *38*, 541–560. [CrossRef]

116. Kadosh, K.C.; Luo, Q.; de Burca, C.; Sokunbi, M.O.; Feng, J.; Linden, D.E.J.; Lau, J.Y.F. Using real-time fMRI to influence effective connectivity in the developing emotion regulation network. *Neuroimage* **2016**, *125*, 616–626. [CrossRef]

117. Krause, E.D.; Vélez, C.E.; Woo, R.; Hoffman, B.; Freres, D.R.; Abenavoli, R.M.; Gillham, J.E. Rumination, Depression, and Gender in Early Adolescence: A Longitudinal Study of a Bidirectional Model. *J. Early Adolesc.* **2017**. [CrossRef]

118. Alloy, L.B.; Hamilton, J.L.; Hamlat, E.J.; Abramson, L.Y. Pubertal development, emotion regulatory styles, and the emergence of sex differences in internalizing disorders and symptoms in adolescence. *Clin. Psychol. Sci.* **2016**, *4*, 867–881. [CrossRef] [PubMed]

119. Wante, L.; Mezulis, A.; Van Beveren, M.-L.; Braet, C. The mediating effect of adaptive and maladaptive emotion regulation strategies on executive functioning impairment and depressive symptoms among adolescents. *Child Neuropsychol.* **2017**, *23*, 935–953. [CrossRef] [PubMed]

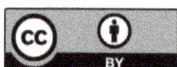

![brain sciences logo] *brain sciences*

MDPI

Review

Maturational Changes in Prefrontal and Amygdala Circuits in Adolescence: Implications for Understanding Fear Inhibition during a Vulnerable Period of Development

Kelsey S. Zimmermann, Rick Richardson and Kathryn D. Baker *

School of Psychology, University of New South Wales (UNSW), Sydney, NSW 2052, Australia·
k.zimmermann@unsw.edu.au (K.S.Z.); r.richardson@unsw.edu.au (R.R.)
* Correspondence: k.baker@unsw.edu.au; Tel.: +61-2-9385-0552

Received: 6 February 2019; Accepted: 14 March 2019; Published: 18 March 2019

Abstract: Anxiety disorders that develop in adolescence represent a significant burden and are particularly challenging to treat, due in no small part to the high occurrence of relapse in this age group following exposure therapy. This pattern of persistent fear is preserved across species; relative to those younger and older, adolescents consistently show poorer extinction, a key process underpinning exposure therapy. This suggests that the neural processes underlying fear extinction are temporarily but profoundly compromised during adolescence. The formation, retrieval, and modification of fear- and extinction-associated memories are regulated by a forebrain network consisting of the prefrontal cortex (PFC), the amygdala, and the hippocampus. These regions undergo robust maturational changes in early life, with unique alterations in structure and function occurring throughout adolescence. In this review, we focus primarily on two of these regions—the PFC and the amygdala—and discuss how changes in plasticity, synaptic transmission, inhibition/excitation, and connectivity (including modulation by hippocampal afferents to the PFC) may contribute to transient deficits in extinction retention. We end with a brief consideration of how exposure to stress during this adolescent window of vulnerability can permanently disrupt neurodevelopment, leading to lasting impairments in pathways of emotional regulation.

Keywords: fear extinction; adolescence; prefrontal cortex; amygdala

---

1. Introduction

Adolescence is a developmental period of "storm and stress," characterised by a host of physical, cognitive, and emotional changes that permit a shift towards achieving independence while simultaneously opening a window of vulnerability to the damaging effects of external stressors [1–3]. Anxiety disorders that emerge during adolescence are a major concern, as they pose more societal burden and treatment cost than those emerging in adulthood [4]. One factor contributing to this burden is that, relative to adults, adolescents are far more prone to relapse following exposure therapy [5,6], the gold standard for treatment for anxiety disorders [7]. Identifying the neurological underpinnings that make adolescents particularly vulnerable to fear relapse will help to inform effective treatment approaches specifically tailored to the developing brain [8]. To this end, characterising the ways in which behaviour, learning, and memory are influenced by dynamic neurodevelopmental processes occurring during adolescence has become a topic attracting burgeoning international interest in recent years (e.g., a special issue devoted to Adolescence in *Neuroscience and Biobehavioral Reviews* in 2016 and a collection on Adolescence in *Nature* in 2018).

Extinction training is commonly used in an experimental setting to model the process of exposure therapy. Briefly, following Pavlovian conditioning, in which a neutral conditioned stimulus (CS; e.g., a white noise) is paired with an aversive unconditioned stimulus (US; e.g., a mild foot shock), an animal will exhibit fear responses to the CS alone. During extinction training, the CS–US contingency is degraded by repeatedly presenting the CS in the absence of the US. Eventually, CS-elicited fear is suppressed as the animal learns that it no longer predicts a threat. Some studies have shown that adolescents (both rodent and human) are delayed in reducing fear during extinction training, referred to as an impairment in within-session extinction [9,10]. Other studies have reported that even when within-session extinction is preserved, adolescents are far more prone to fear relapse than older or younger age groups when tested again at a later time point; that is, adolescents show deficits in extinction *retention* [11–13], reflective of the increased risk of relapse following exposure therapy. Discovering how the neural correlates underlying fear acquisition and extinction change over the course of development is a promising approach to understanding the cognitive and behavioural rigidity associated with aversive learning processes during adolescence.

The neurocircuitry underlying the acquisition and extinction of fear memories in adults has been extensively studied (and reviewed in detail in [14–20]). Two regions of particular interest are the prefrontal cortex (PFC), particularly the medial PFC (mPFC), and the amygdala. These highly interconnected forebrain structures regulate the formation and modification of associative memories, and their contributions to fear learning and extinction have been well established. Both structures undergo significant structural and functional changes over the course of development [21–23] that have the potential to fundamentally alter learning, memory, and behaviour. In this review, we summarise recent research describing developmental changes in PFC and amygdala regional plasticity, synaptic transmission, inhibition/excitation, and connectivity. We incorporate these findings into a structural framework modelling the ways in which these concomitant changes may underlie adolescent-specific deficits in extinction learning and retention, and discuss how behaviour can be impacted when the standard developmental trajectory is disrupted by exposure to external stressors.

2. Plasticity—Dendritic Spines

Developmental changes in neuroplasticity have been well-established; broad convention states that plasticity is highest in early life, when young animals need to quickly process large volumes of information about their environment, and decreases over development until reaching stable levels in adulthood [24]. However, different regions of the brain mature at different rates, meaning that later-developing regions like the PFC [25,26] are still highly plastic when other regions have largely stabilised. Understanding how neuroplasticity changes over development in the PFC and amygdala could help to identify regional imbalances in learning-dependent processes and reveal mechanisms underlying cognitive and behavioural rigidity in adolescence.

One increasingly common approach used to characterise changes in neuroplasticity involves examining the density and stability of dendritic spines. Dendritic spines are the primary sites of glutamatergic synapses on excitatory principal neurons [27], like the pyramidal neurons of the mPFC and basolateral amygdala (BLA). These spines are highly dynamic, and their morphology, density, and stability (i.e., rate of turnover) change rapidly in response to plasticity-inducing forms of stimulation, including learning events. Although data concerning the relationship between learning and spine dynamics is thus far largely correlational (for review see [28]), increases in spine proliferation and reorganisation generally predict enhanced neuroplasticity, while spine elimination signals diminished capacity for change.

2.1. Prefrontal Dendritic Spines

Postnatal development represents a particularly dynamic period of synapse and spine formation and elimination in the cortex across species [29,30]. Post-mortem analyses in humans show that following birth, spines and synapses on excitatory pyramidal neurons in the PFC massively proliferate until levels peak in mid-late childhood. Adolescence represents a period of dendritic pruning as neuronal processes are refined—during this period approximately half of all prefrontal spines and synapses are eliminated until adulthood, when levels stabilise and remain relatively constant [31,32]. This pattern of proliferation and pruning in the PFC is conserved across mammalian species, and has been demonstrated in the mPFC and dorsolateral PFC (dlPFC) of non-human primates [33–35], the mPFC (combined infralimbic [IL] and prelimbic [PL] subregions) of rats [23], and the PL and orbitofrontal cortex (OFC) of mice [36–38]. Importantly, when the PL and IL (rodent homologues of Brodmann Areas 32 and 25, respectively) are examined separately, it appears that the quadratic curve of spine density in the developing mouse mPFC is driven nearly entirely by the PL, with the IL showing little, if any, changes from early adolescence to adulthood [36]. Across regions, this means that in early adolescence, dendritic spine density in the PL is significantly higher than in the IL, whereas in juveniles and adults, densities are comparable between regions. Given that the PL has been associated with fear expression, while the IL has been implicated in extinction [18], this temporary imbalance in plasticity and excitability between these two regions may help to explain the adolescent deficit in extinction retention, a hypothesis discussed in more detail in Section 2.3.

The transition from adolescence to adulthood involves circuit-specific changes in spine dynamics in the PFC which are concurrent with changes in afferent projections (discussed in detail in Section 5), suggesting there may be a relationship between spine fluctuations and the maturation of specific inputs to this region. This idea is supported by findings that transient increases in spine turnover in the PL of early adolescent mice occur in pyramidal neurons located in the same cortical layers that receive input from the ventral hippocampus and BLA (Layers II/III and V). Additionally, this adolescent increase in PL spine density and formation coincides with a peak in PL afferents arising from the ventral hippocampus and BLA [36]. It is likely that the observed reductions in spine plasticity and density in the PL between adolescence and adulthood are influenced by a combination of local changes in excitatory and inhibitory drive and circuit-specific reorganisation of connectivity. We discuss such changes and their implications for fear inhibition in adolescence in more detail in Sections 4 and 5.

2.2. BLA Dendritic Spines

Development of dendritic spines in the amygdala has been studied less extensively than in the PFC, but compelling data from rats suggest that the BLA shows a maturational pattern distinct from the proliferation-pruning trajectory of prefrontal areas. While PFC spines are dramatically eliminated during adolescence, spine density in the BLA shows a relatively linear increase from the juvenile period (childhood) to adulthood [23]. This study also reported slightly different patterns in BLA spine development between males and females; from adolescence to adulthood, there was a modest increase in density in males and an equally modest decrease in females. Concurrent with these changes in BLA spine density are fluctuations in amygdalar volume and the total number of cells within the amygdala. The volume of the lateral, basal, and central nuclei of the amygdala increases from Postnatal Day (P)7 to 35 in rats [39,40] (see Appendix A for a guide to postnatal development in rodents in postnatal days). Thereafter, amygdala volume decreases across adolescence to similar levels as in adulthood by P45 [39]. The decrease in amygdala volume across adolescence is likely due to small decreases in neuron number ([40] but see [39]) and reduced arborisation. It is interesting to note that volumetric analyses of amygdala development in humans appear to parallel the pattern of increasing amygdala volume from preadolescence to early adolescence reported in rats but not the later decreases across adolescence. Instead, the subtle differences between females and males in the trajectory of spine density changes across adolescence in rodents are reflected in the pattern of amygdala volume in human adolescents, although such studies in humans have often lacked the power to detect small sex differences. These studies show a linear increase in amygdala gray matter volume in boys between the ages of 4–18 that begins to slow around age 12, and a subtle quadratic curve for girls, with volume peaking at age 14 before slightly decreasing [41,42]. Results such as these highlight the need for increased research in the area of sex differences in neurodevelopment; this is an understudied topic that requires substantially more attention given the documented differences in prevalence of anxiety between males and females, with women and teenage girls having higher rates of anxiety than men and teenage boys, respectively [43–46]. In addition to more detailed investigations of sex differences in spine density and pruning in prefrontal-amygdala circuits across development (e.g., building on work in adults [47]), future analyses exploring whether there are differential trajectories in distinct populations of BLA neurons (e.g., "fear on" versus "fear off" neurons [48,49]) may provide additional insight into how BLA plasticity impacts fear and extinction across development.

2.3. Implications for Fear Learning and Inhibition

In terms of fear regulation, dendritic spines in the PFC and the BLA show evidence of remodelling following both fear conditioning and extinction in the adult brain [50,51]; however, the direction of the effect (formation vs. elimination of spines) is dependent on the region. In the frontal association cortex, fear conditioning induces spine elimination whereas extinction increases the rate of spine formation [50]. In contrast, fear conditioning is associated with increased spine density in the BLA; this effect is reversed if animals are given extinction training [51]. There may even be individual differences in BLA spine elimination after extinction that reflect the degree of within-session extinction by that animal, given reports that spine density in the BLA is positively correlated with fear expression during extinction, with increased spine density predicting higher levels of fear [52]. Interestingly, the correlation between fear expression and spine density in several brain regions appears to be mediated by stress exposure. Within the amygdala, stress exposure seems to recapitulate the effects of fear conditioning on dendritic spines, in that stressed animals (like fear-conditioned animals) show increased spine density in the BLA [53]. Stress also appears to have a direct impact on the interaction between fear expression and spine density in the mPFC. One study found that fear conditioning plus extinction was associated with decreased spine density in the IL relative to home cage controls [54]. However, when the animals were exposed to acute stress prior to extinction, a protocol that impaired both within-session extinction and extinction retrieval, fear expression during extinction retrieval was negatively correlated with IL spine density [54]. This suggests that increased IL spine density may be a mechanism of stress resilience. Notably, this correlation was not present in non-stressed animals. Although the effects of fear learning and extinction in the PL have not to our knowledge been explored, a similar interaction between dendritic spines and stress resilience is seen in this region; following chronic social defeat, stress-susceptible animals exhibited decreased PL spine density whereas stress-resilient animals showed no changes relative to non-stressed controls [55]. Taken together, it could be argued that spine hypertrophy in the BLA, and hypotrophy in the mPFC, is associated with states of negative emotional valence (i.e., fear and/or stress). As spine density is undergoing a period of growth and proliferation in the adolescent BLA and elimination in the PL (no major changes are detected in the IL), it is possible that the adolescent brain is similar to the brains of high-fear/stress-susceptible adults, rendering them more vulnerable to exaggerated spine loss in the mPFC and excessive hypertrophy in the BLA following adverse experiences. This may bias this age group towards a negatively-valenced state, making them more susceptible to pervasive, inflexible fear memories and more resistant to fear extinction. A novel question for future research is whether extinction in adolescent rats produces the same changes in spine density in the mPFC and BLA that are induced by extinction in adults, and whether such structural changes can be induced in adolescents by interventions that augment extinction retention. A summary of region-specific changes in dendritic spines in response to the conditions described above is provided in Figure 1.

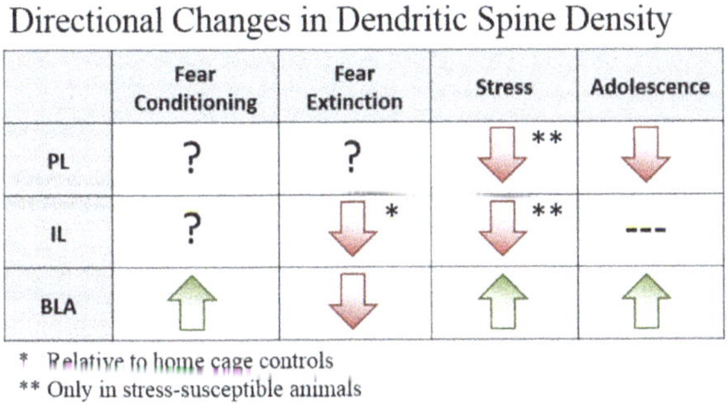

Directional Changes in Dendritic Spine Density

	Fear Conditioning	Fear Extinction	Stress	Adolescence
PL	?	?	⬇ **	⬇
IL	?	⬇ *	⬇ **	---
BLA	⬆	⬇	⬆	⬆

* Relative to home cage controls
** Only in stress-susceptible animals

Figure 1. Summary of directionality of regional dendritic spine changes in response to fear conditioning, extinction, stress, and adolescence.

3. Plasticity—Learning-Dependent Changes in Neural Activity and Excitatory Transmission

Whereas changes in dendritic spine density and turnover in specific regions of the maturing brain can help to explain why adolescents may be biased towards negatively-valenced emotional learning, examination of immediate early genes and physiological indications of synaptic plasticity/long-term potentiation (LTP) in developing animals *around the time of a learning event* (e.g., fear extinction training) can help to identify discrete impairments in different components of memory acquisition, retrieval, and modification. Evidence that the adolescent brain shows altered synaptic plasticity after extinction has been clearly demonstrated by studies examining learning-induced immediate early gene induction and upregulation of protein markers implicated in neuroplasticity. Fear extinction in adults and pre-adolescents causes upregulation of learning-dependent markers of activity and plasticity, for example, c-Fos and phosphorylated mitogen-activated protein kinase (pMAPK) in the mPFC and BLA, that is not seen in adolescent animals [10,12,13]. Such findings indicate that adolescents may be less efficient at recruiting PFC-amygdala pathways during extinction, which may contribute to the extinction retention deficits seen in this age group.

Experience-dependent plasticity in excitatory pyramidal neurons of the PFC and the BLA is widely considered critical for effective storage and expression of fear- and extinction-related memories [56,57] and appears to be dramatically disrupted in adolescence. In juvenile and adult animals, fear conditioning induces an increase in spontaneous excitatory postsynaptic currents (sEPSC) amplitude, EPSC amplitude, c-Fos expression, and AMPA/NMDA ratio in the PL, while extinction training produces the same effects in the IL; none of these patterns is observed in adolescents [10]. EPSC amplitude also appeared to be non-specifically increased in adolescents compared to other age groups in both regions of the mPFC, irrespective of learning condition (i.e., fear conditioning, extinction, or control), creating a ceiling effect that may ostensibly interfere with circuit-specific activation and LTP. Interestingly, this adolescent increase in basal synaptic transmission appears to be specific to the PFC—the same increased activity is not observed in the BLA [58]. However, like the adolescent PFC, the adolescent BLA also fails to show learning-dependent synaptic potentiation following fear conditioning, an effect seen in the juvenile and adult BLA [58]. This suggests that mechanisms other than a ceiling-effect interference with LTP are contributing to adolescent suppression of learning-dependent plasticity.

We have found that, in addition to extended extinction training, treatment with the partial NMDA-agonist D-Cycloserine (DCS) immediately following extinction training can enhance extinction retention in adolescents [11,59]. DCS-mediated improvements in extinction retention were also associated with increased pMAPK in the PFC after extinction training and testing. Further, adolescents also show improved extinction retention and increased pMAPK expression in the mPFC when they receive twice the amount of extinction training [12], suggesting that the lack of prefrontal recruitment during extinction training associated with extinction retention deficits can be overcome. This demonstrates that if an excitatory transmission is pushed above a certain threshold, normal learning-dependent plasticity can be restored in adolescence. It is possible that prefrontal learning-dependent plasticity could be modulated by developing BLA inputs that emerge during adolescence. Evidence for this idea comes from studies in adults demonstrating that direct stimulation of the BLA (or exposure to early life stress) immediately prior to a test of extinction retrieval blocks LTP in the mPFC and causes an increased return of fear [60]. The same study also reported that treatment with the NMDA receptor antagonist MK-801 recapitulated the effects of BLA stimulation/stress exposure on mPFC LTP, while DCS rescued stress-induced impairments in mPFC LTP. Together, these results suggest a model wherein a developmentally-driven increase in BLA→mPFC transmission during adolescence (discussed further in Section 5.1) may disrupt extinction-dependent LTP in the mPFC by dampening NMDA receptor responsivity in the same manner of direct BLA stimulation or previous stress exposure.

4. Development of Inhibitory Networks

Deficits in extinction retention typical of adolescents may also be influenced by shifting excitability and inhibition in fear-modulatory networks over development. Although inhibitory neurons in the BLA and mPFC are composed of several different subpopulations, we will focus primarily on a class of fast-spiking interneurons expressing the calcium-binding protein parvalbumin (PV). Inhibitory PV interneurons are critical for shaping network activity underlying cognition and memory [61]; these GABAergic cells target both pyramidal neurons and other inhibitory interneurons, enabling both direct inhibition as well as disinhibition of excitatory principal neurons [61]. PV interneurons also have a prominent role in generating neuronal oscillations by synchronising the firing patterns of excitatory neurons; in the PL, this process drives fear expression [62], and in the BLA, different PV-coordinated oscillation frequencies drive fear expression vs. fear extinction by changing functional connectivity between the BLA and mPFC [63]. In this section, we review developmental changes in PV interneurons and consider how these changes may impact fear processing in adolescence.

4.1. Prefrontal Inhibition

Levels of PV significantly increase in the mPFC during adolescence [64,65], reflecting a heightened capacity for local inhibition. As the numbers of PV neurons in the PL and IL are similar in juveniles, adolescents, and adults [66,67], this change appears to be driven by increased growth and proliferation of PV cell neurites, meaning that existing interneurons are dramatically arborising and increasing their capacity to integrate signals and regulate activity in pyramidal neurons during adolescence. At the same time, excitatory drive onto this inhibitory population (in the form of both synaptic contacts and glutamatergic transmission) effectively doubles [64,68]. While excitation of inhibitory interneurons in the rat mPFC increases throughout development, it was recently demonstrated that excitatory synapses on inhibitory interneurons in the monkey dlPFC are actually *pruned* over adolescence [69], just as they are on excitatory pyramidal neurons (as discussed in Section 2.1). Though this pattern could be a primate specialisation, it is also possible that development of inhibitory networks may follow different trajectories in later developing prefrontal areas, in which case, one might expect to see pruning of excitatory input to inhibitory neurons in the primate and rodent OFC, though to our knowledge this has not been explored.

The increase in inhibitory tone over the course of adolescence in the mPFC coincides with enhanced GABAergic control of local field potentials. Evidence suggests that relative to adulthood and late adolescence, early adolescence is associated with reduced GABAergic inhibition of glutamatergic pyramidal neurons in the mPFC [70]. This is observed as a failure in the suppression of prefrontal local field potentials in response to high-frequency ventral hippocampal stimulation (20 and 40 Hz) in early adolescence. Ventral hippocampal-mediated long-term depression only emerges in late adolescence, suggesting delayed maturation of GABAergic interneuron function. Other studies have identified signs of increased prefrontal activity in infant and juvenile animals relative to adults (although adolescents were not included) [71], suggesting a linear increase in GABAergic control of prefrontal excitability that stabilises in late adolescence. Importantly, disrupting NMDA receptor-mediated transmission during adolescence (via systemic administration of the antagonist MK-801) from P35–49, but not adulthood, rendered this early adolescent profile of PFC disinhibition long-lasting, such that it was observed well into adulthood [70]. This enduring effect in adult rats after peri-adolescent NMDA receptor disruption was reversed by increasing local GABAergic transmission in the PFC with a single local infusion of the GABAA positive allosteric modulator Indiplon. Evidence suggests that earlier disruption of NMDA signalling (via ketamine or MK-801 during the second-third postnatal week) has similar long-term effects in adulthood, reducing expression of PV, disrupting synaptic properties in interneurons, and causing disinhibition of pyramidal cells [72,73]. Taken together, these findings demonstrate (1) that GABAergic control of prefrontal excitability increases across development before reaching mature functional capacity in late adolescence, and (2) that sustained NMDA receptor transmission is critical for moderating the normal functional development of GABAergic inhibitory networks in the mPFC.

Behaviourally, this developmental trajectory of prefrontal inhibitory networks could significantly affect how memories are acquired, stored, and retrieved at different ages. For instance, transgenic mice bred with a mutation that causes loss of PV neurons in the PFC (but not amygdala or hippocampus) show specific deficits in the extinction of cued fear, but not in its acquisition or expression [74]. Given that extinction retention is intact prior to adolescence when PV neurons are still highly immature, it appears that the mechanisms underlying fear extinction may transition from a PV-independent form in juveniles to a PV-dependent form in adolescence and adulthood, leaving adolescents in a compromised transitional period characterised by impaired extinction processing.

4.2. BLA Inhibition

Although the developmental trajectory of interneuron function in the amygdala has been studied less extensively than in the PFC, the available evidence suggests that PV expression in the rodent basolateral amygdala complex undergoes dynamic changes in periadolescence, and that these changes could have dramatic effects on fear regulation. Berdel and Moryś [75] found that within the magnocellular part of the basal nucleus of the amygdala, the number of PV neurons rapidly increased after P17 and peaked at P21. Density decreased between P21 and P30, and then remained stable through adulthood (P90). In contrast, PV staining in the lateral nucleus of the amygdala was not detected at all at P17 or P21 in this study; it became apparent only at P30 and remained at the same level until P90. Within the basal nucleus, the distribution of PV neurons was largely restricted to the magnocellular region at P17 and P21 and only spread to the parvicellular component at P30 (information about the number of PV neurons in the parvicellular component across development was not provided). It should be noted that using a different antibody than Berdel and Moryś [75], our group detected PV-immunoreactive neurons in the lateral nucleus of juveniles (P24), adolescents (P35–36), and adults (P70), and did not observe changes in the number of labelled cells across development in this region [66]. Within the entirety of the BLA complex (lateral+basal nuclei), we did observe a trend ($p = 0.052$) towards a loss of PV neurons between juveniles and adolescents that appeared to be driven largely by changes in the basal nucleus. Although we did not distinguish between the magnocellular and parvicellular components of the basal nucleus in our study, our results may partially replicate the reduction in PV staining from juvenility to adolescence in the magnocellular basal nucleus found by Berdel and Moryś. It is important to note that the loss of PV staining could reflect a loss of neurons and/or a reduction in PV protein expression. In terms of implications for fear regulation, the anterior magnocellular part of the basal nucleus is connected more prominently to the PL, whereas the IL interacts more with the posterior parvicellular component [49]; differential development of inhibitory networks in these separate regions could therefore create a temporary imbalance between the strength of fear and extinction pathways across development, as the PL-amygdala fear pathway may mature earlier than the IL-amygdala extinction pathway.

Functionally, recent evidence demonstrates that PV interneurons in the BLA have a critical role in modulating relapse of extinguished fear. PV neurons in the BLA are strategically located to modulate PFC activity via BLA to PFC projections. Davis et al. [63] silenced PV interneurons in the BLA using a selective chemogenetic approach coupled with activity-based neuronal-ensemble labelling and electrophysiology. This approach allowed the authors to tag neurons that were active during fear conditioning and examine the effect of PV-silencing specifically on the activity of these identified "fear" neurons. When PV neurons were silenced, BLA fear neurons were disinhibited; as a result, there was also increased activation of neurons in the PL. This BLA-PL fear circuit appears to be important for regulating freezing after extinction, as PL activity associated with BLA dis-inhibition correlated with freezing after extinction (i.e., at an extinction retention test for contextual fear learning). An opposite effect was found in IL, where activity was inhibited following silencing of BLA PV neurons. These findings suggest that impairments in extinction retention could be driven by poor (or immature) functioning of BLA PV neurons, which, in turn, results in disinhibited activation of BLA fear neurons, robust activation of the BLA-PL "fear network", and suppression of the BLA-IL "extinction network". Although this hypothesis (i.e., hypofunctioning of BLA PV neurons during development) has not explicitly been tested, there are indications that inhibitory transmission in the BLA undergoes dramatic changes in adolescence. The mechanisms underlying GABAergic transmission onto BLA pyramidal neurons (i.e., GABA receptor subunit expression, rise/decay time of GABA currents, etc.) are mature in the rat by P28 [76], just at the transition between the juvenile period and adolescence. However, changes in spontaneous inhibitory transmission continue throughout adolescence, suggesting a protracted developmental trajectory for amygdala interneurons. Within the basal nucleus, both spontaneous inhibitory postsynaptic current (sIPSC) frequency and the sIPSC:sEPSC frequency ratio increase from P10 to P30, and then gradually decline into adulthood [77]. In contrast, sEPSC frequency increases sharply between P10 and P15, then remains relatively stable into adulthood. A different pattern is observed in the lateral amygdala; in this nucleus, both sIPSC frequency and the sIPSC:sEPSC frequency ratio increase linearly from infancy through adulthood [78]. As the basal nucleus is the target of prefrontal innervation, it seems likely that some of this periadolescent fine-tuning may be influenced by changing connectivity across development. To explore this possibility further and examine its functional implications, we must consider the postnatal maturation of the robust reciprocal projections between the prefrontal cortex and amygdala.

5. Connectivity

The PFC and the amygdala are strongly connected via robust reciprocal projections. These projections undergo substantial anatomical and functional changes over development that have the potential to dramatically impact the storage and retrieval of fear-related memories. Pyramidal BLA-mPFC projection neurons target both excitatory principal neurons and inhibitory interneurons in the opposite structure, creating complex postsynaptic events that change over the course of development. A summary of pathways established in adult rodents is shown in Figure 2. In this section, we review the anatomical and functional maturation of projections between the mPFC and the BLA, and discuss regulation of this pathway by the ventral hippocampus.

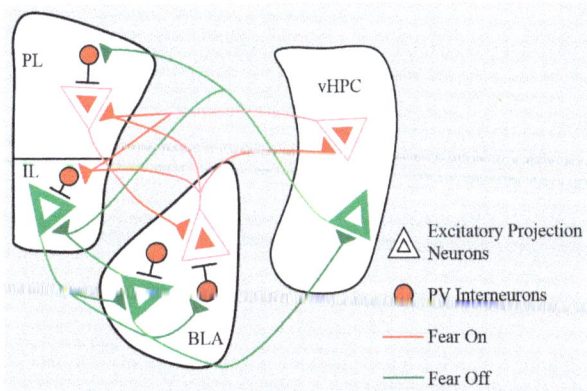

Figure 2. Pathways for Fear and Extinction. Projection neurons in the basolateral amygdala (BLA) and ventral hippocampal (vHPC) target both excitatory neurons and inhibitory interneurons in the medial prefrontal cortex (mPFC). The mPFC targets excitatory and inhibitory cells in the BLA, although innervation of BLA parvalbumin (PV) interneurons comes more strongly from the infralimbic (IL) than the prelimbic (PL). Red pathways represent proposed mechanisms for fear expression, whereas green pathways would promote extinction.

5.1. BLA→mPFC

5.1.1. Anatomical

Infusions of retrograde tracers into the mPFC in developing mice reveal an increase in the density of neurons projecting from the BLA to the PL from juvenility through early adolescence (i.e., from P23 to P30) and a subsequent decrease (at P45) in late adolescence [36]. In the same study, no changes in connectivity were identified between the BLA and IL (p = 0.056), albeit this study had a smaller sample size, suggesting further investigation with larger sample sizes (i.e., >4 per group) might reveal developmental changes in BLA to IL projections. Complementary experiments using anterograde tracers in the BLA show that fibres from the amygdala develop a progressively clear bilaminar pattern with age; fibre density increases in layers II and V of the IL and PL from birth through late adolescence, levelling off in adulthood [79]. This suggests that even as the number of BLA neurons projecting to the mPFC is pruned, the remaining connections continue to mature and strengthen. Cunningham et al. [79] also demonstrated that the percentage of contacts between BLA fibres and the spines, dendrites, and axons of PFC neurons increased linearly with age, while the percentage of fibres making no contacts showed an equal and opposite decrease, providing further evidence that maturing BLA→PFC projections increase in functional capacity with age. It is interesting to consider that while Cunningham et al. [79] reported a linear increase in BLA→mPFC axospinous synapses (excitatory contacts between BLA axon terminals and PFC dendritic spines) over development, synapses, and spines in the PFC overall undergo massive pruning in adolescence, as discussed in Section 2.1. This may suggest that synaptic pruning occurs only in select pathways, presenting opportunities for newly forming patterns of innervation to emerge. As excitatory afferents from distal forebrain sites like the amygdala and hippocampus are slow to arrive in the PFC, one might predict that much of the excitatory innervation of the PFC prior to adolescence is derived from thalamocortical and local corticocortical connectivity, and that these may be the synaptic connections that are more vulnerable to pruning during adolescence.

5.1.2. Functional

Activation of BLA→prefrontal projections induces long-term potentiation (LTP) in the mPFC. This effect is functional by P30 but still maturing, evidenced by larger increases in mPFC local field potentials following BLA stimulation in adults compared to adolescents [80]. This effect was not dependent on GABA, indicating that BLA facilitation of prefrontal LTP is driven by innervation of pyramidal neurons in the mPFC and does not require recruitment of interneurons. It should be noted that these findings do not imply that BLA innervation of prefrontal GABAergic neurons is not biologically or behaviourally relevant; it is entirely possible that discrete activation of BLA subpopulations during complex learning events could selectively stimulate prefrontal GABAergic transmission. For instance, unlike BLA-evoked prefrontal LTP, ventral hippocampal (vHPC) stimulation induces long-term depression (LTD) in the mPFC; this effect emerges later in development (after P55), and is dependent on GABAergic transmission [80]. If inputs from the vHPC and the BLA send axon collaterals to the same PV interneuron, stimulation of that interneuron could drive feedback inhibition onto both inputs, ultimately synchronising the firing pattern of PFC-projecting BLA and vHPFC neurons. Indeed, it has been shown that 1) hippocampal and amygdala afferents converge on neurons in the IL and ventral PL, 2) excitatory responses of these neurons are significantly amplified by simultaneous vHPC+BLA stimulation, and 3) staggered stimulation of BLA and vHPC (separated by 20–40 ms) has an inhibitory effect on the postsynaptic neuron [81]. This suggests that synchronisation of BLA and vHPC firing in the mPFC by PV-mediated feedback inhibition could significantly drive activity and plasticity necessary for the complex integration of cues and context. The fact that desynchronised activity can have inhibitory effects on postsynaptic neurons may also explain the lack of learning-dependent plasticity observed in adolescents (see Section 3). As the PFC is receiving growing input from different brain regions while PV interneurons are still underdeveloped, disorganised excitatory input (while increasing basal synaptic transmission) could actually decrease the probability of action potentials in PFC neurons and blunt learning-dependent changes.

5.2. mPFC→BLA

5.2.1. Anatomical

Neurons in the mPFC that project to the BLA are predominately located in the same layers that receive innervation from the amygdala; BLA-projecting neurons are present in superficial layers II/III and deep layer V across the mPFC [63,82–86]. These neurons receive excitatory inputs from the ventral hippocampus and are subject to inhibitory regulation through local PV interneurons [87]. The number of neurons projecting from the PL and IL appears to be relatively balanced in adults, as infusions of the retrograde tracer CTB in the BLA typically labels similar numbers of neurons in the PL and IL [63]. However, these subregions differ in terms of the types of cells in the BLA that they contact. While projections from the PL and the IL both preferentially innervate the basal nucleus of the BLA, the IL sends stronger inputs to the parvicellular aspects, while the PL more selectively innervates the magnocellular population [49]. In addition, the IL sends more projections to PV BLA interneurons than the PL [63]; given that PV interneurons in the parvicellular division are late to develop (see Section 4.2), this suggests that IL-domination of PV inhibition in the amygdala may not be functionally mature until relatively late in adolescence, and that earlier in development, the balance of control may be tipped more towards the PL.

Unlike bottom-up BLA→mPFC connectivity, top-down projections from the mPFC to the BLA undergo pruning of both fibres and the total number of projection neurons from adolescence through adulthood. Retrograde tracing showed that the number of IL neurons that project to the BLA decreases linearly from juvenility (P25) through adulthood while PL→BLA neurons show a delayed pruning pattern, remaining stable from P25 to late adolescence (P45) before sharply decreasing in number to reach adult levels at P90 [88]. The same study also used anterograde tracing to further examine pathway development, and found that fibres in the BLA originating from the mPFC (PL+IL) maintain a similar density from P25–P45 and are then pruned from late adolescence through adulthood. Another study that examined a broader window of development (six time points from P10–P80) revealed massive mPFC→BLA fibre proliferation between P10 and P30, and confirmed a modest decrease later in adolescence between P45 and adulthood [77]. These results suggest an overall increase in mPFC innervation of the BLA with age, with a discrete period of pruning and reorganisation occurring in late adolescence.

5.2.2. Functional

Stimulation of mPFC afferents in the amygdala coupled with single cell recordings of principal neurons of the BLA (specifically, the basal nucleus) reveal a strengthening of glutamatergic mPFC-amygdala synapses in early development that plateaus by P30 and remains stable through adulthood [77]. However, the same study found that disynaptic inhibitory transmission (i.e., mPFC pyramidal neuron → BLA interneuron → BLA pyramidal neuron) massively increased in amplitude between P21 and P30, and subsided again at P45 and P60. This led to a temporary surge in the IPSC:EPSC amplitude ratio in early adolescence that was more than double the values observed in adulthood, indicating that the mPFC has the capacity to drive substantial GABAergic transmission in the amygdala for a transient period at the onset of adolescence. While the mechanisms for this robust inhibitory potential are as yet unclear, it is possible that the peak in mPFC innervation of the BLA at P30 reflects increased prefrontal targeting of amygdala inhibitory interneurons, and that these synapses are preferentially eliminated between adolescence and adulthood; this could account for the observed reduction in fibre density during this period. Importantly, the findings of Arruda-Carvalho et al. [77] using in vitro stimulation stand in stark contrast to the effects observed using an in vivo stimulation approach. Selleck et al. [89] analysed local field potentials and single-unit recordings in the BLA following electrical stimulation of the mPFC in anaesthetised rats [89]; the findings of this study suggest that prefrontal modulation of amygdala activity is significantly blunted in adolescents compared to adults, contrary to the increased inhibitory control reported by Arruda-Carvalho et al. [77]. In this approach, mPFC stimulation at 10–20 Hz induced local field potential facilitation in the basal nucleus of the BLA of adults, but was ineffective in adolescents (P39). Further analyses showed that in both adolescents and adults, the majority of BLA neurons (~65%) showed an inhibitory response to mPFC stimulation; however, BLA inhibition evoked by stimulation of both the PL and the IL was weaker in adolescents than adults. This pattern of increasing prefrontal inhibitory control of the amygdala from adolescence to adulthood has also been demonstrated in humans [90], and nicely fits the model of compromised emotional regulation in adolescents. Unfortunately, as younger age groups were not included in the in vivo analyses, it is unclear whether the observed impairment in prefrontal regulation of amygdala activity is specific to adolescence or simply a reflection of immature connectivity that would also be observed in juveniles.

Aside from different methodological approaches, what might explain the contradictory findings of Selleck et al. [89] and Arruda-Carvalho et al. [77] concerning mPFC-evoked inhibitory drive in the adolescent BLA? For one, stimulation of the entire mPFC (Selleck et al.) could have more complex downstream effects than discretely driving mPFC terminals within the BLA (Arruda-Carvalho et al.). The former approach would stimulate excitatory and inhibitory cell bodies, dendrites, and afferents within the mPFC and would drive mPFC-BLA network activity in both direct and indirect (i.e., mediated by thalamic or hippocampal relay) pathways. This in vivo approach has obvious advantages in that it reveals how the mPFC coordinates amygdala activity in an intact, biologically-relevant system with information being integrated from multiple networks. However, by excluding all additional activity and honing in on a precise synaptic event, the in vitro approach may reveal more about the precise anatomical and functional development of mPFC-BLA pathways. In any case, when taken together, the results of these two studies show that the mPFC does not effectively inhibit amygdala activity in adolescents under normal conditions, but indicate that it nonetheless has the *capacity* to induce massive inhibition at this developmental stage; this suggests that mPFC→BLA inhibitory transmission is experiencing interference upstream of the BLA during adolescence. Disruption of mPFC-BLA functional connectivity is likely a major contributor to adolescent impairments in extinction retention and future work aimed at facilitating connectivity between these structures may lead to innovative treatment approaches for adolescent-onset anxiety.

5.3. Ventral Hippocampus→mPFC

The BLA-mPFC network obviously does not exist in isolation; as referenced in previous sections, the ventral hippocampus (vHPC) is a critical third node in this fear-regulatory forebrain network. Like the mPFC and the BLA, the vHPC undergoes substantial changes in connectivity across development that critically impact fear- and extinction-related processes.

As previously discussed (Sections 4.1 and 5.1.2), vHPC and BLA inputs into the PFC functionally mature over different developmental time windows (P30 for the BLA and ~P55 for the vHPC) and recruit distinct forms of plasticity in the PFC (LTP for the BLA vs. LTD for the vHPC). The vHPC is a powerful regulator of BLA-mPFC functional connectivity; in adults, stimulation of vHPC inputs with high frequency exerts inhibitory control over BLA drive to the mPFC [91]. Given the late emergence of vHPC-mPFC functional connectivity, this suggests that in early adolescence, the BLA projections to the mPFC are not yet dampened by vHPC regulation; this may contribute to the mPFC being over-responsive to BLA inputs at this age.

In the adult mouse, the vHPC innervates pyramidal neurons situated in both superficial layers II/III and deeper layer V of the IL, but only layer V of the PL [92]. As previously discussed, BLA and vHPC inputs predominantly converge in the IL and the ventral aspects PL. Projections between the vHPC and the PL surge between P23 and P30, peaking in early adolescence before pruning in late adolescence and adulthood [36]. This means that maturation of vHPC→mPFC anatomical connectivity precedes the development of functional connectivity in the form of vHPC-evoked prefrontal LTD and inhibitory control of BLA→mPFC inputs. Like the BLA, the vHPC targets both pyramidal neurons and PV interneurons in the mPFC [87] (see Figure 2). It could be speculated that these early-emerging projections from the vHPC primarily target pyramidal neurons in the PFC, with innervation of interneurons developing later. A simpler (not mutually exclusive) explanation is that prefrontal PV interneurons receive vHPC input in early adolescence but are not yet mature enough to mediate inhibitory transmission at levels sufficient to induce effective vHPC-evoked LTD and synaptic dampening.

vHPC-mediated control of the IL appears to be composed of two functionally disparate pathways: a pro-extinction Brain-Derived Neurotrophic Factor (BDNF)-dependent excitatory pathway and a pro-fear inhibitory pathway. In general, the inhibitory pathway appears to be the default; driving activity in vHPC→IL projections induces PV-mediated feedforward inhibition onto IL pyramidal neurons, and both broad activation of the vHPC and selective activation of vHPC→IL projections results in increased recovery of fear [87]. In contrast, extinction training induces BDNF production in the vHPC, which has been shown to increase the firing rates of IL (but not PL) neurons and facilitate acquisition and retention of extinction [93,94]. Notably, Rosas-Vidal et al. [93] found that while most of the neurons recorded in the PL showed no change in response to vHPC BDNF, approximately 30% were inhibited (compared to the excitatory effect on IL neurons). However, recordings appear to have been taken from both deep and superficial layers of the PL, with a slight bias towards superficial layers II/III; if recordings were restricted to layer V (which receives the majority of vHPC inputs), it is possible that a more consistent inhibitory response would have been observed in the PL. Inactivating the vHPC prior to extinction has also been shown to impair extinction acquisition and retention [95]. This suggests that while inhibition may be the dominant force mediating vHPC-IL interactions, during extinction learning hippocampal BDNF selectively facilitates activity in an excitatory vHPC-IL pathway that is necessary for fear suppression. vHPC-mediated control of the PL is also prominently regulated by BDNF. Inhibiting BDNF activity in the vHPC during adolescence both impairs extinction learning and causes diminished vHPC innervation of the PL (but not the IL) in adulthood [96]. Taken together, these findings demonstrate that the vHPC can differentially modulate activity in the mPFC to either promote fear expression or facilitate extinction. Delayed functional development of the pro-extinction BDNF-dependent pathways relative to the vHPC→IL pro-fear inhibitory pathway may be a contributing factor driving increased fear relapse in adolescence, but this remains a question for future research.

6. Disruption by Chronic Stress

Considering the massive changes in brain structure and function discussed above, it is no great surprise that adolescence represents a significant window of vulnerability that renders the developing animal particularly sensitive to environmental insults. These potential insults are wide-ranging and include poor diet, drugs of abuse, and many other damaging influences, but for the purposes of this discussion we will focus on the effects of chronic stress. Here we focus on how exposure to external stressors during adolescence disrupts the normative developmental trajectory and results in persistent changes to behaviour such as fear regulation. However, neurodevelopment and emotional behaviour are affected by adverse experiences throughout the lifespan, including prior to conception [97], prenatal [98] and early postnatal periods [99], and so we direct the reader to excellent reviews on those topics.

In terms of effects on fear extinction in adolescence, chronic stressor exposure by restraint or social instability in adolescence impairs the acquisition or retention of extinction memories when tested in adolescence relative to non-stressed controls [100–102]. Adolescence appears to be a particularly stress-sensitive developmental period in terms of fear regulation because animals are more susceptible to extinction deficits when stress occurs during adolescence compared to when it occurs in the juvenile period [103] or adulthood [102,104]. Further, such deficits induced by adolescent stress are long-lasting, persisting into adulthood [104]. The consequences of adolescent stress on fear extinction are important clinically when considering strategies for chronically stressed youth presenting for treatment of anxiety disorders. This is because chronic exposure to the stress hormone corticosterone in adolescence reduces the benefit of two approaches that augment extinction retention in adolescent rats, namely extra extinction training [103,104] and pharmacological augmentation by DCS [103]. Such results suggest that a history of chronic stress could further reduce the efficacy of anxiety treatments in adolescents.

The enduring effects of adolescent stress may be caused by maladaptive developmental trajectories of subcortical and cortical emotion regulation systems. In support of this claim, there is evidence that human adolescents with traumatic stress exposure (in late childhood or adolescence) have weaker PFC-amygdala connectivity (reviewed by [2]). Further, in rodents, chronic exogenous corticosterone exposure in adolescence diminishes neuronal activity in the mPFC via a down-regulation of glutamatergic receptors (e.g., NMDA receptors [105]), which are essential for extinction consolidation, and induces structural changes by simplifying hippocampal dendritic structure and altering neuronal spine density in the IL, OFC, hippocampus, and amygdala [106]. Specifically, adolescent corticosterone exposure (for 20 days in mice aged between 5 and 7 weeks old) reduces spine density on pyramidal neurons in the IL (in deep layers), OFC, and hippocampus but has the opposite effect in the amygdala [106]. Although some of these changes were transient and recovered once stressor exposure ended, others such as spine reductions in the OFC and dendritic arborisation in the CA1 were long-term effects that persisted after the stressor had ended.

Earlier onset of chronic stress may induce more persistent, and opposite, effects on BLA spine density. For example, one study reported both immediate and long-term reductions in spine density of BLA pyramidal neurons following restraint stress during juvenility and early adolescence (i.e., 2 h daily restraint from P21 to P35; [107]). The reduction in spinogenesis in the BLA from chronic stress in the juvenile-adolescent period contrasts with reports of increased spinogenesis and dendritic hypertrophy resulting from stress later in adolescent development (described above [106]) or adulthood [108]. Further, chronic restraint stressor exposure in adolescence can induce changes in dendritic morphology in the dorsal mPFC that are layer specific [107], suggesting that synaptic communication of specific afferents (e.g., from the BLA) could be impaired.

The transition from juvenility to adolescence is also a time of maturation of prefrontal and amygdala perineuronal net (PNN) maturation around PV inhibitory interneurons [66] and so it is not surprising that chronic stress occurring during this time reduces inhibitory neuron expression in the PL [109] and alters PNN expression in the PFC (in the OFC) [110]. The stress-induced loss of PV interneurons may reduce local inhibition of pyramidal neurons in the PL and shift this region towards a more "pro-fear" state. Other work links adolescent stress-induced deficits to impaired function of the IL. For instance, chronic unpredictable and chronic restraint stress in adolescence impair fear extinction in adulthood through reductions in basal levels of BDNF and activation of its principal receptor (i.e., pTrkB) and downstream pMAPK signalling in the IL [111]. These cellular mechanisms in the PL and IL may therefore lead to increased fear despite extended extinction training in stress-exposed male adolescent animals [104]. Taken together, the findings discussed in this section illustrate that chronic stress in adolescence alters pyramidal cell and interneuron structure and function, developmental trajectories of PNN maturation, and suggest potential mechanisms by which adolescent stress might impair extinction. Future studies could further investigate the functional consequences of stress in adolescence, such as whether there is reduced synaptic plasticity in reciprocal connections between the BLA and PFC during extinction, and whether the neural and behavioural effects of adolescent stress can be prevented or rescued.

7. Conclusions

In this review, we summarise developmental changes in neuroplasticity, inhibition, and connectivity that occur within and between the mPFC and amygdala in adolescent animals, see Figure 3. We suggest ways in which these changes may influence the characteristic deficits in extinction retention displayed by adolescents, and consider how these delicately-modulated neural processes may be influenced by exposure to stress. It should be noted that the developmental differences discussed here are by no means comprehensive; many other variables, including (but not limited to) dopaminergic infiltration of the PFC, exposure to sex hormones, and changing levels of neurotrophins/neurotrophin receptors likely have dramatic impacts on fear learning and memory in adolescence. Creating a comprehensive roadmap of the complex and dynamic mechanisms underlying emotional processing in the adolescent brain continues to be a massive undertaking; however, increasing interest in the field means that the body of knowledge in this area is swiftly proliferating. Thanks to valuable research contributions like those described above, we are steadily advancing towards the development of targeted treatment approaches designed to meet the storm and stress of adolescence head-on.

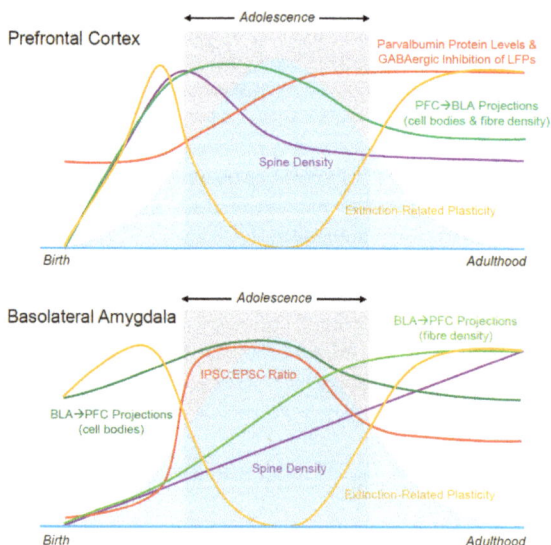

Figure 3. Summary of Neuroanatomical Changes Across Development. Blue bell curve represents fear relapse following extinction. Key: PFC, prefrontal cortex; BLA, basolateral amygdala; LFPs, local field potentials; I/EPSC, inhibitory/excitatory postsynaptic current.

Funding: This research was funded by a Project Grant from the National Health and Medical Research Council to R.R. and KB (NHMRC; APP1086855), an Australian Research Council Discovery Early Career Researcher Award (DE170100392) to K.D.B., and a Sir Keith Murdoch Fellowship from the American Australian Association to K.S.Z.

Conflicts of Interest: The authors declare no conflict of interest. The funders had no role in the writing of the manuscript.

Abbreviations

BDNF	Brain-Derived Neurotrophic Factor
CS	Conditioned stimulus
(m)PFC	(medial) Prefrontal Cortex
IL	Infralimbic
PL	Prelimbic
OFC	Orbitofrontal Cortex
dlPFC	Dorsolateral Prefrontal Cortex
BLA	Basolateral Nucleus of the Amygdala
vHPC	Ventral Hippocampus
PV	Parvalbumin
LTP	Long-Term Potentiation
LTD	Long-Term Depression
(s)EPSC	(spontaneous) Excitatory Postsynaptic Current
(s)IPSC	(spontaneous) Inhibitory Postsynaptic Current
AMPA	Alpha-Amino-3-Hydroxy-5-Methyl-4-Isoxazolepropionic Acid
NMDA	N-Methyl-D-aspartic acid
DCS	D-Cycloserine
GABA	Gamma-Aminobutyric Acid
P	Postnatal Day
PNN	Perineuronal Nets
UCS	Unconditioned stimulus

Appendix A Guide to Rodent Development in (Approximate) Postnatal Days

<7—Perinatal
P7–21—Infancy
P22–P27—Juvenility
P28–P35—Early Adolescence
P36–P41—Mid-Adolescence
P42–P55—Late Adolescence
>P60—Adulthood
*See [30,112]. Values are based on rat development, but a similar trajectory is observed in mice.

References

1. Malter Cohen, M.; Tottenham, N.; Casey, B.J. Translational developmental studies of stress on brain and behavior: Implications for adolescent mental health and illness? *Neuroscience* **2013**, *249*, 53–62. [CrossRef] [PubMed]
2. Tottenham, N.; Galvan, A. Stress and the adolescent brain: Amygdala-prefrontal cortex circuitry and ventral striatum as developmental targets. *Neurosci. Biobehav. Rev.* **2016**, *70*, 217–227. [CrossRef] [PubMed]
3. Casey, B.J.; Duhoux, S.; Malter Cohen, M. Adolescence: What Do Transmission, Transition, and Translation Have to Do with It? *Neuron* **2010**, *67*, 749–760. [CrossRef]
4. Lee, F.S.; Heimer, H.; Giedd, J.N.; Lein, E.S.; Šestan, N.; Weinberger, D.R.; Casey, B.J. Adolescent mental health-Opportunity and obligation. *Science* **2014**, *346*, 547–549. [CrossRef]
5. DiMauro, J.; Domingues, J.; Fernandez, G.; Tolin, D.F. Long-term effectiveness of CBT for anxiety disorders in an adult outpatient clinic sample: A follow-up study. *Behav. Res. Ther.* **2013**, *51*, 82–86. [CrossRef]
6. Ginsburg, G.S.; Becker, E.M.; Keeton, C.P.; Sakolsky, D.; Piacentini, J.; Albano, A.M.; Compton, S.N.; Iyengar, S.; Sullivan, K.; Caporino, N.; et al. Naturalistic follow-up of youths treated for pediatric anxiety disorders. *JAMA Psychiatry* **2014**, *71*, 310–318. [CrossRef] [PubMed]

7. Craske, M.G.; Stein, M.B. Anxiety. *Lancet* **2016**, *388*, 3048–3059. [CrossRef]
8. Casey, B.J.; Glatt, C.E.; Lee, F.S. Treating the developing versus developed brain: Translating preclinical mouse and human studies. *Neuron* **2015**, *86*, 1358–1368. [CrossRef]
9. Hefner, K.; Holmes, A. Ontogeny of fear-, anxiety- and depression-related behavior across adolescence in C57BL/6J mice. *Behav. Brain Res.* **2007**, *176*, 210–215. [CrossRef]
10. Pattwell, S.S.; Duhoux, S.; Hartley, C.A.; Johnson, D.C.; Jing, D.; Elliott, M.D.; Ruberry, E.J.; Powers, A.; Mehta, N.; Yang, R.R.; et al. Altered fear learning across development in both mouse and human. *Proc. Natl. Acad. Sci. USA* **2012**, *109*, 16318–16323. [CrossRef]
11. McCallum, J.; Kim, J.H.; Richardson, R. Impaired extinction retention in adolescent rats: Effects of D-cycloserine. *Neuropsychopharmacology* **2010**, *35*, 2134–2142. [CrossRef] [PubMed]
12. Kim, J.H.; Li, S.; Richardson, R. Immunohistochemical analyses of long-term extinction of conditioned fear in adolescent rats. *Cereb. Cortex* **2011**, *21*, 530–538. [CrossRef] [PubMed]
13. Baker, K.D.; Richardson, R. Forming competing fear learning and extinction memories in adolescence makes fear difficult to inhibit. *Learn. Mem.* **2015**, *22*, 537–543. [CrossRef]
14. Sevenster, D.; Visser, R.M.; D'Hooge, R. A translational perspective on neural circuits of fear extinction: Current promises and challenges. *Neurobiol. Learn. Mem.* **2018**, *155*, 113–126. [CrossRef] [PubMed]
15. Orsini, C.A.; Maren, S. Neural and cellular mechanisms of fear and extinction memory formation. *Neurosci. Biobehav. Rev.* **2012**, *36*, 1773–1802. [CrossRef] [PubMed]
16. Maren, S. Out with the old and in with the new: Synaptic mechanisms of extinction in the amygdala. *Brain Res.* **2015**, *1621*, 231–238. [CrossRef] [PubMed]
17. Marek, R.; Sun, Y.; Sah, P. Neural circuits for a top-down control of fear and extinction. *Psychopharmacology* **2018**. [CrossRef] [PubMed]
18. Milad, M.R.; Quirk, G.J. Fear extinction as a model for translational neuroscience: Ten years of progress. *Annu. Rev. Psychol.* **2012**, *63*, 129–151. [CrossRef]
19. Arruda-Carvalho, M.; Clem, R.L. Prefrontal-amygdala fear networks come into focus. *Front. Syst. Neurosci.* **2015**, *9*, 145. [CrossRef]
20. Krabbe, S.; Grundemann, J.; Luthi, A. Amygdala Inhibitory Circuits Regulate Associative Fear Conditioning. *Biol. Psychiatry* **2017**. [CrossRef] [PubMed]
21. Caballero, A.; Granberg, R.; Tseng, K.Y. Mechanisms contributing to prefrontal cortex maturation during adolescence. *Neurosci. Biobehav. Rev.* **2016**, *70*, 4–12. [CrossRef]
22. Jalbrzikowski, M.; Larsen, B.; Hallquist, M.N.; Foran, W.; Calabro, F.; Luna, B. Development of White Matter Microstructure and Intrinsic Functional Connectivity Between the Amygdala and Ventromedial Prefrontal Cortex: Associations With Anxiety and Depression. *Biol. Psychiatry* **2017**, *82*, 511–521. [CrossRef] [PubMed]
23. Koss, W.A.; Belden, C.E.; Hristov, A.D.; Juraska, J.M. Dendritic remodeling in the adolescent medial prefrontal cortex and the basolateral amygdala of male and female rats. *Synapse* **2014**, *68*, 61–72. [CrossRef]
24. Oberman, L.; Pascual-Leone, A. Changes in plasticity across the lifespan: Cause of disease and target for intervention. *Prog. Brain Res.* **2013**, *207*, 91–120. [CrossRef]
25. Gogtay, N.; Giedd, J.N.; Lusk, L.; Hayashi, K.M.; Greenstein, D.; Vaituzis, A.C.; Nugent, T.F.; Herman, D.H.; Clasen, L.S.; Toga, A.W.; et al. Dynamic mapping of human cortical development during childhood through early adulthood. *Proc. Natl. Acad. Sci. USA* **2004**, *101*, 8174–8179. [CrossRef]
26. Giedd, J.N.; Raznahan, A.; Alexander-Bloch, A.; Schmitt, E.; Gogtay, N.; Rapoport, J.L. Child Psychiatry Branch of the National Institute of Mental Health Longitudinal Structural Magnetic Resonance Imaging Study of Human Brain Development. *Neuropsychopharmacology* **2015**, *40*, 43–49. [CrossRef]
27. Alvarez, V.A.; Sabatini, B.L. Anatomical and physiological plasticity of dendritic spines. *Annu. Rev. Neurosci.* **2007**, *30*, 79–97. [CrossRef] [PubMed]
28. Segal, M. Dendritic spines: Morphological building blocks of memory. *Neurobiol. Learn. Mem.* **2017**, *138*, 3–9. [CrossRef] [PubMed]
29. Moyer, C.E.; Zuo, Y. Cortical dendritic spine development and plasticity: Insights from in vivo imaging. *Curr. Opin. Neurobiol.* **2018**, *53*, 76–82. [CrossRef]
30. Spear, L.P. The adolescent brain and age-related behavioral manifestations. *Neurosci. Biobehav. Rev.* **2000**, *24*, 417–463. [CrossRef]
31. Huttenlocher, P.R. Synaptic density in human frontal cortex — Developmental changes and effects of aging. *Brain Res.* **1979**, *163*, 195–205. [CrossRef]

32. Petanjek, Z.; Judaš, M.; Šimić, G.; Rašin, M.R.; Uylings, H.B.M.; Rakic, P.; Kostović, I. Extraordinary neoteny of synaptic spines in the human prefrontal cortex. *Proc. Natl. Acad. Sci. USA* **2011**, *108*, 13281–13286. [CrossRef]

33. Bourgeois, J.-P.; Goldman-Rakic, P.S.; Rakic, P. Synaptogenesis in the Prefrontal Cortex of Rhesus Monkeys. *Cereb. Cortex* **1994**, *4*, 78–96. [CrossRef]

34. Rakic, P.; Bourgeois, J.-P.; Goldman-Rakic, P.S. Synaptic development of the cerebral cortex: Implications for learning, memory, and mental illness. In *Progress in Brain Research*, Van Pelt, J., Corner, M.A., Uylings, H.B.M., Lopes Da Silva, F.H., Eds.; Elsevier: Amsterdam, the Netherlands, 1994; Volume 102, pp. 227–243.

35. Anderson, S.A.; Classey, J.D.; Condé, F.; Lund, J.S.; Lewis, D.A. Synchronous development of pyramidal neuron dendritic spines and parvalbumin-immunoreactive chandelier neuron axon terminals in layer III of monkey prefrontal cortex. *Neuroscience* **1995**, *67*, 7–22. [CrossRef]

36. Pattwell, S.S.; Liston, C.; Jing, D.; Ninan, I.; Yang, R.R.; Witztum, J.; Murdock, M.H.; Dincheva, I.; Bath, K.G.; Casey, B.J.; et al. Dynamic changes in neural circuitry during adolescence are associated with persistent attenuation of fear memories. *Nat. Commun.* **2016**, *7*, 11475. [CrossRef]

37. Gourley, S.L.; Olevska, A.; Warren, M.S.; Taylor, J.R.; Koleske, A.J. Arg Kinase Regulates Prefrontal Dendritic Spine Refinement and Cocaine-Induced Plasticity. *J. Neurosci.* **2012**, *32*, 2314–2323. [CrossRef] [PubMed]

38. DePoy, L.M.; Noble, B.; Allen, A.G.; Gourley, S.L. Developmentally divergent effects of Rho-kinase inhibition on cocaine- and BDNF-induced behavioral plasticity. *Behav. Brain Res.* **2013**, *243*, 171–175. [CrossRef]

39. Kraszpulski, M.; Dickerson, P.A.; Salm, A.K. Prenatal stress affects the developmental trajectory of the rat amygdala. *Stress* **2006**, *9*, 85–95. [CrossRef]

40. Rubinow, M.J.; Juraska, J.M. Neuron and glia numbers in the basolateral nucleus of the amygdala from preweaning through old age in male and female rats. A stereological study. *J. Comp. Neurol.* **2009**, *512*, 717–725. [CrossRef]

41. Giedd, J.N.; Vaituzis, A.C.; Hamburger, S.D.; Lange, N.; Rajapakse, J.C.; Kaysen, D.; Vauss, Y.C.; Rapoport, J.L. Quantitative MRI of the temporal lobe, amygdala, and hippocampus in normal human development: Ages 4–18 years. *J. Comp. Neurol.* **1996**, *366*, 223–230. [CrossRef]

42. Hu, S.; Pruessner, J.C.; Coupé, P.; Collins, D.L. Volumetric analysis of medial temporal lobe structures in brain development from childhood to adolescence. *NeuroImage* **2013**, *74*, 276–287. [CrossRef]

43. McEvoy, P.M.; Grove, R.; Slade, T. Epidemiology of anxiety disorders in the Australian general population: Findings of the 2007 Australian National Survey of Mental Health and Wellbeing. *Aus. NZJ Psychiatry* **2011**, *45*, 957–967. [CrossRef] [PubMed]

44. McLean, C.P.; Asnaani, A.; Litz, B.T.; Hofmann, S.G. Gender differences in anxiety disorders: Prevalence, course of illness, comorbidity and burden of illness. *J. Psychiatr Res.* **2011**, *45*, 1027–1035. [CrossRef] [PubMed]

45. Li, S.H.; Graham, B.M. Why are women so vulnerable to anxiety, trauma-related and stress-related disorders? The potential role of sex hormones. *Lancet Psychiatry* **2017**, *4*, 73–82. [CrossRef]

46. Kessler, R.C.; Avenevoli, S.; Costello, E.J.; Georgiades, K.; Green, J.G.; Gruber, M.J.; He, J.-P.; Koretz, D.; McLaughlin, K.A.; Petukhova, M.; et al. Prevalence, persistence, and sociodemographic correlates of DSM-IV disorders in the National Comorbidity Survey Replication Adolescent Supplement. *Arch. Gen. Psychiatry* **2012**, *69*, 372–380. [CrossRef] [PubMed]

47. Gruene, T.M.; Roberts, E.; Thomas, V.; Ronzio, A.; Shansky, R.M. Sex-specific neuroanatomical correlates of fear expression in prefrontal-amygdala circuits. *Biol. Psychiatry* **2015**, *78*, 186–193. [CrossRef]

48. Herry, C.; Ciocchi, S.; Senn, V.; Demmou, L.; Muller, C.; Luthi, A. Switching on and off fear by distinct neuronal circuits. *Nature* **2008**, *454*, 600–606. [CrossRef]

49. Kim, J.; Pignatelli, M.; Xu, S.; Itohara, S.; Tonegawa, S. Antagonistic negative and positive neurons of the basolateral amygdala. *Nat. Neurosci.* **2016**, *19*, 1636–1646. [CrossRef]

50. Lai, C.S.; Franke, T.F.; Gan, W.B. Opposite effects of fear conditioning and extinction on dendritic spine remodelling. *Nature* **2012**, *483*, 87–91. [CrossRef]

51. Heinrichs, S.C.; Leite-Morris, K.A.; Guy, M.D.; Goldberg, L.R.; Young, A.J.; Kaplan, G.B. Dendritic structural plasticity in the basolateral amygdala after fear conditioning and its extinction in mice. *Behav. Brain Res.* **2013**, *248*, 80–84. [CrossRef]

52. Maroun, M.; Ioannides, P.J.; Bergman, K.L.; Kavushansky, A.; Holmes, A.; Wellman, C.L. Fear extinction deficits following acute stress associate with increased spine density and dendritic retraction in basolateral amygdala neurons. *Eur. J. Neurosci.* **2013**, *38*, 2611–2620. [CrossRef]

53. Vyas, A.; Jadhav, S.; Chattarji, S. Prolonged behavioral stress enhances synaptic connectivity in the basolateral amygdala. *Neuroscience* **2006**, *143*, 387–393. [CrossRef]

54. Moench, K.M.; Maroun, M.; Kavushansky, A.; Wellman, C. Alterations in neuronal morphology in infralimbic cortex predict resistance to fear extinction following acute stress. *Neurobiol. Stress* **2016**, *3*, 23–33. [CrossRef] [PubMed]

55. Qu, Y.; Yang, C.; Ren, Q.; Ma, M.; Dong, C.; Hashimoto, K. Regional differences in dendritic spine density confer resilience to chronic social defeat stress. *Acta Neuropsychiatr.* **2018**, *30*, 117–122. [CrossRef]

56. Kim, J.J.; Jung, M.W. Neural circuits and mechanisms involved in Pavlovian fear conditioning: A critical review. *Neurosci. Biobehav. Rev.* **2006**, *30*, 188–202. [CrossRef] [PubMed]

57. Yizhar, O.; Klavir, O. Reciprocal amygdala prefrontal interactions in learning. *Curr. Opin. Neurobiol.* **2018**, *52*, 149–155. [CrossRef]

58. Pattwell, S.S.; Bath, K.G.; Casey, B.J.; Ninan, I.; Lee, F.S. Selective early-acquired fear memories undergo temporary suppression during adolescence. *Proc. Natl. Acad. Sci. USA* **2011**, *108*, 1182–1187. [CrossRef] [PubMed]

59. Baker, K.D.; Richardson, R. Pharmacological evidence that a failure to recruit NMDA receptors contributes to impaired fear extinction retention in adolescent rats. *Neurobiol. Learn. Mem.* **2017**, *143*, 18–26. [CrossRef]

60. Inoue, S.; Kamiyama, H.; Matsumoto, M.; Yanagawa, Y.; Hiraide, S.; Saito, Y.; Shimamura, K.; Togashi, H. Synaptic Modulation via Basolateral Amygdala on the Rat Hippocampus–Medial Prefrontal Cortex Pathway in Fear Extinction. *J. Pharmacol. Sci.* **2013**, *123*, 267–278. [CrossRef]

61. Lucas, E.K.; Clem, R.L. GABAergic interneurons: The orchestra or the conductor in fear learning and memory? *Brain Res. Bull.* **2017**. [CrossRef] [PubMed]

62. Courtin, J.; Chaudun, F.; Rozeske, R.R.; Karalis, N.; Gonzalez-Campo, C.; Wurtz, H.; Abdi, A.; Baufreton, J.; Bienvenu, T.C.; Herry, C. Prefrontal parvalbumin interneurons shape neuronal activity to drive fear expression. *Nature* **2014**, *505*, 92–96. [CrossRef] [PubMed]

63. Davis, P.; Zaki, Y.; Maguire, J.; Reijmers, L.G. Cellular and oscillatory substrates of fear extinction learning. *Nat. Neurosci.* **2017**, *20*, 1624–1633. [CrossRef] [PubMed]

64. Caballero, A.; Flores-Barrera, E.; Cass, D.K.; Tseng, K.Y. Differential regulation of parvalbumin and calretinin interneurons in the prefrontal cortex during adolescence. *Brain Struct. Funct.* **2014**, *219*, 395–406. [CrossRef]

65. Caballero, A.; Tseng, K.Y. GABAergic Function as a Limiting Factor for Prefrontal Maturation during Adolescence. *Trends Neurosci.* **2016**, *39*, 441–448. [CrossRef] [PubMed]

66. Baker, K.D.; Gray, A.R.; Richardson, R. The Development of Perineuronal Nets Around Parvalbumin GABAergic Neurons in the Medial Prefrontal Cortex and Basolateral Amygdala of Rats. *Behav. Neurosci.* **2017**, *131*, 289–303. [CrossRef]

67. Brenhouse, H.C.; Andersen, S.L. Nonsteroidal anti-inflammatory treatment prevents delayed effects of early life stress in rats. *Biol. Psychiatry* **2011**, *70*, 434–440. [CrossRef] [PubMed]

68. Cunningham, M.G.; Bhattacharyya, S.; Benes, F.M. Increasing Interaction of Amygdalar Afferents with GABAergic Interneurons between Birth and Adulthood. *Cereb. Cortex* **2008**, *18*, 1529–1535. [CrossRef] [PubMed]

69. Chung, D.W.; Wills, Z.P.; Fish, K.N.; Lewis, D.A. Developmental pruning of excitatory synaptic inputs to parvalbumin interneurons in monkey prefrontal cortex. *Proc. Natl. Acad. Sci. USA* **2017**, *114*, E629–E637. [CrossRef]

70. Thomases, D.R.; Cass, D.K.; Tseng, K.Y. Periadolescent exposure to the NMDA receptor antagonist MK-801 impairs the functional maturation of local GABAergic circuits in the adult prefrontal cortex. *J. Neurosci.* **2013**, *33*, 26–34. [CrossRef] [PubMed]

71. Jia, M.; Travaglia, A.; Pollonini, G.; Fedele, G.; Alberini, C.M. Developmental changes in plasticity, synaptic, glia, and connectivity protein levels in rat medial prefrontal cortex. *Learn. Mem.* **2018**, *25*, 533–543. [CrossRef]

72. Jeevakumar, V.; Kroener, S. Ketamine Administration During the Second Postnatal Week Alters Synaptic Properties of Fast-Spiking Interneurons in the Medial Prefrontal Cortex of Adult Mice. *Cereb. Cortex* **2016**, *26*, 1117–1129. [CrossRef] [PubMed]

73. Murueta-Goyena, A.; Ortuzar, N.; Gargiulo, P.A.; Lafuente, J.V.; Bengoetxea, H. Short-Term Exposure to Enriched Environment in Adult Rats Restores MK-801-Induced Cognitive Deficits and GABAergic Interneuron Immunoreactivity Loss. *Mol. Neurobiol.* **2018**, *55*, 26–41. [CrossRef] [PubMed]

74. Bissonette, G.B.; Bae, M.H.; Suresh, T.; Jaffe, D.E.; Powell, E.M. Prefrontal cognitive deficits in mice with altered cerebral cortical GABAergic interneurons. *Behav. Brain Res.* **2014**, *259*, 143–151. [CrossRef]

75. Berdel, B.; Moryś, J. Expression of calbindin-D28k and parvalbumin during development of rat's basolateral amygdaloid complex. *Int. J. Dev. Neurosci.* **2000**, *18*, 501–513. [CrossRef]

76. Ehrlich, D.E.; Ryan, S.J.; Hazra, R.; Guo, J.D.; Rainnie, D.G. Postnatal maturation of GABAergic transmission in the rat basolateral amygdala. *J. Neurophysiol.* **2013**, *110*, 926–941. [CrossRef]

77. Arruda-Carvalho, M.; Wu, W.C.; Cummings, K.A.; Clem, R.L. Optogenetic Examination of Prefrontal-Amygdala Synaptic Development. *J. Neurosci.* **2017**, *37*, 2976–2985. [CrossRef] [PubMed]

78. Bosch, D.; Ehrlich, I. Postnatal maturation of GABAergic modulation of sensory inputs onto lateral amygdala principal neurons. *J. Physiol.* **2015**, *593*, 4387–4409. [CrossRef]

79. Cunningham, M.G.; Bhattacharyya, S.; Benes, F.M. Amygdalo-cortical sprouting continues into early adulthood: Implications for the development of normal and abnormal function during adolescence. *J. Comp. Neurol.* **2002**, *453*, 116–130. [CrossRef]

80. Caballero, A.; Thomases, D.R.; Flores-Barrera, E.; Cass, D.K.; Tseng, K.Y. Emergence of GABAergic-dependent regulation of input-specific plasticity in the adult rat prefrontal cortex during adolescence. *Psychopharmacology* **2014**, *231*, 1789–1796. [CrossRef]

81. Ishikawa, A.; Nakamura, S. Convergence and Interaction of Hippocampal and Amygdalar Projections within the Prefrontal Cortex in the Rat. *J. Neurosci.* **2003**, *23*, 9987–9995. [CrossRef] [PubMed]

82. Little, J.P.; Carter, A.G. Synaptic mechanisms underlying strong reciprocal connectivity between the medial prefrontal cortex and basolateral amygdala. *J. Neurosci.* **2013**, *33*, 15333–15342. [CrossRef] [PubMed]

83. Ferreira, A.N.; Yousuf, H.; Dalton, S.; Sheets, P.L. Highly differentiated cellular and circuit properties of infralimbic pyramidal neurons projecting to the periaqueductal gray and amygdala. *Front. Cell Neurosci.* **2015**, *9*. [CrossRef] [PubMed]

84. Bouwmeester, H.; Smits, K.; Van Ree, J.M. Neonatal development of projections to the basolateral amygdala from prefrontal and thalamic structures in rat. *J. Comp. Neurol.* **2002**, *450*, 241–255. [CrossRef] [PubMed]

85. Gabbott, P.L.; Warner, T.A.; Jays, P.R.; Salway, P.; Busby, S.J. Prefrontal cortex in the rat: Projections to subcortical autonomic, motor, and limbic centers. *J. Comp. Neurol.* **2005**, *492*, 145–177. [CrossRef] [PubMed]

86. Hirai, Y.; Morishima, M.; Karube, F.; Kawaguchi, Y. Specialized Cortical Subnetworks Differentially Connect Frontal Cortex to Parahippocampal Areas. *J. Neurosci.* **2012**, *32*, 1898–1913. [CrossRef] [PubMed]

87. Marek, R.; Jin, J.; Goode, T.D.; Giustino, T.F.; Wang, Q.; Acca, G.M.; Holehonnur, R.; Ploski, J.E.; Fitzgerald, P.J.; Lynagh, T.; et al. Hippocampus-driven feed-forward inhibition of the prefrontal cortex mediates relapse of extinguished fear. *Nat. Neurosci.* **2018**, *21*, 384–392. [CrossRef] [PubMed]

88. Cressman, V.L.; Balaban, J.; Steinfeld, S.; Shemyakin, A.; Graham, P.; Parisot, N.; Moore, H. Prefrontal cortical inputs to the basal amygdala undergo pruning during late adolescence in the rat. *J. Comp. Neurol.* **2010**, *518*, 2693–2709. [CrossRef] [PubMed]

89. Selleck, R.A.; Zhang, W.; Samberg, H.D.; Padival, M.; Rosenkranz, J.A. Limited prefrontal cortical regulation over the basolateral amygdala in adolescent rats. *Sci. Rep.* **2018**, *8*, 17171. [CrossRef] [PubMed]

90. Gee, D.G.; Humphreys, K.L.; Flannery, J.; Goff, B.; Telzer, E.H.; Shapiro, M.; Hare, T.A.; Bookheimer, S.Y.; Tottenham, N. A Developmental Shift from Positive to Negative Connectivity in Human Amygdala–Prefrontal Circuitry. *J. Neurosci.* **2013**, *33*, 4584–4593. [CrossRef]

91. Thomases, D.R.; Cass, D.K.; Meyer, J.D.; Caballero, A.; Tseng, K.Y. Early adolescent MK-801 exposure impairs the maturation of ventral hippocampal control of basolateral amygdala drive in the adult prefrontal cortex. *J. Neurosci.* **2014**, *34*, 9059–9066. [CrossRef] [PubMed]

92. Liu, X.; Carter, A.G. Ventral Hippocampal Inputs Preferentially Drive Corticocortical Neurons in the Infralimbic Prefrontal Cortex. *J. Neurosci.* **2018**, *38*, 7351–7363. [CrossRef] [PubMed]

93. Rosas-Vidal, L.E.; Do-Monte, F.H.; Sotres-Bayon, F.; Quirk, G.J. Hippocampal-prefrontal BDNF and memory for fear extinction. *Neuropsychopharmacology* **2014**, *39*, 2161–2169. [CrossRef] [PubMed]

94. Rosas-Vidal, L.E.; Lozada-Miranda, V.; Cantres-Rosario, Y.; Vega-Medina, A.; Melendez, L.; Quirk, G.J. Alteration of BDNF in the medial prefrontal cortex and the ventral hippocampus impairs extinction of avoidance. *Neuropsychopharmacology* **2018**, *43*, 2636–2644. [CrossRef] [PubMed]

95. Sierra-Mercado, D.; Padilla-Coreano, N.; Quirk, G.J. Dissociable roles of prelimbic and infralimbic cortices, ventral hippocampus, and basolateral amygdala in the expression and extinction of conditioned fear. *Neuropsychopharmacology* **2011**, *36*, 529–538. [CrossRef]

96. Giza, J.I.; Kim, J.; Meyer, H.C.; Anastasia, A.; Dincheva, I.; Zheng, C.I.; Lopez, K.; Bains, H.; Yang, J.; Bracken, C.; et al. The BDNF Val66Met Prodomain Disassembles Dendritic Spines Altering Fear Extinction Circuitry and Behavior. *Neuron* **2018**, *99*, 163–178. [CrossRef] [PubMed]

97. Keenan, K.; Hipwell, A.E.; Class, Q.A.; Mbayiwa, K. Extending the developmental origins of disease model: Impact of preconception stress exposure on offspring neurodevelopment. *Dev. Psychol. Biol.* **2018**, *60*, 753–764. [CrossRef]

98. van den Bergh, B.R.H.; Dahnke, R.; Mennes, M. Prenatal stress and the developing brain: Risks for neurodevelopmental disorders. *Dev. Psychopathol.* **2018**, *30*, 743–762. [CrossRef] [PubMed]

99. Cowan, C.S.; Callaghan, B.L.; Kan, J.M.; Richardson, R. The lasting impact of early-life adversity on individuals and their descendants: Potential mechanisms and hope for intervention. *Genes Brain Behav.* **2016**, *15*, 155–168. [CrossRef] [PubMed]

100. McCormick, C.M.; Mongillo, D.L.; Simone, J.J. Age and adolescent social stress effects on fear extinction in female rats. *Stress* **2013**, *16*, 678–688. [CrossRef] [PubMed]

101. Negrón-Oyarzo, I.; Pérez, M.Á.; Terreros, G.; Muñoz, P.; Dagnino-Subiabre, A. Effects of chronic stress in adolescence on learned fear, anxiety, and synaptic transmission in the rat prelimbic cortex. *Behav. Brain Res.* **2014**, *259*, 342–353. [CrossRef] [PubMed]

102. Zhang, W.; Rosenkranz, J.A. Repeated restraint stress enhances cue-elicited conditioned freezing and impairs acquisition of extinction in an age-dependent manner. *Behav. Brain Res.* **2013**, *248*, 12–24. [CrossRef]

103. Stylianakis, A.A.; Richardson, R.; Baker, K.D. Timing is everything: Developmental differences in the effect of a chronic stressor on extinction retention. *Behav. Neurosci.*. under review.

104. Den, M.L.; Altmann, S.R.; Richardson, R. A comparison of the short- and long-term effects of cortico- sterone exposure on extinction in adolescence versus adulthood. *Behav. Neurosci.* **2014**, *128*, 722–735. [CrossRef]

105. Yuen, E.Y.; Wei, J.; Liu, W.; Zhong, P.; Li, X.; Yan, Z. Repeated stress causes cognitive impairment by suppressing glutamate receptor expression and function in prefrontal cortex. *Neuron* **2012**, *73*, 962–977. [CrossRef] [PubMed]

106. Gourley, S.L.; Swanson, A.M.; Koleske, A.J. Corticosteroid-induced neural remodeling predicts behavioral vulnerability and resilience. *J. Neurosci.* **2013**, *33*, 3107–3112. [CrossRef] [PubMed]

107. Pinzon-Parra, C.; Vidal-Jimenez, B.; Camacho-Abrego, I.; Flores-Gomez, A.A.; Rodriguez-Moreno, A.; Flores, G. Juvenile stress causes reduced locomotor behavior and dendritic spine density in the prefrontal cortex and basolateral amygdala in Sprague-Dawley rats. *Synapse* **2019**, *73*, e22066. [CrossRef] [PubMed]

108. Vyas, A.; Mitra, R.; Shankaranarayana Rao, B.S.; Chattarji, S. Chronic Stress Induces Contrasting Patterns of Dendritic Remodeling in Hippocampal and Amygdaloid Neurons. *J. Neurosci.* **2002**, *22*, 6810–6818. [CrossRef]

109. Page, C.E.; Coutellier, L. Adolescent Stress Disrupts the Maturation of Anxiety-related Behaviors and Alters the Developmental Trajectory of the Prefrontal Cortex in a Sex- and Age-specific Manner. *Neuroscience* **2018**, *390*, 265–277. [CrossRef]

110. De Araujo Costa Folha, O.A.; Bahia, C.P.; de Aguiar, G.P.S.; Herculano, A.M.; Coelho, N.L.G.; de Sousa, M.B.C.; Shiramizu, V.K.M.; de Menezes Galvao, A.C.; de Carvalho, W.A.; Pereira, A. Effect of chronic stress during adolescence in prefrontal cortex structure and function. *Behav. Brain Res.* **2017**, *326*, 44–51. [CrossRef] [PubMed]

111. Deng, J.H.; Yan, W.; Han, Y.; Chen, C.; Meng, S.Q.; Sun, C.Y.; Xu, L.Z.; Xue, Y.X.; Gao, X.J.; Chen, N.; et al. Predictable Chronic Mild Stress during Adolescence Promotes Fear Memory Extinction in Adulthood. *Sci. Rep.* **2017**, *7*, 7857. [CrossRef]

112. Cowan, C.S.M.; Richardson, R. A Brief Guide to Studying Fear in Developing Rodents: Important Considerations and Common Pitfalls. *Curr. Protoc. Neurosci.* **2018**, *83*, e44. [CrossRef] [PubMed]

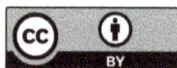

![brain sciences logo] **brain sciences**

MDPI

Article

Impaired Fear Extinction Recall in Serotonin Transporter Knockout Rats Is Transiently Alleviated during Adolescence

Pieter Schipper [1], Paola Brivio [2], David de Leest [1], Leonie Madder [1], Beenish Asrar [1], Federica Rebuglio [1], Michel M. M. Verheij [1], Tamas Kozicz [3], Marco A. Riva [2], Francesca Calabrese [2], Marloes J. A. G. Henckens [1] and Judith R. Homberg [1,*]

[1] Department of Cognitive Neuroscience, Donders Institute for Brain, Cognition and Behaviour, Radboud University Medical Center, Kapittelweg 29, 6525 EN Nijmegen, The Netherlands; ptrschipper@gmail.com (P.S.); deLeest@gmail.com (D.d.L.); Madder@hotmail.com (L.M.); beenish.phdns4@iiu.edu.pk (B.A.); frederica.rebuglio@unimi.it (F.R.); Michel.Verheij@radboudumc.nl (M.M.M.V.); Marloes.Henckens@radboudumc.nl (M.J.A.G.H.)
[2] Department of Pharmacological and Biomolecular Sciences, Universita' degli Studi di Milano, 20133 Milan, Italy; paola.brivio@unimi.it (P.B.); m.riva@unimi.it (M.A.R.); francesca.calabrese@unimi.it (F.C.)
[3] Department of Clinical Genomics, Mayp Clinic, Rochester, MN 55905, USA; Tamas.Kozicz@radboudumc.nl
[*] Correspondence: Judith.Homberg@radboudumc.nl; Tel.: +31-24-361-0906

Received: 27 March 2019; Accepted: 21 May 2019; Published: 22 May 2019

Abstract: Adolescence is a developmental phase characterized by emotional turmoil and coincides with the emergence of affective disorders. Inherited serotonin transporter (5-HTT) downregulation in humans increases sensitivity to these disorders. To reveal whether and how *5-HTT* gene variance affects fear-driven behavior in adolescence, we tested wildtype and serotonin transporter knockout (5-HTT$^{-/-}$) rats of preadolescent, adolescent, and adult age for cued fear extinction and extinction recall. To analyze neural circuit function, we quantified inhibitory synaptic contacts and, through RT-PCR, the expression of c-Fos, brain-derived neurotrophic factor (BDNF), and NDMA receptor subunits, in the medial prefrontal cortex (mPFC) and amygdala. Remarkably, the impaired recall of conditioned fear that characterizes preadolescent and adult 5-HTT$^{-/-}$ rats was transiently normalized during adolescence. This did not relate to altered inhibitory neurotransmission, since mPFC inhibitory immunoreactivity was reduced in 5-HTT$^{-/-}$ rats across all ages and unaffected in the amygdala. Rather, since mPFC (but not amygdala) c-Fos expression and NMDA receptor subunit 1 expression were reduced in 5-HTT$^{-/-}$ rats during adolescence, and since PFC c-Fos correlated negatively with fear extinction recall, the temporary normalization of fear extinction during adolescence could relate to altered plasticity in the developing mPFC.

Keywords: serotonin transporter; rat; fear extinction; medial prefrontal cortex; NMDA; BDNF; adolescence; age

---

1. Introduction

Adolescence is a period of physical and brain maturation that is characterized by emotional turmoil and an increase in pervasive fears, and coincides with the emergence of anxiety and other affective disorders [1–7]. Recent data implicates organizational changes of the cognitive control circuitry regulating emotional behavior in this vulnerability during adolescence. More specifically, there is evidence for relative immaturity of the medial prefrontal cortex (mPFC) and its top-down control over subcortical areas mediating emotion and motivation such as the amygdala, whose development precedes that of the PFC [3]. According to the developmental mismatch hypothesis, the delayed maturation of the PFC in comparison to the amygdala results in a temporary imbalance between emotion and its regulatory processes [8]. However, there are substantial individual differences [9] in this transient "imbalance" during adolescence, and the underlying mechanisms and factors influencing the maturation process are not yet clear. As the PFC-amygdala circuit is dysfunctional in anxiety disorders [10] that frequently emerge during adolescence and often persist into adulthood [11], the understanding of the maturation of the PFC-amygdala circuit in healthy subjects is expected to inform the pathophysiology of stress-related neuropsychiatric disorders.

Appropriate PFC-amygdala circuit balance is critical for adequate extinction of fear. Previous research demonstrated that fear extinction is diminished in pre-adolescents and adolescents compared to adults, in both humans and animals [12–14]. This phenomenon only applies to fear that is cue-dependent and thus involving the PFC, whose activity—as assessed by c-Fos immunoreactivity—has been found to be reduced during adolescence compared to preadolescence and adulthood [12]. In contrast, improved extinction of contextual fear, as mediated by the hippocampus, is observed in adolescence compared to preadolescence and adulthood [15].

GABAergic inhibitory signaling plays an important role in this regulation of fear. The excitability of the basolateral amygdala (BLA), the amygdalar subnucleus responsible for maintaining the learned fear-association [16], is regulated by inhibitory signaling of local GABAergic interneurons [17], a mechanism by which fear and anxiety are attenuated [18]. Similarly, top-down control as mediated by the infralimbic cortex (IL) is modulated by GABAergic inhibition. The infralimbic cortex (IL) contributes to the inhibition of the fear response in the central amygdala (CeA) after successful fear extinction via its glutamatergic excitatory projections to the intercalated cells of the amygdala. IL function is regulated by excitatory inputs from several regions, including the BLA [19–21]. Although these projections are glutamatergic, their stimulation in vivo primarily inhibits neural activity in the PFC [22,23], which has been suggested to be caused by robust feedforward inhibition mediated by GABAergic interneurons [23,24]. Similar to the amygdala, some hippocampal projections may preferentially target IL interneurons, inhibiting IL output to downstream targets [25]. Besides this local inhibition, the IL also receives inhibitory innervations from the dorsal raphe nucleus (DRN) [26] as well as the basal forebrain [27]. Patients suffering from post-traumatic stress disorder, a disorder of aberrant fear extinction, are characterized by abnormalities in GABAergic signaling within the prefrontal cortex [28], implicating this local inhibitory circuit in its pathology. However, as of yet, the exact contribution of these inhibitory circuits to the impaired fear extinction in adolescents remains to be investigated.

Glutamate receptors represent another signaling system critical for the consolidation of extinction memories. Previous studies have demonstrated that the partial NMDA receptor agonist D-cycloserine (DCS) improves extinction retention in adolescent rats [13,29]. This implies that besides alterations in GABAergic signaling, a failure to recruit N-methyl-D-aspartate (NMDA) receptors may contribute to the impaired fear extinction during adolescence as well [12].

Brain-derived neurotrophic factor (BDNF) has also been implicated in fear circuitry maturation [30]. BDNF levels in the hippocampus peak during adolescence, suggesting that BDNF plays a key role in the maturation of subcortical regions. Furthermore, developmental studies utilizing a genetic *BDNF* single nucleotide polymorphism (Val66Met) knock-in mouse indicate that BDNF$^{Met/Met}$ mice tested in preadolescence and early adolescence do not differ from wild-type controls regarding fear extinction, but show an impairment during adulthood. These results indicate that the impairment in cued fear extinction in BDNF$^{Met/Met}$ mice emerges in a time frame corresponding to the transition from adolescence to adulthood and that BDNF may thus be critical in this developmental stage for appropriate circuit development.

Interestingly, the adolescent behavioral and supposed neural phenotype shows striking similarities to those seen in carriers of the low activity variant short (s) allele of the serotonin transporter linked polymorphic region (5-HTTLPR) in humans. Adult s-allele carriers, which presumably display increased extracellular serotonin levels, show increased acquisition [31] and reduced extinction [32] of conditioned fear, together with amygdala hyper-reactivity [33] and attenuated anatomical and functional coupling between the mPFC and amygdala [34,35]. Thus, the behavioral and brain phenotypes seen in adult carriers of the s-allele of the 5-HTTLPR may also imply a cortical-subcortical functional imbalance. Serotonin acts as a neurotrophic factor during development, and variations in serotonin availability occurring due to a limited availability of 5-HTT are thought to affect the development of circuits involved in the regulation of emotional behavior [36–38]. This poses the hypothesis that 5-HTTLPR may affect the development of the cortical-subcortical circuit, such that the transitions from preadolescence to adolescence, and from adolescence to adulthood are altered in 5-HTTLPR s-allele carriers.

Serotonin transporter knockout (5-HTT$^{-/-}$) rats are used as a model organism for the 5-HTTLPR s-allele in humans and show many phenotypical similarities, both adaptive and maladaptive, to s-allele carriers [39]. Similar to humans and rodents during adolescence, as well as adult 5-HTTLPR s-allele carriers, 5-HTT$^{-/-}$ rodents display impaired fear extinction (recall) [40–46]. Since 5-HTT$^{-/-}$ rats display decreased inhibitory GABAergic control over excitatory neurons in the cortex during preadolescence [47], reduced expression of BDNF and GABA system components across development [48], altered NMDA receptor subunit expression in the PFC at adulthood [49], and an association with impaired fear extinction-reduced c-Fos expression in the IL [46], it is possible that the 5-HTT genotype affects the development of the PFC–amygdala circuitry and thereby fear extinction recall across developmental stages.

Here, we employed a cued fear extinction paradigm to evaluate how differential 5-HTT expression affects the development of fear extinction learning and recall across adolescence using homozygous (5-HTT$^{-/-}$) and heterozygous (5-HTT$^{+/-}$) serotonin transporter knockout rats and compared them to wildtype animals (5-HTT$^{+/+}$). We assessed the population of inhibitory cells in the IL and BLA by measuring the number of synaptic contacts expressing the inhibitory markers glutamic acid decarboxylase 65 and 67 (GAD65/67). Additionally, we assessed expression levels of BDNF, NMDA receptor subunits, and c-Fos in the PFC and amygdala at baseline and after fear extinction and fear extinction recall across ages in 5-HTT$^{+/+}$ and 5-HTT$^{-/-}$ rats.

2. Materials and Methods

2.1. Animals

All experiments were approved by the Committee for Animal Experiments of the Radboud University Nijmegen Medical Centre, Nijmegen, the Netherlands, and all efforts were made to minimize animal suffering and to reduce the number of animals used. Serotonin transporter knockout rats (Slc6a41Hubr) were generated on a Wistar background by N-ethyl-N-nitrosurea (ENU)-induced mutagenesis [50]. Experimental animals were derived from crossing heterozygous 5-HT transporter knockout (5-HTT$^{+/-}$) rats that were outcrossed for at least 12 generations with wildtype Wistar rats obtained from Harlan Laboratories (Horst, the Netherlands). Ear punches were taken at the age of 21 days for genotyping, which was done by Kbiosciences (Hoddesdon, United Kingdom. Male adult 5-HTT$^{-/-}$, 5-HTT$^{+/-}$, and wildtype (5-HTT$^{+/+}$) rats entered the experiment at p24 (preadolescent), p35 (adolescent), or p70 (adult). The adult animals were housed in pairs, while the adolescent and preadolescent animals were housed three per cage, in open cages. All animals had ad libitum access to food and water. A 12 h light–dark cycle was maintained, with lights on at 8:00 a.m. All behavioral experiments were performed between 8:00 a.m. and 6:00 p.m.

2.2. Apparatus

A 30.5 × 24.1 × 21 cm operant conditioning chamber (Model VFC-008, Med Associates) was used for fear conditioning and sham conditioning. The box was housed within a sound-attenuating cubicle and contained a white LED stimulus light, a white and near infrared house light, as well as a speaker capable of producing an 85 dB 2.8 kHz tone. The metal grid floor of the apparatus was connected to a scrambled shock generator (model ENV-412, Med Associates) configured to deliver shocks at 0.6

mA intensity. Fear extinction and extinction recall were tested in a novel context, in a novel room. The novel context consisted of a 25 × 25 × 30 cm Plexiglas cage, the bottom of which was covered with a +/− 0.5-cm-thick layer of black bedding. In this context, 85 dB (measured at the center of the floor) 2.8 kHz auditory stimuli were delivered through a set of external speakers.

2.3. Procedure

In total, 329 rats were exposed to behavioral testing. As genotypes of the animals at some ages were only known after completion of the protocol, relatively more 5-HTT$^{+/-}$ animals were tested compared to 5-HTT$^{+/+}$ and 5-HTT$^{-/-}$ rats ($n_{5\text{-HTT}}{}^{+/+}$-p24 = 26, $n_{5\text{-HTT}}{}^{+/+}$-p35 = 30, $n_{5\text{-HTT}}{}^{+/+}$-p70 = 35, $n_{5\text{-HTT}}{}^{+/-}$-p24 = 51, $n_{5\text{-HTT}}{}^{+/-}$-p35 = 79, $n_{5\text{-HTT}}{}^{+/-}$-p70 = 32, $n_{5\text{-HTT}}{}^{-/-}$-p24 = 25, $n_{5\text{-HTT}}{}^{-/-}$-p35 = 21, $n_{5\text{-HTT}}{}^{-/-}$-p70 = 30). On the day on which the animals entered the experiment (p24 for the preadolescent group, p35 for the adolescent group, and p70 for the adult group), the animals were habituated to the conditioning context for 10 minutes. Twenty-four hours after habituation, animals were given a cued fear conditioning session. Fear conditioning began with a 2-minute habituation period, followed by 5 instances of a 30-second 85 dB 2.8 kHz auditory stimulus co-terminating with a 1-second 0.6 mA foot shock, followed by a 1-minute inter-trial interval. Twenty-four, 48, and 72 hours after conditioning, fear extinction and two sessions of extinction recall were given, respectively. Thus, extinction learning and extinction recall (2×) were assessed on three consecutive days. In each of these sessions, rats were exposed to a 2-minute habituation period, after which 24 20-second presentations of the auditory stimulus were given, with an inter-trial interval of 5 seconds. Sessions were recorded, and freezing was automatically assessed by a software program (see below). For the conditioning and the habituation to the fear conditioning chamber, the apparatus was cleaned before and after each animal using a tissue slightly dampened with 70% EtOH. Water was used for cleaning in between the extinction and extinction recall sessions.

2.4. Assessment of Behavior

Time spent freezing during the conditioning session was not assessed, as previous work as indicated no differences between genotypes in the acquisition of fear memory [46]. For assessing the time spent freezing during extinction learning and both extinction recall sessions, we used the Ethovision 9.0 behavioral software package (Noldus Information Technology B.V., Wageningen, the Netherlands). Freezing was determined using the Activity Monitor feature of the software package. The threshold for pixel change between frames was set between 0.05 and 0.09% (depending on the specific camera in use, but not different between groups). Automatic assessment was compared to manually scored samples in in total 696 samples of 20 seconds, derived from 29 extinction sessions by two different observers blind to the genotype of the animal, and proved to be a reliable assessment of freezing behavior (correlation between manual and automatic outcomes: r = 0.7397). To analyze fear extinction learning, extinction sessions were divided into 6 blocks representing the average freezing responses to 4 auditory cue presentations each. Average freezing to all auditory cue presentations during the recall sessions was used as index for fear extinction recall.

Since 5-HTT$^{+/-}$ and 5-HTT$^{+/+}$ showed a comparable behavioral profile, we focused on 5-HTT$^{-/-}$ and 5-HTT$^{+/+}$ rats during subsequent histological and molecular studies aiming to understand the mechanisms underlying the genotype × age effects.

2.5. GAD65/67 Immunostaining

The immunostaining procedure was adopted from Olivier et al. (2008) and Nonkes et al. (2010) [51,52]. Ninety minutes following either the extinction learning session or the second extinction recall session, a subset of the rats (n = 5, randomly selected) were anesthetized and perfused transcardially with 0.1 mol/L PBS, pH 7.3, followed by 4% paraformaldehyde dissolved in 0.1 mol/L phosphate buffer (PB), pH 7.2. The pressure of the perfusion was reduced for the preadolescent rats. Perfusion continued until signs of successful perfusion were observed (shaking limbs, stiff cheeks, etc.). Subsequently, the brains were removed from the skull and post-fixed overnight in 4%

paraformaldehyde at 4 °C. Before sectioning, the brains were cryoprotected with 30% sucrose in 0.1 mol/L PB. Forty-micrometer-thick brain sections were cut on a freezing microtome and collected in six parallel series in 0.1 mol/L PBS containing 0.1% sodium azide. One series from each rat was used for every staining. The free-floating sections were washed three times in PBS and preincubated with 0.3% perhydrol (30% H2O2, Merck, Darmstadt, Germany) for 30 min. After washing three times in PBS, the sections were presoaked for 30 min in an incubation medium consisting of PBS with 0.1% bovine serum albumin and 0.5% Triton X-100. The sections were then incubated with goat anti-GAD65/67, 1:2000 (Santa Cruz Biotechnology Inc., Santa Cruz, CA, USA), overnight on a shaker, at room temperature, and consecutively incubated for 90 min at room temperature with biotinylated donkey-anti-goat (Jackson Immuno Research Laboratories, West Grove, PA, USA) diluted 1:1500 in incubation medium and for 90 min at room temperature with ABC-elite, diluted 1:800 in PB (Vector Laboratories, Burlingame, CA, USA). Between incubations, sections were rinsed three times with PBS. The GAD65/67–antibody peroxidase complex was made visible using 3,3-diaminobenzidine tetrahydrochloride staining. Sections were incubated for 10 min in a chromogen solution consisting of 0.02% 3,3-diaminobenzidine tetrahydrochloride and 0.03% nickel–ammonium sulfate in 0.05 mol/L Tris-buffer (pH 7.6) and subsequently for 10 min in chromogen solution containing 0.006% hydrogen peroxide. This resulted in a blue–black staining. The sections were then rinsed three times in PBS and mounted on gelatin chrome alum-coated glass slides, dried overnight in a stove at 37 °C, dehydrated in an increased series of ethanol, cleared in xylene, embedded with Entellan (Merck), and coverslipped.

2.6. Quantification

Numbers of GAD65/67-immunopositive granules, representing inhibitory synaptic contacts, were quantified using the software program Fiji ImageJ, a public domain image-processing program (http://rsb.info.nih.gov/ij/) [53]. Granules were counted in the IL in equally framed sections across groups at 2.20 from Bregma at ×40 magnification using an Axio Imager.A2 microscope (Zeiss, Oberkochen, Germany). BLA GAD65/67 immunoreactivity was measured in sections at −1.88 mm from Bregma at ×40 magnification. The results for each subject are expressed as the total amount of immunopositive granules counted in a standardized sample area measuring 281.6 × 211.2 um within each section.

2.7. Gene Expression Analyses

The remaining animals were sacrificed by rapid decapitation at 90 minutes following either the extinction learning session or the second extinction recall session. Brains were rapidly removed from the skull and quick-frozen on dry ice and stored at −80 °C until further processing.

Brains from WT and 5-HTT$^{-/-}$ rats were sectioned into 220 μm coronal slices on a Leica CM3050 S Research Cryostat (Leica Biosystems, Amsterdam, the Netherlands), with a chamber temperature of −12 °C and an object temperature of −10 °C, after which regions of interest were punched out. To be able to relate gene expression profiles following extinction (recall) to basal gene expression patterns, additional naïve control WT and 5-HTT$^{-/-}$ brains were obtained and processed in a similar fashion ($n_{5\text{-HTT}}{}^{+/+}$-p24 = 6, $n_{5\text{-HTT}}{}^{+/+}$-p35 = 7, $n_{5\text{-HTT}}{}^{+/+}$-p70 = 7, $n_{5\text{-HTT}}{}^{-/-}$-p24 = 7, $n_{5\text{-HTT}}{}^{-/-}$-p35 = 7, $n_{5\text{-HTT}}{}^{-/-}$-p70 = 6). Medial prefrontal cortex punches were taken bilaterally with a 1.0 mm diameter hollow needle from 8 subsequent slices (Bregma ≈ 3.70:2.20 mm), for a total of 32 punches (prelimbic and infralimbic cortex were punched bilaterally and punches combined to obtain sufficient amounts of material for gene expression analyses). Likewise, 8–10 1.0 mm diameter punches were taken from the bilateral amygdala (Bregma ≈ −2.30: −3.30 mm).

Total RNA was isolated by a single step of guanidinium isothiocyanate/phenol extraction using PureZol RNA isolation reagent (Bio-Rad Laboratories, Italy) according to the manufacturer's instructions and quantified by spectrophotometric analysis. Following total RNA extraction, the samples were processed for real-time polymerase chain reaction (RT-PCR) to assess total BDNF, NR1, NR2A, and c-Fos mRNA expression. An aliquot of each sample was treated with DNase to avoid DNA contamination. RNA was analyzed by TaqMan qRT-PCR instrument (CFX384 real time system,

Bio-Rad Laboratories, Segrate, Italy) using the iScriptTM one-step RT-PCR kit for probes (Bio-Rad Laboratories, Segrate, Italy). Samples were run in 384 well formats in triplicate as multiplexed reactions with a normalizing internal control (β-actin). Primers sequences (Table 1) used were purchased from Eurofins MWG-Operon.

Table 1. Sequences of forward and reverse primers and probes used in real-time PCR analyses and purchased from Eurofins MWG-Operon.

Gene	Forward Primer	Reverse Primer	Probe
BDNF tot	AAGTCTGCATTACATTCCTCGA	GTTTTCTGAAAGAGGGACAGTTTAT	TGTGGTTTGTTGCCGTTGCCAAG
NR1	TCATCTCTAGCCAGGTCTACG	CAGAGTAGATGGACATTCGGG	TGGGAGTGAAGTGGTCGTTGGG
NR2A	GCACCAGTACATGACCAGATTC	ACCAGTTTACAGCCTTCATCC	CGTCCAACTTCCCGGTTTTCAAGC
c-Fos	TCCTTACGGACTCCCCAC	CTCCGTTTCTCTTCCTCTTCAG	TGCTCTACTTTGCCCCTTCTGCC
β-actin	CACTTTCTACAATGAGCTGCG	CTGGATGGCTACGTACATGG	TCTGGGTCATCTTTTCACGGTTGGC

Thermal cycling was initiated with an incubation at 50 °C for 10 min (RNA retrotranscription) and then at 95 °C for 5 min (TaqMan polymerase activation). After this initial step, 39 cycles of PCR were performed. Each PCR cycle consisted of heating the samples at 95 °C for 10 s to enable the melting process and then for 30 s at 60 °C for the annealing and extension reactions. A comparative cycle threshold method was used to calculate the relative target gene expression [54]

2.8. Statistics

All statistical analyses were performed using SPSS Statistics version 24.0 (SPSS Inc., IBM, Armonk, NY, USA). Data are presented as mean ± standard error of the mean (SEM). Behavioral data were analyzed using a repeated measures analysis of variance (ANOVA), whereas the immunohistochemical and gene expression were analyzed using a 2-way ANOVA, with genotype and age (preadolescent, adolescent, adult) as between-subject factors. Statistical testing on the latter was performed on obtained deltaCT values, whereas data are plotted as fold-change expression levels relative to the preadolescent 5-HTT$^{+/+}$ group. For Pearson correlation analyses between freezing and neural measures, we averaged freezing rates observed during all cue presentations to a single measure. Probability *p*-values of less than 0.05 were considered significant. Bonferroni correction was applied to correct for multiple testing in post hoc tests.

3. Results

3.1. Freezing Behavior

Baseline freezing. To measure baseline freezing, we assessed freezing during the 2-minute stimulus free period preceding the first extinction session. Freezing in response to the novel context was significantly affected by age ($F_{(2,319)} = 41.016$, $p < 0.001$), but not genotype ($F_{(2,319)} = 1.745$, $p = 0.176$), and no significant genotype × age interaction was found ($F_{(4,319)} < 1$) (Figure 1). Bonferroni post hoc analysis revealed that adolescent animals froze more upon novel context exposure than adult animals ($p < 0.001$), while preadolescent animals froze more than adolescent and adult animals (both $p < 0.001$).

Fear extinction learning. In the extinction learning session, freezing during the cue presentations reduced over blocks ($F_{(5,324)} = 145.945$, $p < 0.001$), and this reduction (i.e. The speed of extinction learning) was dependent on both age (block × age interaction; $F_{(10,650)} = 3.607$, $p < 0.001$) and genotype (block × genotype interaction; $F_{(20,650)} = 3.458$, $p < 0.001$), but not on a genotype × age interaction ($F_{(20,1308)} < 1$) (Figure 1). Exploration of the genotype effect through post hoc tests revealed that 5-HTT$^{-/-}$ rats showed slower extinction learning than both 5-HTT$^{+/-}$ and 5-HTT$^{+/+}$ rats (both $p < 0.001$), whereas 5-HTT$^{+/-}$ and 5-HTT$^{+/+}$ animals showed similar extinction rates ($p = 0.653$). Exploration of the age effect revealed significant differences in extinction learning curves between all three ages, which seemed to be driven by slower extinction in pre-adolescent compared to adolescent rats ($p = 0.006$) and lower initial freezing (in block 1) of adult rats compared to preadolescent rats ($p = 0.008$). There were no age effects within the genotypes ($p > 0.1$).

First fear extinction recall. Total freezing during the first extinction recall session was used as a behavioral indicator of the recall of the extinction memory acquired during the first fear extinction learning session. We observed a main effect of genotype ($F_{(2,144)} = 4.051$, $p = 0.019$), a trend-level significant main effect of age ($F_{(2,144)} = 2.910$, $p = 0.058$) and a genotype $\times$ age interaction for this parameter ($F_{(4,144)} = 2.747$, $p = 0.031$) (Figure 1). The latter appeared to be driven by a significant effect of genotype in the preadolescent ($F_{(2,46)} = 6.016$, $p = 0.005$), but not the adolescent ($F_{(2,52)} = 1.401$, $p = 0.255$) and adult animals ($F_{(2,46)} = 2.254$, $p = 0.116$). The genotype effect in the preadolescent group was driven by 5-HTT$^{-/-}$ rats, which froze significantly more than 5-HTT$^{+/-}$ ($p = 0.012$) and 5-HTT$^{+/+}$ ($p = 0.007$) animals, while freezing was not different between 5-HTT$^{+/-}$ and 5-HTT$^{+/+}$ animals ($p = 1.000$). When comparing age effects in genotype groups we observed that fear extinction recall was significantly affected by age in 5-HTT$^{-/-}$ rats ($F_{(2,35)} = 60.527$, $p = 0.004$), but not 5-HTT$^{+/+}$ ($F_{(2,35)} < 1$) and 5-HTT$^{+/-}$ ($F_{(2,74)} < 1$ rats. The age effect in 5-HTT$^{-/-}$ rats was attributed to improved recall during adolescence compared to preadolescence ($p = 0.004$) and adulthood ($p = 0.049$), in the absence of a difference between the latter two groups ($p = 0.471$).

Second fear extinction recall. We found a main effect of genotype ($F_{(2,142)} = 8.601$, $p < 0.001$), age ($F_{(2,142)} = 10.756$, $p < 0.001$), and genotype $\times$ age interaction ($F_{(4,142)} = 2.921$, $p = 0.023$) in freezing behavior during the second extinction recall session (Figure 1). Here, we found a significant effect of genotype in the preadolescent ($F_{(2,44)} = 7.334$, $p = 0.002$) and the adult group ($F_{(2,46)} = 6.115$, $p = 0.004$), but again not in the adolescent animals ($F_{(2,52)} < 1$). 5-HTT$^{-/-}$ rats froze more than 5-HTT$^{+/-}$ and 5-HTT$^{+/+}$ animals in both the preadolescent ($p = 0.001$ and $p = 0.016$, respectively) and the adult ($p = 0.005$ and $p = 0.057$ respectively) age groups, while freezing between 5-HTT$^{+/-}$ and wildtype animals was not different in either age group (both p-values = 1.000). When comparing age effects in genotype groups, we observed that fear extinction recall was significantly affected by age in 5-HTT$^{-/-}$ rats ($F_{(2,35)} = 75.819$, $p = 0.002$), but not 5-HTT$^{+/+}$ rats ($F_{(2,35)} = 1.286$, $p = 0.289$). In 5-HTT$^{-/-}$ rats, reduced freezing was observed during adolescence as compared to preadolescence ($p = 0.002$), but not adulthood ($p = 0.125$), whereas freezing at these latter two ages did not differ significantly ($p = 0.125$). In 5-HTT$^{+/-}$ rats, a significant effect of age was found ($F_{(2,72)} = 20.583$, $p = 0.037$), caused by improved fear extinction with age (resulting in a significant difference in freezing during recall in preadolescence vs. adulthood ($p = 0.036$), whereas the other comparisons were non-significant (all p-values > 0.27)). As all significant genotype effects were driven by aberrant behavior of the 5-HTT$^{-/-}$ rats, further neural analyses focused on the comparison of these genotypes with their 5-HTT$^{+/+}$ counterparts.

In Figure S1, the freezing per genotype across the three ages is depicted, and Figure S2 depicts the freezing across blocks during the recall sessions.

3.2. GAD65/67 Immunoreactivity

Infralimbic cortex. The number of GAD65/67 immunopositive granules in the IL was significantly affected by genotype ($F_{(1,24)} = 14.326$, $p = 0.001$), but not age ($F_{(2,24)} = 2.110$, $p = 0.143$), and no genotype $\times$ age interaction could be detected ($F_{(2,24)} = 1.222$, $p = 0.312$, Figure 2). The number of granules expressing GAD65/67 was significantly reduced in 5-HTT$^{-/-}$ animals compared to 5-HTT$^{+/+}$ animals ($p = 0.001$). Although the effect of genotype did not significantly differ between age groups, post hoc testing revealed the most prominent effects of genotype in preadolescent rats ($p < 0.001$), whereas adolescent and adult rats did not display significant differences between genotypes (p-values > 0.3).

Basolateral amygdala. No effects of genotype ($F_{(1,24)} < 1$) or age ($F_{(1,24)} < 1$), nor a genotype $\times$ age interaction ($F_{(2,24)} = 1.583$, $p = 0.226$), were found in the number of GAD65/67 immuno-positive granules in the BLA (Figure 2).

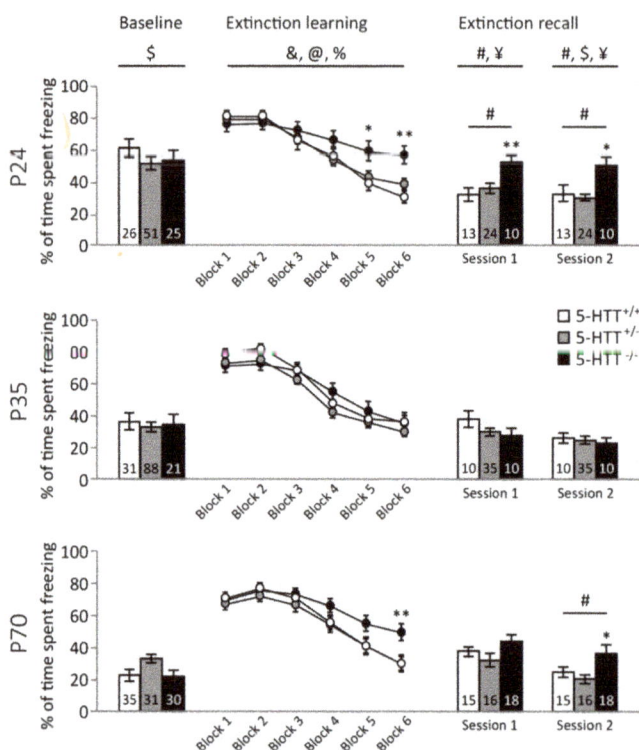

Figure 1. Fear conditioning behavioral data across extinction learning and the two extinction recall sessions. Freezing during the 2-minute stimulus free baseline period preceding extinction learning decreased across age in all genotypes. Fear extinction learning is impaired in preadolescent 5-HTT$^{-/-}$ rats, normalized in this genotype during adolescence, and impaired again in adulthood. Fear extinction recall is impaired in preadolescent 5-HTT$^{-/-}$ rats, normalized in this genotype during adolescence, and impaired again in adulthood. Data are expressed as the mean % of time spent freezing during stimulus presentations ± standard error of the mean. #: a significant effect of genotype ($p < 0.05$); $: a significant effect of age ($p < 0.05$); ¥: a significant age × genotype interaction ($p < 0.05$); *: a significant post hoc difference between 5-HTT$^{-/-}$ vs. 5-HTT$^{+/-}$ and/or 5-HTT$^{+/+}$ rats ($p < 0.05$); **: a significant post hoc difference between 5-HTT$^{-/-}$ vs. 5-HTT$^{+/-}$ and/or 5-HTT$^{+/+}$ rats ($p < 0.05$); &: a significant effect of extinction block ($p < 0.05$); @ a significant age × block interaction ($p < 0.05$); % a significant genotype × block interaction ($p < 0.05$).

3.3. Gene Expression Levels Neuronal Plasticity and Activity Genes

Basal expression. mPFC. In the mPFC of naive control animals (Figure 3, upper panel), c-Fos expression was affected by genotype ($F_{(1,32)} = 16.321$, $p < 0.001$) and age ($F_{(2,32)} = 3.502$, $p = 0.042$), but not by a genotype × age interaction ($F_{(2,32)} = 1.828$, $p = 0.177$). These effects appeared to be driven by significantly lower c-Fos expression levels in 5-HTT$^{-/-}$ compared to 5-HTT$^{+/+}$ rats ($p < 0.001$), whereas adolescent animals tended to display increased expression compared to pre-adolescent ($p = 0.036$), but not adult ($p = 0.236$) rats. BDNF expression was also dependent on genotype ($F_{(1,33)} = 29.072$, $p < 0.001$) and age ($F_{(2,33)} = 27.108$, $p < 0.001$), without displaying a genotype × age interaction ($F_{(2,33)} < 1$). Additionally, BDNF levels were significantly lower in 5-HTT$^{-/-}$ compared to 5-HTT$^{+/+}$ rats ($p < 0.001$), whereas adolescent rats displayed the highest expression (both *p*-values < 0.001), whereas adult rats displayed higher levels than preadolescent rats ($p = 0.007$). NR1 levels only depended on the age of the rat ($F_{(2,33)} = 71.644$, $p < 0.001$), with again the adolescent rats displaying the highest expression (both *p*-values < 0.001), and adult rats displaying higher levels than preadolescent rats ($p = 0.020$). NR2A levels were characterized by a main effect of age ($F_{(2,32)} = 113.835$, $p < 0.001$) and a genotype × age interaction ($F_{(2,32)} = 8.020$, $p = 0.002$). Similarly to NR1 and BDNF, NR2A expression levels were highest in adolescence (both *p*-values < 0.001), and adult rats showed higher NR2A expression than pre-adolescent rats ($p = 0.001$). Moreover, in adolescence, 5-HTT$^{-/-}$ rats displayed significantly higher NR2A expression levels compared to 5-HTT$^{+/+}$ rats ($p < 0.001$), whereas no differences between genotypes were observed at preadolescence ($p = 0.165$) and adulthood ($p = 0.666$).

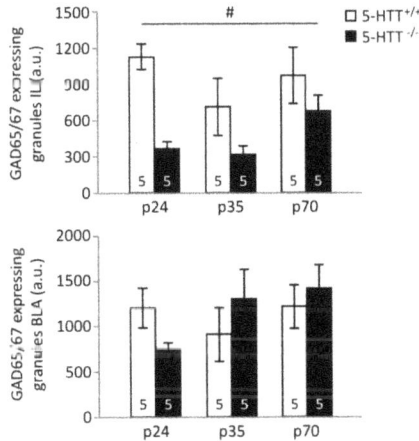

Figure 2. GAD65/67 immunoreactivity in the infralimbic cortex (IL) and basolateral amygdala (BLA) of preadolescent (p24), adolescent (p35), and adult (p70) 5-HTT$^{-/-}$ and 5-HTT$^{+/+}$ rats. GAD 65/67 immunoreactivity is significantly reduced in preadolescent, adolescent, and adult 5-HTT$^{-/-}$ animals in the IL, but not BLA. #: a significant effect of genotype ($p < 0.05$).

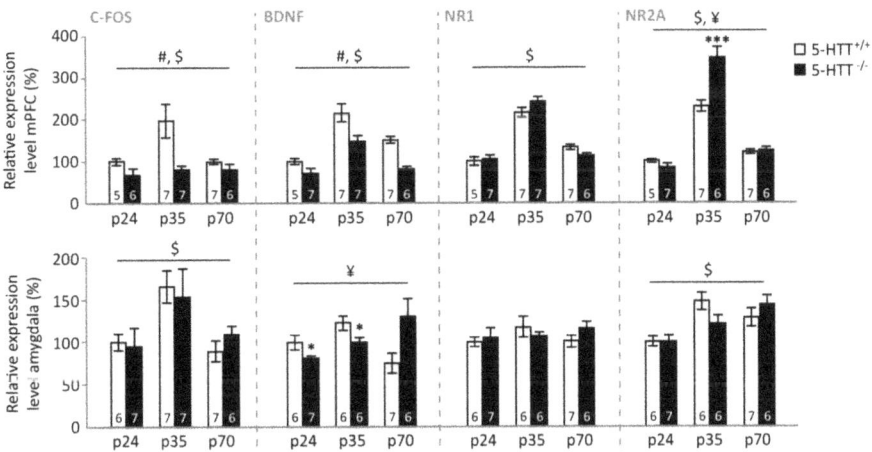

Figure 3. Relative expression levels of c-Fos, BDNF, NR1, and NR2A in the medial prefrontal cortex (mPFC) and amygdala of naive preadolescent (p24), adolescent (p35), and adult (p70) 5-HTT$^{-/-}$ and 5-HTT$^{+/+}$ rats. #: a significant effect of genotype ($p < 0.05$); $: a significant effect of age ($p < 0.05$); ¥: a significant age × genotype interaction ($p < 0.05$); *: a significant post hoc difference between 5-HTT$^{-/-}$ vs. age-matched 5-HTT$^{+/+}$ rats (* $p < 0.05$; *** $p < 0.001$).

Amygdala. In the amygdala (Figure 3, lower panel), c-Fos expression was modulated by age ($F_{(2,34)} = 7.090$, $p = 0.003$), but not genotype ($F_{(1,34)} < 1$) nor a genotype × age interaction ($F_{(2,34)} = 1.171$, $p = 0.322$). This age effect was driven by a significantly higher expression in adolescent compared to preadolescent ($p = 0.005$) and adult rats ($p = 0.011$), whereas no differences between these latter age groups were found ($p = 1.000$). BDNF expression in the amygdala was modulated by a genotype × age interaction ($F_{(2,32)} = 6.067$, $p = 0.006$), but no main effects (both p-values > 0.2). Further testing suggested that this interaction was driven by lower amygdala BDNF expression in pre-adolescent and adolescent 5-HTT$^{-/-}$ rats compared to WTs ($p = 0.041$ and $p = 0.046$ respectively), whereas adult 5-HTT$^{-/-}$ rats tended to display increased amygdala BDNF expression ($p = 0.069$). Amygdala NR1 expression was not modulated by genotype, age (both F-values < 1), or a genotype × age interaction ($F_{(2,32)} = 1.059$, $p = 0.359$), whereas NR2A expression was different for the distinct age groups ($F_{(2,32)} = 11.156$, $p < 0.001$), without a significant effect of genotype ($F_{(1,32)} < 1$) or genotype × age interaction ($F_{(2,32)} = 2.371$. $p = 0.110$). Further testing revealed that pre-adolescent rats displayed lower amygdala NR2A expression compared to adolescent and adult rats (both p-values = 0.001), whereas the latter two age groups were not different ($p = 1.000$).

3.4. Gene Expression following Fear Extinction Learning

mPFC. Levels of c-Fos expression in the mPFC following extinction learning (Figure 4, upper panel) were dependent on the rats' age ($F_{(2,36)} = 6.182$, $p = 0.005$), but not on genotype ($F_{(1,36)} = 1.032$, $p = 0.317$) or on the genotype × age interaction ($F_{(2,36)} < 1$). Preadolescent rats showed lower c-Fos expression than adolescent ($p = 0.014$) and adult ($p = 0.002$) animals, whereas adolescent and adult animals displayed similar levels ($p = 0.850$). mPFC BDNF expression following extinction was also dependent on age ($F_{(2,39)} = 7.507$, $p = 0.002$) and showed a trend towards an effect of genotype ($F_{(1,39)} = 3.107$, $p = 0.086$), without displaying a genotype × age interaction ($F_{(2,39)} = 1.185$, $p = 0.316$). Similar to naïve animals, BDNF levels were highest in adolescent rats ($p < 0.001$ and $p = 0.003$ compared to preadolescent and adult rats, respectively), whereas no differences were observed between adult and preadolescent rats ($p = 0.502$). Adolescent 5-HTT$^{-/-}$ rats showed lower mPFC BDNF expression than 5-HTT$^{+/+}$ rats ($p = 0.014$), while no significant differences were observed at the other ages (both p-values > 0.5). NR1 levels only depended on the age of the rat ($F_{(2,40)} = 30.131$, $p < 0.001$), with again the adolescent rats displaying the highest expression (both p-values < 0.001), and levels in preadolescent and adult rats not differing ($p = 0.206$). Similarly, mPFC NR2A expression following extinction was characterized by a main effect of age ($F_{(2,39)} = 36.840$, $p < 0.001$), but no effect of genotype or genotype × age interaction (both F-values < 1). Again, expression levels were highest in adolescence (both p-values < 0.001), and adult rats showed higher NR2A expression than pre-adolescent rats ($p = 0.031$). No correlations were observed between basal or cue-induced freezing and mPFC expression levels.

Amygdala. In the amygdala (Figure 4, lower panel), c-Fos expression following extinction learning was modulated by age ($F_{(2,40)} = 5.918$, $p = 0.006$) and a genotype × age interaction ($F_{(2,40)} = 3.870$, $p = 0.029$), whereas the main effect of genotype did not reach significance ($F_{(1,40)} = 3.092$, $p = 0.086$). This age effect was driven by a higher expression in the adolescent compared to preadolescent amygdala ($p = 0.017$), whereas neither age group significantly differed from adults ($p = 0.547$ and $p = 0.379$ respectively). The interaction was driven by a significant genotype effect in preadolescent rats, with WTs showing lower expression ($p = 0.047$), whereas no differences were observed at the other ages (both p-values > 0.22). Amygdala BDNF expression was also dependent on age ($F_{(2,37)} = 5.158$, $p = 0.011$), without the effect of genotype nor the interaction (both F-values < 1). BDNF levels were higher in the adult compared to the preadolescent ($p = 0.053$) and adolescent ($p = 0.006$) amygdala, whereas the latter were not different from each other ($p = 1.000$). Similarly, amygdala NR1 expression following extinction depended on age ($F_{(2,40)} = 4.992$, $p = 0.012$), but not genotype or a genotype × age interaction (both F-values < 1), with adult rats displaying the same expression levels as the preadolescent rats ($p = 0.149$) but higher levels compared to adolescent rats ($p = 0.007$). These groups did not differ from each other ($p = 0.927$)). Amygdala NR2A expression was not affected by age, genotype, or their interaction (all F-values < 1).

Correlational analyses across all ages and genotypes related both amygdala BDNF and NR1 levels to basal anxiety, with lower expression levels following testing being related to higher freezing during the habituation period (BDNF: $r(43) = 0.307$, $p = 0.045$; NR1: $r(46) = 0.310$, $p = 0.036$) (Figure S3). Moreover, amygdala BDNF was negatively related to cue-induced freezing during the extinction session ($r(43) = 0.440$, $p = 0.003$) (Figure S3).

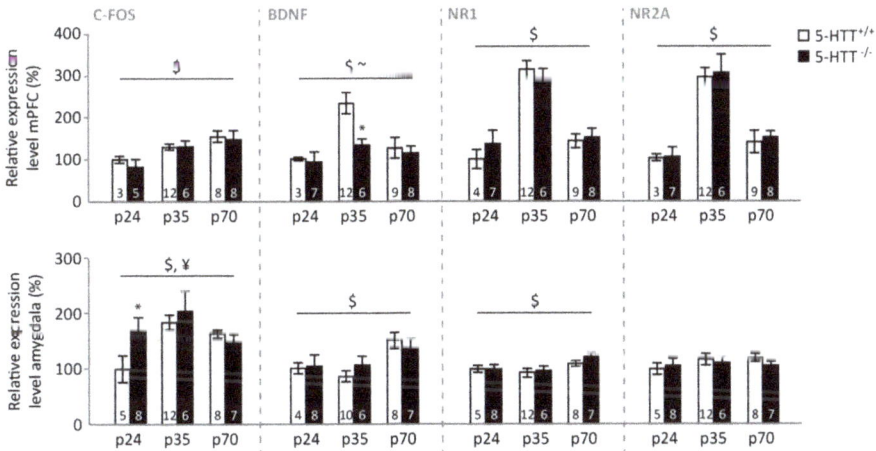

Figure 4. Relative expression levels of c-Fos, BDNF, NR1, and NR2A in the medial prefrontal cortex (mPFC) and amygdala of 5-HTT$^{-/-}$ and 5-HTT$^{+/+}$ rats following fear extinction learning during preadolescence (p24), adolescence (p35), and adulthood (p70). #: a significant effect of genotype ($p < 0.05$); ~: a trend-level significant effect of genotype ($p = 0.086$); \$: a significant effect of age ($p < 0.05$); ¥: a significant age × genotype interaction ($p < 0.05$); *: a significant post hoc difference between 5-HTT$^{-/-}$ vs. age-matched 5-HTT$^{+/+}$ rats ($p < 0.05$).

3.5. Gene Expression following Fear Extinction Recall

mPFC. Following the last fear extinction recall session, expression levels of c-Fos in the mPFC (Figure 5, upper panel) were modulated by the rats' age ($F_{(2,25)} = 4.993$, $p = 0.015$), genotype ($F_{(1,25)} = 13.612$, $p = 0.001$), and a genotype × age interaction ($F_{(2,25)} = 4.046$, $p = 0.030$). Further testing revealed that WT rats showed highest expression levels in adolescence ($p < 0.001$ and $p = 0.001$ compared to preadolescent and adult animals, respectively) and higher levels in adult compared to preadolescent rats ($p = 0.043$). No such effect of age was observed in 5-HTT$^{-/-}$ rats (all p-values = 1.000), resulting in significantly higher mPFC c-Fos expression in WT compared to 5-HTT$^{-/-}$ rats during adolescence ($p = 0.013$), but not preadolescence ($p = 0.778$) or adulthood ($p = 0.075$). mPFC BDNF expression following extinction recall was modulated by a genotype × age interaction ($F_{(2,28)} = 5.397$, $p = 0.010$), without the main effects of age (F < 1) or genotype ($F_{(1,28)} - 1.084$, $p = 0.307$). This interaction was caused by a significant effect of age in 5-HTT$^{+/+}$ rats ($F_{(2,13)} = 6.174$, $p = 0.013$) that was absent in 5-HTT$^{-/-}$ rats ($F_{(2,15)} = 1.672$, $p = 0.221$), resulting in a significant effect of genotype only at adult age ($p = 0.005$, other p-values > 0.2), with 5-HTT$^{+/+}$ rats displaying lower BDNF expression. Additionally, mPFC NR1 levels following extinction recall were modulated in a genotype × age manner ($F_{(2,28)} = 4.034$, $p = 0.029$), without main effects of age or genotype (both F-values < 1). Preadolescents ($p = 0.960$) of both genotypes showed similar NR1 expression. Adolescent 5-HTT$^{-/-}$ rats were characterized by lower NR1 expression compared to their 5-HTT$^{+/+}$ counterparts ($p = 0.048$), whereas adult 5-HTT$^{-/-}$ rats tended to show higher expression ($p = 0.081$). NR2A expression levels were characterized by a genotype × age interaction as well ($F_{(2,28)} = 4.080$, $p = 0.028$), without significant effects of age ($F < 1$) or genotype ($F_{(1,28)} = 1.920$, $p = 0.177$). Post hoc testing only revealed a significant effect of genotype during adulthood, when mPFC NR2A expression in response to extinction recall was significantly increased in 5-HTT$^{-/-}$ compared to 5-HTT$^{+/+}$ rats ($p = 0.034$). No significant differences were found during preadolescence and adolescence between 5-HTT$^{-/-}$ compared to WT rats ($p = 0.106$ and $p = 0.137$, respectively).

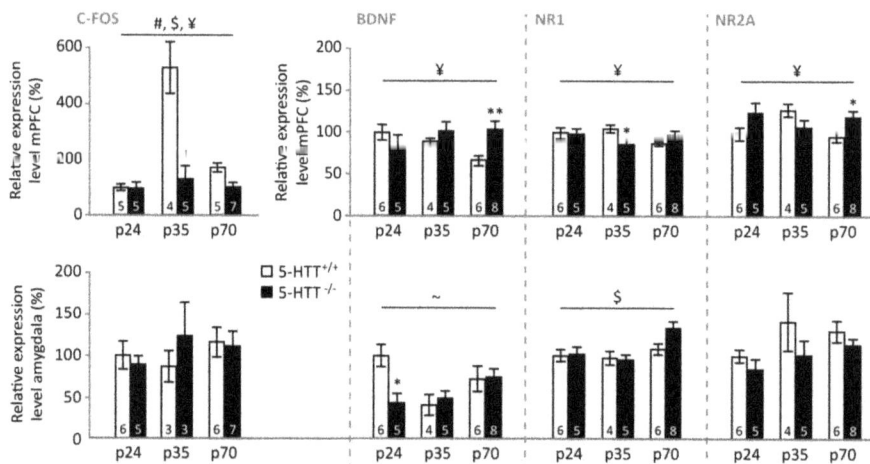

Figure 5. Relative expression levels of c-Fos, BDNF, NR1, and NR2A in the medial prefrontal cortex (mPFC) and amygdala of 5-HTT$^{-/-}$ and 5-HTT$^{+/+}$ rats following the second session of fear extinction recall during preadolescence (p24), adolescence (p35), and adulthood (p70). #: a significant effect of genotype ($p < 0.05$); $: a significant effect of age ($p < 0.05$); ¥: a significant age × genotype interaction ($p < 0.05$); ~: a trend-level significant age × genotype interaction ($p = 0.054$); *: a significant post hoc difference between 5-HTT$^{-/-}$ vs. age-matched 5-HTT$^{+/+}$ rats (* $p < 0.05$; ** $p < 0.01$).

Correlational analyses across all ages and genotypes revealed that mPFC c-Fos expression was significantly related to the amount of cue-induced freezing during this last extinction recall session ($r(31) = 0.366$, $p = 0.043$), with reduced c-Fos levels relating to increased freezing, reflecting impaired extinction recall (Figure S3).

Amygdala. In the amygdala (Figure 5, lower panel), c-Fos expression following extinction recall was not modulated by age, genotype, or a genotype × age interaction (all F-values < 1). Amygdala BDNF expression revealed a trend towards an age × genotype interaction ($F_{(2,28)} = 3.242$, $p = 0.054$), without a main effect of genotype ($F_{(1,28)} = 1.111$, $p = 0.301$) or age ($F_{(2,28)} = 2.450$, $p = 0.105$). Exploratory post hoc tests revealed a significant reduction in amygdala BDNF expression during preadolescence in 5-HTT$^{-/-}$ compared to 5-HTT$^{+/+}$ rats ($p = 0.017$) that was not observed at other ages (p-values > 0.6). Amygdala NR1 expression following extinction recall only revealed a significant effect of age ($F_{(2,28)} = 5.178$, $p = 0.012$), but not of genotype ($F_{(1,28)} = 1.106$, $p = 0.302$) or of their interaction ($F_{(2,28)} = 1.403$, $p = 0.262$), with adult rats displaying higher expression levels compared to preadolescent ($p = 0.035$) and adolescent rats ($p = 0.015$), whereas these latter groups did not differ from each other ($p = 1.000$). Amygdala NR2A expression only revealed trends for a reduced expression in 5-HTT$^{-/-}$ rats across ages ($F_{(1,28)} = 3.871$, $p = 0.056$) and an increase with age ($F_{(2,28)} = 2.662$, $p = 0.087$), without interaction ($F < 1$). No significant correlations between amygdala gene expression levels and freezing during extinction recall were observed.

4. Discussion

Here, we confirm that fear extinction recall is impaired in 5-HTT$^{-/-}$ rats, an established and often replicated phenomenon [44,45,55,56], as is extinction learning in rats of this genotype [46]. Strikingly, an effect of age on fear extinction recall was seen only in 5-HTT$^{-/-}$ rats, which enjoyed a transient normalization (i.e. improvement) of fear extinction recall during adolescence. Whereas augmented fear extinction learning seems to be responsible for the improved fear extinction recall observed in 5-HTT$^{-/-}$ rats during adolescence, age × genotype effects on learning rates failed to reach significance. The number of GAD65/67 positive synaptic contacts, indicative of inhibitory regulation, was decreased in the IL of 5-HTT$^{-/-}$ rats, regardless of age, and no clear effect of age or genotype were seen on the number of GAD65/67 positive synaptic contacts in the BLA. In naïve rats, we observed increases in BDNF, NR1, and NR2A expression levels in the mPFC, and in c-Fos in the mPFC and amygdala, during adolescence. Furthermore, BDNF levels were reduced in 5-HTT$^{-/-}$ rats across all ages. While no genotype × age interactions were observed following fear extinction learning, fear extinction recall was associated with a genotype × age interaction for NR1, NR2A, and c-Fos in the mPFC. These data suggest that specifically (glutamatergic) plasticity changes in the mPFC contribute to the temporary normalization of fear extinction recall in 5-HTT$^{-/-}$ rats during adolescence.

A number of developmental abnormalities arising from 5-HTT abolishment have been described in the literature. The development of several motor and sensory functions, namely reflexes, motor coordination and olfactory discrimination, is delayed in 5-HTT$^{-/-}$ rats but normalized upon reaching adulthood [57]. Remarkably, other deficiencies seen in adult 5-HTT$^{-/-}$ animals, i.e. impaired object recognition, object directed behavior, and sensorimotor gating, do not arise until after adolescence [57]. The present results suggest that the abnormal emotional profile seen in 5-HTT$^{-/-}$ rats is subject to a nonlinear developmental trajectory as well, implying that 5-HTT abolishment influences neural maturation depending on the developmental phase and locus. The finding of the transiently alleviated recall of fear extinction during adolescence in 5-HTT$^{-/-}$ rats suggests that the pacing of development of cortical and subcortical regions may be altered in these rats. Congruent with our findings, a study in 5-HTT$^{-/-}$ mice has demonstrated that increased anxiety, another hallmark trait of the 5-HTT$^{-/-}$ rodent phenotype, is not present during adolescence [58].

This study does not replicate findings from other studies that suggest fear extinction recall deficits in adolescent animals and humans with normal 5-HTT expression [12,13], as our results indicate that, in 5-HTT$^{+/+}$ animals, fear extinction recall is not significantly affected by age. We corroborate findings of another study, in which extinction learning was found to be similar between adolescent and adult C57BL/6J mice [59]. Differences in the details of the experimental procedures may crucially determine whether an effect of age presents itself. For instance, the experiments may differ in the degree to which contextual cues from the conditioning session are present during the extinction, which determines the additional involvement of the hippocampus on fear expression and extinction [60]. This variability in the reported findings necessitates additional investigation towards the exact circumstances under which adolescent fear extinction (recall) is impaired.

The inhibitory immunoreactivity in the IL as assessed by immunohistochemistry is reduced in 5-HTT$^{-/-}$ rats across all age groups. This finding is in line with previous observations of reduced inhibitory synapses onto cortical excitatory neurons in preadolescent 5-HTT$^{-/-}$ rats [47]. Previous work has, however, associated *increased* inhibitory synaptic transmission onto IL projection neurons with impaired retrieval of extinction memory by inhibiting the consolidation of extinction [61], which contrasts our observation of reduced inhibition in the genotype group with poorest extinction recall. Yet, here we did not determine the class of neurons targeted by these inhibitory contacts, leaving the possibility of reduced inhibition of local interneurons in 5-HTT$^{-/-}$ rats open. In any case, the observed reduction in inhibitory synapses appears to remain stable across the development from preadolescence to adulthood, making it unlikely that altered development of prefrontal inhibition contributing to the remarkable development of fear extinction behavior seen in these animals.

Under basal conditions, in naive rats, c-Fos, BDNF, NR1, and NR2A gene expression levels in the mPFC were highest during adolescence, indicating that adolescence is indeed a critical period of mPFC development. For NR2A, we additionally observed that levels were highest during adolescence in 5-HTT$^{-/-}$ rats. The peak in NMDA receptor expression may relate to pruning (removal of synapses), known to occur during adolescence and to be NMDA-receptor-dependent [62]. Increased c-Fos expression levels in the PFC during adolescence may reflect a compensatory attempt of the mPFC to retain control over the amygdala, while the lower c-Fos expression levels in 5-HTT$^{-/-}$ rats across ages may correspond to the reduced prefrontal cortical top-down control over the amygdala as reported for human 5-HTTLPR s-allele carriers [34]. The peak in BDNF levels during adolescence is in line with previous observations [30]. We also replicated previous observations of reduced BDNF expression in the PFC of 5-HTT$^{-/-}$ regardless of age [48,63,64]. In the amygdala, c-Fos levels were found to peak during adolescence, which potentially reflects the increased activity of this area due to reduced prefrontal top-down control [4]. However, c-Fos remained high during adulthood, which might reflect the completion of amygdala maturation during adolescence. Amygdala BDNF levels were reduced in 5-HTT$^{-/-}$ rats during preadolescence and adolescence, in line with the overall decreased BDNF levels in these rats found previously [48,63,64], but BDNF levels tended to be increased in 5-HTT$^{-/-}$ rats during adulthood. For NR1, no genotype and age effects were observed, and for NR2A there was a decrease in expression in preadolescent rats. These data show that the mPFC and amygdala mature at different paces and through different plasticity routes.

BDNF, NR1, and NR2A expression levels in the mPFC after fear extinction learning largely recapitulated the baseline findings in naive rats, suggesting that extinction learning does not change the expression of these plasticity factors. During the recall test, however, we observed that (over all animals and ages combined) c-Fos expression in the mPFC was negatively correlated with cue-induced freezing. This implies that impaired extinction recall is associated with reduced prefrontal cortex activity and thereby cognitive control over the emotional response. This finding is in line with the study of Patwell et al. [12] reporting a link between impaired extinction recall and reduced c-Fos expression in the IL in adolescent animals. Nonetheless, the increased mPFC c-Fos expression in 5-HTT$^{+/+}$ adolescents is quite remarkable. It is important to note that we combined IL and PrL tissue for gene expression analyses, raising the possibility that the increase in c-Fos expression in adolescent 5-HTT$^{+/+}$ rats is due to increased c-Fos expression in the PrL. The function of this is open to speculation. As this observation does not result in lower freezing levels in adolescent 5-HTT$^{-/-}$ rats, other neuroplasticity changes in the mPFC or amygdala might counteract this effect. BDNF and NR2A were increased in adult 5-HTT$^{-/-}$ rats specifically, which thereby seem to be unrelated to the temporary improvement in fear extinction in adolescent 5-HTT$^{-/-}$ rats. We furthermore observed that adolescent 5-HTT$^{-/-}$ rats display lower levels of NR1 in the mPFC. The essential NR1 subunit of the NMDA receptor expressed in excitatory prefrontal cortical neurons has been shown to decrease fear generalization [65]. If NMDAR-dependent neural signaling in the mPFC is a component of a neural mechanism for disambiguating the meaning of fear signals, our finding may point towards a temporary improvement in the interpretation of the fear-predicting cue during adolescence in 5-HTT$^{-/-}$ rats, allowing the animals to discriminate the fear and safety better. We did not explicitly assess fear generalization in this study, but the measure that comes closest is baseline freezing observed prior to the tone presentations in the extinction recall sessions. Interestingly, baseline freezing prior to extinction recall was modulated by genotype, with 5-HTT$^{-/-}$ rats displaying higher freezing than the other groups (Figure S2). Thus, 5-HTT$^{-/-}$ rats showed higher baseline freezing levels as well as reduced mPFC NR1 expression in adulthood. However, these measures did not significantly correlate ($p > 0.15$), leaving our interpretation still speculative. In the amygdala, c-Fos expression tended to peak in adolescence independently of genotype, which thereby follows the pattern observed in the mPFC. None of the other genes assessed displayed an expression pattern that followed the age- and genotype-dependent changes in freezing during extinction learning. This implies that the amygdala does not play a key role in the temporary disappearance of genotype effects on freezing during extinction learning in adolescence. We did observe that BDNF and NR1 expression significantly correlated with baseline freezing behavior. Specifically, lower expression of both NR1 and BDNF in the amygdala was associated with more freezing during the habituation period. Furthermore, amygdala BDNF was negatively related to cue-induced freezing during the extinction session. Amygdala BDNF has been demonstrated to facilitate fear learning [66], which appears incongruent with our observation. Potentially, lower BDNF levels in the amygdala mediated unconditioned fear in this study. Overall, our data suggest that the temporary normalization of fear extinction recall in 5-HTT$^{-/-}$ rats during adolescence relates to neuroplasticity changes in the mPFC, whereas the amygdala seems to exert more generalized (genotype-independent) effects on the freezing response.

Some limitations of the study require attention. The quantified granules in the IL are hypothesized to represent synaptic contacts. However, without performing a functional tracer study, it is not possible to determine the source of the GABAergic inputs. In addition, it is not certain that these synaptic terminals interface with neurons that are functional within the circuitry driving fear expression and extinction. In addition, animals that had undergone one and three days of fear extinction were pooled to determine GAD65/67 immunoreactivity in the IL and BLA to obtain sufficient statistical power for a comparison. Since GAD65/67 expression is influenced by recent fear conditioning, it is possible that levels of expression were affected by this variation in time between conditioning and sacrifice of the animal. However, all GAD65/67 positive synaptic contacts were included in the assessment regardless of expression level; given the high signal to the background ratio of the DAB-Ni, variations in expression due to the varying regimes of fear conditioning is unlikely to have affected the findings. Furthermore, because CT values were too different between the obtained from the naïve, extinction learning, and extinction recall group, we did not express the gene expression changes after extinction as the percentage of baseline gene expression in the naïve animals. For RT-PCR, we punched the whole mPFC, while we studied the IL part of the mPFC in the immunohistochemical study. This was necessary to obtain a sufficient amount of tissue for the PCRs and to reduce gene expression variance due to variations in the precise positioning of the punch needle. As a consequence, it is possible that differential gene expression in the IL and PrL diluted the effects we observed for the whole mPFC. Another limitation is that we did not measure freezing during conditioning during acquisition. We previously observed no genotype differences during fear conditioning in adults [46]. However, we do not know whether genotype differences are also absent during preadolescence and adulthood. Since freezing during Blocks 1–4 was not different between genotypes during the fear memory recall/extinction session, it is not likely there were genotype differences in freezing during conditioning. As yet another limitation, visual observation of Figure 1 implies that the increased freezing during Session 2 and 3 is due to an extinction learning deficit during Session 1. However, the observed age × genotype effects as observed during the extinction recall sessions seemed to result from altered recall of extinction. Nonetheless, additional differences in extinction learning between genotypes and ages cannot be ruled out. Finally, housing conditions varied between the age groups; although no animals were kept in isolation, preadolescent and adolescent animals were housed with more cage mates than adults for practical and ethical reasons. Although this aspect is often overlooked in animal research concerning stress and psychiatric illness, social elements in housing conditions have been shown to influence emotional behavior [67] and are known to be especially influential and instrumental to psychiatric wellbeing during adolescence [68].

5. Conclusions

In conclusion, the present findings show that the influence of genetic reduction of *5-HTT* expression on the development of fear extinction recall manifests in a non-linear pattern, temporarily normalizing during adolescence, to become deficient again at adulthood. This discovery raises as many questions as it answers; delayed or aberrant maturation of cortical or subcortical regions or interconnecting tracts is a likely cause but exploiting this finding for therapeutic benefit will require further specification of their nature and functional implications. The anatomical and functional development of excitatory neurons in the IL projecting to the amygdala are of particular interest for future study. An in vivo electrophysiology or calcium imaging study in which single neurons or populations of neurons are followed across the different stages from fear conditioning to extinction and extinction recall would be enlightening. As it stands, the data suggest that reduced inhibitory signaling within the IL and temporary altered excitatory signaling in the mPFC represent potential causes for the impaired control over the amygdala seen in individuals with reduced expression of 5-HTT and its temporary normalization during adolescence.

Supplementary Materials: The following are available online at http://www.mdpi.com/2076-3425/9/5/118/s1, Figure S1: Fear conditioning behavioral data across extinction learning and the two extinction recall sessions, sorted on genotype, Figure S2: Fear conditioning behavioral data across extinction learning and the two extinction recall sessions, including baseline, Figure S3: Correlational plots showing associations between brain gene expression levels and behavioral freezing.

Author Contributions: Conceptualization: P.S., J.R.H., and M.J.A.G.H.; methodology: P.S., J.R.H., M.J.A.G.H., and F.C.; validation: P.S., P.B., D.d.L., L.M., D.A., T.R., and M.M.M.V.; formal analysis: P.S. and M.J.A.G.H.; writing—original draft preparation: P.S., M.J.A.G.H., and J.R.H.; writing—review and editing: P.S., M.M.M.V., T.K., M.A.R., F.C., M.J.A.G.H., and J.R.H.; visualization: M.J.A.G.H.; supervision: M.J.A.G.H. and J.R.H.; funding acquisition: M.J.A.G.H. and J.R.H.

Funding: M.J.A.G.H. is the recipient of VENI grant 863.15.008. This work was supported by Era-Net NEURON grant "RESPOND" and VIDI grant 864.10.003 awarded to J.R.H. Funding organizations had no further role in the design of the study or in the collection, analysis, and interpretation of data.

Acknowledgments: We thank Anthonieke Middelman for the breeding and genotyping of the animals, and Jana van Luttikhuizen and Jos Dederen for their assistance with the immunostainings.

Conflicts of Interest: There are no conflicts of interest.

References

1. Somerville, L.H.; Kelley, W.M.; Heatherton, T.F. Self-esteem Modulates Medial Prefrontal Cortical Responses to Evaluative Social Feedback. *Cereb. Cortex* **2010**, *20*, 3005–3013. [CrossRef] [PubMed]
2. Pine, D.S.; Coplan, J.D.; Papp, L.A.; Klein, R.G.; Martinez, J.M.; Kovalenko, P.; Tancer, N.; Moreau, D.; Dummit, E.S.; Shaffer, D.; et al. Ventilatory Physiology of Children and Adolescents With Anxiety Disorders. *Arch. Gen. Psychiatry* **1998**, *55*, 123–129. [CrossRef] [PubMed]
3. Somerville, L.H.; Casey, B. Developmental neurobiology of cognitive control and motivational systems. *Curr. Opin. Neurobiol.* **2010**, *20*, 236–241.
4. Somerville, L.H.; Jones, R.M.; Casey, B.J. A time of change: Behavioral and neural correlates of adolescent sensitivity to appetitive and aversive environmental cues. *Brain Cogn.* **2010**, *72*, 124–133. [CrossRef]
5. Dahl, R.E. Adolescent brain development: A period of vulnerabilities and opportunities. Keynote address. *Ann. N. Y. Acad. Sci.* **2004**, *1021*, 1–22. [CrossRef]
6. Steinberg, L. Cognitive and affective development in adolescence. *Trends Cogn. Sci.* **2005**, *9*, 69–74. [CrossRef]
7. Britton, J.C.; Lissek, S.; Grillon, C.; Norcross, M.A.; Pine, D.S. Development of anxiety: The role of threat appraisal and fear learning. *Depress. Anxiety* **2011**, *28*, 5–17. [CrossRef]
8. Heller, A.S.; Cohen, A.O.; Dreyfuss, M.F.W.; Casey, B.J. Changes in cortico-subcortical and subcortico-subcortical connectivity impact cognitive control to emotional cues across development. *Soc. Cogn. Affect. Neurosci.* **2016**, *11*, 1910–1918. [CrossRef] [PubMed]
9. Hare, T.A.; Tottenham, N.; Galvan, A.; Voss, H.U.; Glover, G.H.; Casey, B. Biological substrates of emotional reactivity and regulation in adolescence during an emotional go-nogo task. *Biol. Psychiatry* **2008**, *63*, 927–934. [CrossRef]
10. Shin, L.M.; Liberzon, I. The neurocircuitry of fear, stress, and anxiety disorders. *Neuropsychopharmacology* **2010**, *35*, 169–191. [CrossRef]
11. Kim-Cohen, J.; Caspi, A.; Moffitt, T.E.; Harrington, H.; Milne, B.J.; Poulton, R. Prior juvenile diagnoses in adults with mental disorder: Developmental follow-back of a prospective-longitudinal cohort. *Arch. Gen. Psychiatry* **2003**, *60*, 709–717. [CrossRef]

12. Pattwell, S.S.; Duhoux, S.; Hartley, C.A.; Johnson, D.C.; Jing, D.; Elliott, M.D.; Ruberry, E.J.; Powers, A.; Mehta, N.; Yang, R.R.; et al. Altered fear learning across development in both mouse and human. *Proc. Natl. Acad. Sci. USA* **2012**, *109*, 16318–16323. [CrossRef] [PubMed]

13. McCallum, J.; Kim, J.H.; Richardson, R. Impaired Extinction Retention in Adolescent Rats: Effects of D-Cycloserine. *Neuropsychopharmacology* **2010**, *35*, 2134–2142. [CrossRef] [PubMed]

14. Baker, K.D.; Bisby, M.A.; Richardson, R. Impaired fear extinction in adolescent rodents: Behavioural and neural analyses. *Neurosci. Biobehav. Rev.* **2016**, *70*, 59–73. [CrossRef]

15. Pattwell, S.S.; Bath, K.G.; Casey, B.J.; Ninan, I.; Lee, F.S. Selective early-acquired fear memories undergo temporary suppression during adolescence. *Proc. Natl. Acad. Sci. USA* **2011**, *108*, 1182–1187. [CrossRef]

16. LeDoux, J.; Cicchetti, P.; Xagoraris, A.; Romanski, L. The lateral amygdaloid nucleus: Sensory interface of the amygdala in fear conditioning. *J. Neurosci.* **1990**, *10*, 1062–1069. [CrossRef]

17. Saffari, R.; Teng, Z.; Zhang, M.; Kravchenko, M.; Hohoff, C.; Ambrée, O.; Zhang, W. NPY^{+-}, but not PV^{+-} GABAergic neurons mediated long-range inhibition from infra- to prelimbic cortex. *Transl. Psychiatry* **2016**, *6*, e736. [CrossRef]

18. Ehrlich, I.; Humeau, Y.; Grenier, F.; Ciocchi, S.; Herry, C.; Lüthi, A. Amygdala Inhibitory Circuits and the Control of Fear Memory. *Neuron* **2009**, *62*, 757–771. [CrossRef]

19. Krettek, J.E.; Price, J.L. Projections from the amygdaloid complex to the cerebral cortex and thalamus in the rat and cat. *J. Comp. Neurol.* **1977**, *172*, 687–722. [CrossRef] [PubMed]

20. Little, J.P.; Carter, A.G. Synaptic Mechanisms Underlying Strong Reciprocal Connectivity between the Medial Prefrontal Cortex and Basolateral Amygdala. *J. Neurosci.* **2013**, *33*, 15333–15342. [CrossRef]

21. Little, J.P.; Carter, A.G. Subcellular Synaptic Connectivity of Layer 2 Pyramidal Neurons in the Medial Prefrontal Cortex. *J. Neurosci.* **2012**, *32*, 12808–12819.

22. Floresco, S.B.; Tse, M.T. Dopaminergic Regulation of Inhibitory and Excitatory Transmission in the Basolateral Amygdala-Prefrontal Cortical Pathway. *J. Neurosci.* **2007**, *27*, 2045–2057.

23. Dilgen, J.; Tejeda, H.A.; O'Donnell, P. Amygdala inputs drive feedforward inhibition in the medial prefrontal cortex. *J. Neurophysiol.* **2013**, *110*, 221–229.

24. McGarry, L.M.; Carter, A.G. Inhibitory Gating of Basolateral Amygdala Inputs to the Prefrontal Cortex. *J. Neurosci.* **2016**, *36*, 9391–9406.

25. Sotres-Bayon, F.; Sierra-Mercado, D.; Pardilla-Delgado, E.; Quirk, G.J. Gating of fear in prelimbic cortex by hippocampal and amygdala inputs. *Neuron* **2012**, *76*, 804–812. [CrossRef]

26. Bang, S.J.; Commons, K.G. Forebrain GABAergic Projections From the Dorsal Raphe Nucleus Identified by Using GAD67–GFP Knock-In Mice. *J. Comp. Neurol.* **2012**, *520*, 4157–4167. [CrossRef]

27. Henny, P.; Jones, B.E. Projections from basal forebrain to prefrontal cortex comprise cholinergic, GABAergic and glutamatergic inputs to pyramidal cells or interneurons. *Eur. J. Neurosci.* **2008**, *27*, 654–670.

28. Michels, L.; Schulte-Vels, T.; Schick, M.; O'Gorman, R.L.; Zeffiro, T.; Hasler, G.; Mueller-Pfeiffer, C. Prefrontal GABA and glutathione imbalance in posttraumatic stress disorder: Preliminary findings. *Psychiatry Res. Neuroimaging* **2014**, *224*, 288–295. [CrossRef]

29. Baker, K.D.; Richardson, R. Pharmacological evidence that a failure to recruit NMDA receptors contributes to impaired fear extinction retention in adolescent rats. *Neurobiol. Learn Mem.* **2017**, *143*, 18–26. [CrossRef]

30. Dincheva, I.; Lynch, N.B.; Lee, F.S. The Role of BDNF in the development of fear learning. *Depress. Anxiety* **2016**, *33*, 907–916. [CrossRef]

31. Garpenstrand, H.; Annas, P.; Ekblom, J.; Oreland, L.; Fredrikson, M. Human fear conditioning is related to dopaminergic and serotonergic biological markers. *Behav. Neurosci.* **2001**, *115*, 358–364. [CrossRef] [PubMed]

32. Klucken, T.; Alexander, N.; Schweckendiek, J.; Merz, C.J.; Kagerer, S.; Osinsky, R.; Walter, B.; Vaitl, D.; Hennig, J.; Stark, R. Individual differences in neural correlates of fear conditioning as a function of 5 HTTLPR and stressful life events. *Soc. Cogn. Affect. Neurosci.* **2013**, *8*, 318–325. [CrossRef]

33. Hariri, A.R.; Mattay, V.S.; Tessitore, A.; Kolachana, B.; Fera, F.; Goldman, D.; Egan, M.F.; Weinberger, D.R. Serotonin transporter genetic variation and the response of the human amygdala. *Science* **2002**, *297*, 400–403. [CrossRef]

34. Pezawas, L.; Meyer-Lindenberg, A.; Drabant, E.M.; A Verchinski, B.; E Munoz, K.; Kolachana, B.S.; Egan, M.F.; Mattay, V.S.; Hariri, A.R.; Weinberger, D.R. 5-HTTLPR polymorphism impacts human cingulate-amygdala interactions: A genetic susceptibility mechanism for depression. *Nat. Neurosci.* **2005**, *8*, 828–834. [CrossRef]

35. Pacheco, J.; Beevers, C.G.; Benavides, C.; McGeary, J.; Stice, E.; Schnyer, D.M. Frontal-Limbic White Matter Pathway Associations with the Serotonin Transporter Gene Promoter Region (5-HTTLPR) Polymorphism. *J. Neurosci.* **2009**, *29*, 6229–6233. [CrossRef]

36. Witteveen, J.S.; Middelman, A.; Van Hulten, J.A.; Martens, G.J.M.; Homberg, J.R.; Kolk, S.M.; Martens, G.J.M. Lack of serotonin reuptake during brain development alters rostral raphe-prefrontal network formation. *Front. Cell. Neurosci.* **2013**, *7*, 143. [CrossRef]

37. Gaspar, P.; Cases, O.; Maroteaux, L. The developmental role of serotonin: news from mouse molecular genetics. *Nat. Rev. Neurosci.* **2003**, *4*, 1002–1012. [CrossRef]

38. Homberg, J.R.; Schubert, D.; Gaspar, P. New perspectives on the neurodevelopmental effects of SSRIs. *Trends Pharmacol. Sci.* **2010**, *31*, 60–65. [CrossRef]

39. Homberg, J.R.; Lesch, K.-P. Looking on the Bright Side of Serotonin Transporter Gene Variation. *Biol. Psychiatry* **2011**, *69*, 513–519. [CrossRef]

40. Narayanan, V.; Heiming, R.S.; Jansen, F.; Lesting, J.; Sachser, N.; Pape, H.-C.; Seidenbecher, T. Social Defeat: impact on Fear Extinction and Amygdala-Prefrontal Cortical Theta Synchrony in 5-HTT Deficient Mice. *PLoS ONE* **2011**, *6*, e22600. [CrossRef] [PubMed]

41. Pang, R.D.; Wang, Z.; Klosinski, L.P.; Guo, Y.; Herman, D.H.; Celikel, T.; Dong, H.W.; Holschneider, D.P. Mapping Functional Brain Activation Using [14C]-Iodoantipyrine in Male Serotonin Transporter Knockout Mice. *PLoS ONE* **2011**, *6*, e23869. [CrossRef]

42. Hartley, C.A.; McKenna, M.C.; Salman, R.; Holmes, A.; Casey, B.J.; Phelps, E.A.; Glatt, C.E. Serotonin transporter polyadenylation polymorphism modulates the retention of fear extinction memory. *Proc. Natl. Acad. Sci. USA* **2012**, *109*, 5493–5498. [CrossRef]

43. Wellman, C.L.; Izquierdo, A.; Garrett, J.E.; Martin, K.P.; Carroll, J.; Millstein, R.; Lesch, K.-P.; Murphy, D.L.; Holmes, A. Impaired Stress-Coping and Fear Extinction and Abnormal Corticolimbic Morphology in Serotonin Transporter Knock-Out Mice. *J. Neurosci.* **2007**, *27*, 684–691. [CrossRef]

44. Shan, L.; Schipper, P.; Nonkes, L.J.P.; Homberg, J.R. Impaired Fear Extinction as Displayed by Serotonin Transporter Knockout Rats Housed in Open Cages Is Disrupted by IVC Cage Housing. *PLoS ONE* **2014**, *9*, e91472. [CrossRef]

45. Nonkes, L.J.; De Pooter, M.; Homberg, J.R. Behavioural therapy based on distraction alleviates impaired fear extinction in male serotonin transporter knockout rats. *J. Psychiatry Neurosci.* **2012**, *37*, 224–230. [CrossRef]

46. Shan, L.; Guo, H.-Y.; Heuvel, C.N.A.M.V.D.; Van Heerikhuize, J.; Homberg, J.R. Impaired fear extinction in serotonin transporter knockout rats is associated with increased 5-hydroxymethylcytosine in the amygdala. *CNS Neurosci. Ther.* **2018**, *24*, 810–819. [CrossRef]

47. Miceli, S.; Kasri, N.N.; Joosten, J.; Huang, C.; Kepser, L.; Proville, R.; Selten, M.M.; Van Eijs, F.; Azarfar, A.; Homberg, J.R.; et al. Reduced Inhibition within Layer IV of Sert Knockout Rat Barrel Cortex is Associated with Faster Sensory Integration. *Cereb. Cortex* **2017**, *27*, 933–949. [CrossRef]

48. Calabrese, F.; Guidotti, G.; Middelman, A.; Racagni, G.; Homberg, J.; Riva, M.A. Lack of Serotonin Transporter Alters BDNF Expression in the Rat Brain During Early Postnatal Development. *Mol. Neurobiol.* **2013**, *48*, 244–256. [CrossRef]

49. Karel, P.; Calabrese, F.; Riva, M.; Brivio, P.; van der Veen, B.; Reneman, L.; Verheij, M.; Homberg, J. D-Cycloserine enhanced extinction of cocaine-induced conditioned place preference is attenuated in serotonin transporter knockout rats. *Addict. Biol.* **2018**, *23*, 120–129. [CrossRef]

50. Smits, B.M.G.; Mudde, J.B.; Van De Belt, J.; Verheul, M.; Olivier, J.; Homberg, J.; Guryev, V.; Cools, A.R.; A Ellenbroek, B.; A Plasterk, R.H.; et al. Generation of gene knockouts and mutant models in the laboratory rat by ENU-driven target-selected mutagenesis. *Pharmacogenetics Genom.* **2006**, *16*, 159–169.

51. Olivier, J.; Van Der Hart, M.; Van Swelm, R.; Dederen, P.; Homberg, J.; Cremers, T.; Deen, P.; Cuppen, E.; Cools, A.; Ellenbroek, B. A study in male and female 5-HT transporter knockout rats: An animal model for anxiety and depression disorders. *Neuroscience* **2008**, *152*, 573–584. [CrossRef]

52. Nonkes, L.J.; Tomson, K.; Mærtin, A.; Dederen, J.; Maes, J.R.; Homberg, J. Orbitofrontal cortex and amygdalar over-activity is associated with an inability to use the value of expected outcomes to guide behaviour in serotonin transporter knockout rats. *Neurobiol. Learn. Mem.* **2010**, *94*, 65–72. [CrossRef]

53. Schindelin, J.; Arganda-Carreras, I.; Frise, E.; Kaynig, V.; Longair, M.; Pietzsch, T.; Preibisch, S.; Rueden, C.; Saalfeld, S.; Schmid, B.; et al. Fiji: An open-source platform for biological-image analysis. *Nat. Methods* **2012**, *9*, 676–682. [CrossRef]

54. Livak, K.J.; Schmittgen, T.D. Analysis of relative gene expression data using real-time quantitative PCR and the 2(-Delta Delta C(T)) Method. *Methods* **2001**, *25*, 402–408. [CrossRef]

55. Schipper, P.; Kiliaan, A.J.; Homberg, J.R. A mixed polyunsaturated fatty acid diet normalizes hippocampal neurogenesis and reduces anxiety in serotonin transporter knockout rats. *Behav. Pharmacol.* **2011**, *22*, 324–334. [CrossRef]

56. Schipper, P.; Nonkes, L.J.; Karel, P.; Kiliaan, A.J.; Homberg, J.R. Serotonin transporter genotype x construction stress interaction in rats. *Behav. Brain* **2011**, *223*, 169–175. [CrossRef]

57. Kroeze, Y.; Dirven, B.; Janssen, S.; Kröhnke, M.; Barte, R.M.; Middelman, A.; Van Bokhoven, H.; Zhou, H.; Homberg, J.R. Perinatal reduction of functional serotonin transporters results in developmental delay. *Neuropharmacology* **2016**, *109*, 96–111. [CrossRef]

58. Sakakibara, Y.; Kasahara, Y.; Hall, F.S.; Lesch, K.-P.; Murphy, D.L.; Uhl, G.R.; Sora, I. Developmental alterations in anxiety and cognitive behavior in serotonin transporter mutant mice. *Psychopharmacology* **2014**, *231*, 4119–4133. [CrossRef]

59. Hefner, K.; Holmes, A. Ontogeny of fear-, anxiety- and depression-related behavior across adolescence in C57BL/6J mice. *Behav. Brain Res.* **2007**, *176*, 210–215. [CrossRef]

60. Maren, S.; Phan, K.L.; Liberzon, I. The contextual brain: Implications for fear conditioning, extinction and psychopathology. *Nat. Rev. Neurosci.* **2013**, *14*, 417–428. [CrossRef]

61. Vollmer, L.L.; Schmeltzer, S.; Schurdak, J.; Ahlbrand, R.; Rush, J.; Dolgas, C.M.; Baccei, M.L.; Sah, R. Neuropeptide Y Impairs Retrieval of Extinguished Fear and Modulates Excitability of Neurons in the Infralimbic Prefrontal Cortex. *J. Neurosci.* **2016**, *36*, 1306–1315. [CrossRef]

62. Henson, M.A.; Tucker, C.J.; Zhao, M.; Dudek, S.M. Long-term depression-associated signaling is required for an in vitro model of NMDA receptor-dependent synapse pruning. *Neurobiol. Learn Mem.* **2017**, *138*, 39–53. [CrossRef]

63. Molteni, R.; Cattaneo, A.; Calabrese, F.; Macchi, F.; Olivier, J.D.; Racagni, G.; Ellenbroek, B.A.; Gennarelli, M.; Riva, M.A. Reduced function of the serotonin transporter is associated with decreased expression of BDNF in rodents as well as in humans. *Neurobiol. Dis.* **2010**, *37*, 747–755. [CrossRef]

64. Guidotti, G.; Calabrese, F.; Auletta, F.; Olivier, J.; Racagni, G.; Homberg, J.; Riva, M.A. Developmental influence of the serotonin transporter on the expression of npas4 and GABAergic markers: Modulation by antidepressant treatment. *Neuropsychopharmacology* **2012**, *37*, 746–758. [CrossRef]

65. Vieira, P.A.; Corches, A.; Lovelace, J.W.; Westbrook, K.B.; Mendoza, M.; Korzus, E. Prefrontal NMDA receptors expressed in excitatory neurons control fear discrimination and fear extinction. *Neurobiol. Learn. Mem.* **2015**, *119*, 52–62. [CrossRef]

66. Endres, T.; Lessmann, V. Age-dependent deficits in fear learning in heterozygous BDNF knock-out mice. *Learn. Mem.* **2012**, *19*, 561–570. [CrossRef]

67. Hunter, A.S. The effects of social housing on extinction of fear conditioning in rapid eye movement sleep-deprived rats. *Exp. Brain* **2014**, *232*, 1459–1467. [CrossRef]

68. Crone, E.A.; Dahl, R.E. Understanding adolescence as a period of social–affective engagement and goal flexibility. *Nat. Rev. Neurosci.* **2012**, *13*, 636–650. [CrossRef]

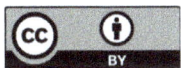

MDPI
St. Alban-Anlage 66
4052 Basel
Switzerland
Tel. +41 61 683 77 34
Fax +41 61 302 89 18
www.mdpi.com

Actuators Editorial Office
E-mail: actuators@mdpi.com
www.mdpi.com/journal/actuators

www.ingramcontent.com/pod-product-compliance
Lightning Source LLC
Chambersburg PA
CBHW051855210326
41597CB00033B/5906